# HANDBOOK OF EXPERIENTIAL
PSYCHOTHERAPY

# HANDBOOK
# OF EXPERIENTIAL
# PSYCHOTHERAPY

Edited by

Leslie S. Greenberg
Jeanne C. Watson
Germain Lietaer

THE GUILFORD PRESS
New York   London

© 1998 The Guilford Press
A Division of Guilford Publications, Inc.
72 Spring Street, New York, NY 10012
http://www.guilford.com

Printed in the United States of America

This book is printed on acid-free paper.

Last digit is print number: 9  8  7  6  5  4  3  2  1

**Library of Congress Cataloging-in-Publication Data**

Handbook of experiential psychotherapy / edited by Leslie S. Greenberg, Jeanne C. Watson, Germain Lietaer.
    p.    cm.
    Includes bibliographical references and index.
    ISBN 1–57230–374–3
    1. Experiential psychotherapy—Handbooks, manuals, etc.
  2. Existential psychotherapy—Handbooks, manuals, etc.
  I. Greenberg, Leslie S.  II. Watson, Jeanne C.  III. Lietaer, G.
(Germain)
    [DNLM:  1. Psychotherapy—methods.  WM 420H2313 1998]
RC489.E96H36   1998
  616.89'14—dc21
DNLM/DLC
for Library of Congress

*To Laura North Rice,*
*our friend and mentor,*
*and to the influence of Gene Gendlin*

# Contributors

**Eva-Maria Biermann-Ratjen, Dipl.Psych.**, Psychiatrische Universität-sklinik Hamburg–Eppendorf, Hamburg, Germany

**Arthur C. Bohart, PhD**, Department of Psychology, California State University—Dominguez Hills, Carson, CA

**Kenneth L. Davis, PhD**, Department of Psychology, University of Toledo, Toledo, OH

**Jochen Eckert, PhD**, Psychologisches Institut III, Universität Hamburg, Hamburg, Germany

**Robert Elliott, PhD**, Department of Psychology, University of Toledo, Toledo, OH

**Rhonda Goldman, PhD**, Illinois School of Professional Psychology, Chicago, IL

**Leslie S. Greenberg, PhD**, Department of Psychology and Psychotherapy Research Center, York University, North York, Ontario, Canada

**M. Katherine Hudgins, PhD, TEP**, The Center for Experiential Learning, Ltd., Charlottesville, VA

**Mia Leijssen, PhD**, Counseling Centrum, Katholieke Universiteit te Leuven, Leuven, Belgium

**Germain Lietaer, PhD**, Department of Psychology, Katholieke Universiteit te Leuven, Leuven, Belgium

**Alvin R. Mahrer, PhD**, School of Psychology, University of Ottawa, Ottawa, Canada

**Joseph Melnick, PhD**, Editor in Chief, *The Gestalt Review*, Portland, ME

**Sandra March Nevis, PhD**, *The Gestalt Review*, Portland, ME

**Garry Prouty, PhD**, Midwestern University, Downer's Grove, IL

**Rainer Sachse, PhD,** Ruhr-Universität Bochum, Fakultat fur Psychologie, Bochum, Germany

**Kirk J. Schneider, PhD,** Saybrook Institute, San Francisco, CA

**Patti Sigl, PsyD candidate,** American School of Professional Psychology—Virginia Branch, Arlington, VA

**Emil Slatick, MA,** Department of Psychology, University of Toledo, Toledo, OH

**Gert-Walter Speierer, MD,** Medizinische Psychologie, Universität Regensburg, Postfach, Germany

**Karen Tallman, PhD candidate,** Department of Educational Psychology, University of Southern California, Los Angeles, CA

**Greet Vanaerschot, PhD,** private practice, Erps-Kwerps, Belgium

**Richard Van Balen, PhD,** Professor Emeritus, Katholieke Universiteit te Leuven, Leuven, Belgium

**Wim van Kessel, psychologist–psychotherapist,** private practice, De Bilt, The Netherlands

**Margaret S. Warner, PhD,** Illinois School of Professional Psychology

**Jeanne C. Watson, PhD,** Department of Adult Education, Community Development and Counselling Psychology, University of Toronto, Toronto, Canada

**Barry E. Wolfe, PhD,** American School of Professional Psychology—Virginia Campus, Arlington, VA

**Gary Yontef, PhD, FAClinP,** Gestalt Therapy Institute of Los Angeles, Santa Monica, CA

# Preface

*The influence of the* humanistic approaches to psychotherapy has waned since their prominence in the sixties and seventies. The so called "third force" that swept North America in this period with a positive view of human nature and the promise of a revolution in human well-being has given way to more structured and directive treatments. The pendulum swung away from a process-oriented approach to facilitating in-session change in experience, back toward more modificational, homework-based, cognitive approaches, and to more interpretive, brief dynamic approaches.

Despite their disappearance from center stage, the experientially oriented therapies have continued to develop in small pockets in North America and more extensively in Europe. These approaches have generated new theoretical perspectives on human functioning, drawing on advances in emotion and cognitive science, and on continued research on the process of change. This has led to the development of more focused approaches to process-oriented treatment and to the development of differential brief experiential treatment approaches to a number of different populations. Having championed a growth and actualization model over a disease model and having eschewed the use of diagnosis, out of a concern for the possible stigma of pathological labels, the humanistic approaches were often seen by many as not being appropriate for more distressed populations. We will suggest in this book that the experiential approaches are useful not only for the "worried well" but also for a variety of diagnostic groups.

We believe that the "third force" has an important contribution to make in the treatment of human suffering and are concerned that it has not received the amount of attention it deserves, both in academic training programs and in the mainstream of psychotherapeutic practice. We hope with this book to begin to remedy this problem by providing under one cover some of the latest developments in this approach. We invited leading European and North American writers who shared certain fundamental assumptions common to experiential therapy to contribute chapters. The authors all agreed on the importance of awareness and choice in healthy functioning and have all theorized on the importance of both the therapeutic relationship and the evocation and symbolization of new experience in the therapy session, in facilitating psychotherapeutic change.

We have, in this book, for the first time, integrated approaches such as client-centered, Gestalt, existential, and psychodrama under the overarching title of experiential psychotherapy, a name that has become more and more common in North America in referring to the third force approaches. This is the name we suggest for integrating a variety of humanistic approaches that emphasize the promotion of deeper in-session experience as a means of facilitating therapeutic change. Experiential approaches all see people as experiencing agents who, by symbolizing and reflecting on their experience, construct new meaning and choose courses of action.

In the chapters that follow we present a comprehensive view of experiential therapy as it approaches the new millennium. The first section of this book presents an overview of the history and current developments in practice as well as a chapter on a current theory of experiential therapy. This is followed by a section on the fundamental principles of an experiential approach including empathy, awareness and dialogue, experiential focusing, the client as active agent, the interpersonal process, the existential dimension, and the importance of translating in-session change to extra-sessional change. This is followed by a section on differential brief treatment approaches. We present evidence-based experiential approaches to the treatment of depression, posttraumatic stress, psychosomatic and borderline disorders as well as highly developed approaches to anxiety disorders, sexual abuse, fragile personality, and hallucinatory disorders. In addition, two chapters on experiential perspectives on psychopathology and diagnosis are included. The final chapter synthesizes the contributions to the book to offer a view on the current status and future directions of an experiential therapy for the new millennium. We trust that this book will facilitate your experiencing, promote symbolization and reflection, help you create new meaning, and encourage you to adopt some of our suggested approaches to helping people change.

# Contents

# III  DIFFERENTIAL TREATMENT APPLICATIONS

# IV  CONCLUSION

# HANDBOOK OF EXPERIENTIAL PSYCHOTHERAPY

# I

*****

# HISTORY AND THEORY

# 1

*****

# The Experiential Paradigm Unfolding
## RELATIONSHIP AND EXPERIENCING IN THERAPY

Jeanne C. Watson
Leslie S. Greenberg
Germain Lietaer

*T*his chapter focuses on the history of the practice of experientially oriented therapy. We will trace its development historically and explicate its major current forms. Experiential therapy has its roots in client-centered, existential, and Gestalt approaches to psychotherapy. These humanistic approaches emphasize that clients are aware, subjective beings and self-reflective agents (Heidegger, 1962; Jaspers, 1963; Lietaer, 1990; F. S. Perls, 1973; Polster & Polster, 1973; Taylor, 1975; Tiryakian, 1962; Rennie, 1998; Rice & Greenberg, 1992; Rogers, 1951, 1959; Schneider & May, 1995). The main objective of experiential therapy is working with clients' awareness, both by focusing on subjective experience and by promoting reflexivity and a sense of agency. Despite the changes in emphasis in the evolution of praxis over time, two important foci can be identified as the cornerstones of experiential approaches: the first focus is on the importance of the therapeutic relationship in facilitating change in clients, and the second is on the importance of clients' experiencing in therapy, consisting of clients' representation and examination of their inner subjective worldviews, including feelings, perceptions, goals, values and constructs (Gendlin, 1964).

We trace the development of experiential therapy through its client-centered, Gestalt, and existential roots to its most recent conceptualization and form based on these two basic principles. In the practice of experiential therapy a genuine empathic and confirming relationship is seen as a crucial curative factor in its own right as well as facilitative of the other main task of this approach—that of deepening clients' experiencing in therapy (Gendlin, 1996; Greenberg, Rice, & Elliott, 1993). We distinguish between the therapeutic relationship and the experiencing tasks to anchor and differentiate among the different major approaches to experiential therapy. We also trace the development and distinguish between the more intrapsychic and more interpersonal perspectives to practice to capture the evolution of experiential therapy from its original focus on the client as the primary source of change to its current interpersonal focus that includes both the growth forces within the individual as well as the confirming presence of the therapist as contributing to the change process.

# EVOLUTION

## Client-Centered Therapy

The practice of client-centered therapy (Rogers, 1942, 1951) has evolved through a number of different stages, each of which has emphasized slightly different ways for therapists to interact with their clients. The first phase emphasized that therapists should be *nondirective* with their clients. During this phase Rogers hypothesized that counselors promoted change by avoiding advice and interpretation and by consistently recognizing and accepting clients' feelings. As he developed this view he concentrated on identifying specific techniques, for example, reflections, that would facilitate clients' growth and development. Rogers later came to see the emphasis on specific techniques as too mechanistic and as impeding the development of a real authentic relationship with clients. Instead of techniques Rogers began to emphasize the *relationship conditions* of empathy, unconditional positive regard, and congruence (1957). This view emphasized sensitive immersion in clients' worlds, accompanied by a prizing of clients so as to enable them to become aware of their feelings in the session. This requires that therapists continually check their ongoing understanding of their clients' inner worlds with them and that they not hide behind masks of professionalism but reveal their experience when it is deemed helpful to do so. During this phase Rogers concentrated on understanding clients' processes of change, and it was from this examination that client's experiencing in therapy emerged as a critical component of therapeutic work. In the later third stage of his development, as he began to work with schizophrenics, groups, and the larger sociopolitical context, Rogers increasingly emphasized the need for therapists to be *genuine* with their clients in order to facilitate the change process. With experience came a growing recognition that it was important for the therapist to be appreciated as a person in the relationship and to be trusted just as the client is trusted. Toward the end of his life Rogers emphasized that therapists operating with full awareness can use their inner capacities so that their presence will be releasing of the growth capacity in others (Rogers, 1980).

## Existential Therapy

Existential therapy is concerned with people realizing their potential. It emphasizes working with the whole person and not losing their wholeness in concepts such as drives, conditioning, or archetypes. As with other experiential approaches, a therapeutic relationship that is genuine or authentic is seen as fundamental to the work of psychotherapy. Two strands of experiential therapy have emerged since World War II: the existential–humanistic approach and the transpersonal (Bugenthal & McBeath, 1995). The existential–humanistic approach holds that as people develop they build self and world construct systems (SAWCS) based on their experience of themselves in the world. As they develop they must confront the givens of existence including the inevitability of death, the conflict between freedom and the limits of existence, existential isolation, and the meaninglessness of existence (Schneider & May, 1995). How people confront these concerns is partly determined by their SAWCS. If their SAWCS are challenged or somehow inadequate to cope with the exigencies of existence that everybody confronts then they may need to be revised. Revision of clients' SAWCS is one of the primary tasks of existential therapy. The transpersonal approach emphasizes people's spirituality and their higher order consciousness. The primary objective is to make people more aware not only of their own inner subjective and intuitive knowledge but also to become more aware of themselves as spiritual beings with access to different levels of consciousness (Bugenthal & McBeath, 1995).

## Gestalt Therapy

Gestalt therapy is currently seen as being based on three fundamental principles (Resnick, 1995): field theory, emphasizing that everything is relational and in flux; phenomenology, which emphasizes subjective experience and the creation of meaning; and dialogue, involving open engagement between the client and therapist for therapeutic purposes. The practice of Gestalt therapy has evolved from a more individualistic form, one that emphasized the development of self-support, to a more interpersonal view of practice that emphasizes the importance of field support and interdependence (Wheeler, 1991). Gestalt therapy early on referred to the "here and now" and "I and Thou" as the two legs on which the approach stood, but the relationship was not of particular interest in the actual practice of the approach. In the 1960s Frederick S. Perls emphasized awareness, experiencing, and the Gestalt experiment. A recent shift to a more dialogic form of

Gestalt therapy has brought the "I–Thou" dialogue into the foreground as the foundation of practice.

Early on in North America, Gestalt therapy split into two streams. One focused on visceral experience and emphasized the active experiment, getting clients to do things, often in groups, that helped them experience rather than talk about their concerns (F. S. Perls, 1969). The other stream is based on the analysis of the organism's contact with the environment and involved following the moment-by-moment process of making experiential contact with the actual situation (L. Perls, 1976). This approach views awareness of the moments of the contact formation as essential to healthy functioning and concentrated on helping people become aware of the stages and process of contact formation and how they were interrupted. In this approach awareness of interruptions and the reestablishment of contact rather than the relationship itself were seen as curative.

Recently all the varied parts of Gestalt therapy have been synthesized to form a more dialogic Gestalt therapy (Wheeler, 1991; Yontef, 1991). In this approach the interpersonal relationship has been given a more central role alongside phenomenological focusing and the human encounter as important sources of growth. As a result there has been more of a focus on the therapeutic relationship and specifically the type of contacts between clients and therapists and less use of active experimentation.

## Experiential Therapy

Recently two other versions of experiential therapy have been proposed, one by Gendlin (1981) and the other by Greenberg et al. (1993). Gendlin developed focusing as a way of helping clients access their experience by having them attend to their bodily felt sense. To this end he leads clients through different stages from clearing a space to attending to and symbolizing their felt sense. Greenberg and colleagues (1993) articulated a process-experiential approach to therapy that essentially represents a merger of client-centered, existential, and Gestalt approaches. Drawing on Rice's (1983) distinction, process-experiential therapists distinguish between the relational conditions and the working conditions of therapy, and see each as contributing uniquely to client change. With respect to the working conditions, following Rogers and Perls this approach emphasizes the need for clients to become aware of their inner experience in therapy. The primary objective in process-experiential therapy is to help clients integrate information from their emotional and cognitive systems to facilitate a more satisfactory adjustment to their environment. Process-experiential therapists emphasize the role of emotion in personal development and functioning. According to this view the growth tendency is based on adaptive emotional experience. Emotions are seen as being important to people's well-being to the extent that they enhance orientation and problem solving (Greenberg et al., 1993; Watson & Greenberg, 1996a).

# THE IMPORTANCE OF
# THE THERAPEUTIC RELATIONSHIP

## Client-Centered Therapy

### *The Nondirective Approach*

Initially Rogers (1942) saw the therapeutic relationship as an essential vehicle for facilitating clients' change processes. He suggested that therapists be nondirective with their clients so that the latter could acquire insight into themselves and their situation at their own pace (Hart, 1970). By nondirective Rogers meant that therapists should provide a structured but permissive and nonauthoritarian environment for their clients so that they would feel free to engage in self-exploration without having to be defensive or concerned about their therapists' reaction. This view emphasized the use of reflections as opposed to interpretations and questions to further clients' self-exploration and growth. The goal of this approach was for clients to develop strategies for positive, self-initiated actions as a result of new self-understanding. During this stage of the development of his theory Rogers was trying to differentiate nondirective counseling from the other two approaches that were popular at the time, a psychoanalytic approach and a more directive counseling approach. The latter was designed to help clients find solutions to career difficulties (Zimring & Raskin, 1992).

Subsequently Rogers' emphasis on the therapeutic relationship as the primary vehicle of change became formulated in terms of the three therapist conditions of empathy, unconditional positive regard, and congruence. These were viewed as the necessary and sufficient conditions of therapeutic change. According to this formulation, if therapists were empathic to their clients' experiences and tried to see the world through their eyes, without judgment of either a positive or negative nature, then clients would not only be able to reveal themselves candidly and freely in therapy but they would independently come to attend to their own inner experience and use it as a valid source of information. In addition, through the process of validating their experiences, clients would come to use their experience as a means of evaluating things for themselves and then use it as a guide to future action. In this way they would develop their own internal locus of control so that they would no longer be dependent on the introjected values of others.

### *The Classical Client-Centered Approach*

In this view therapist attitudes are seen as central to promoting change. Later client-centered theorists continued to deemphasize techniques in favor of the relationship (Bozarth, 1990; Brodley, 1990; Raskin & Rogers, 1989). Bozarth (1990) suggested that it did not matter so much what client-centered therapists did or what the precise nature of their responses were. The only requirement was that they provide the client with time, freedom to explore, and their undivided attention in order for clients to solve the problems that brought them into therapy. Brodley (1990), writing in a similar vein, emphasized that the therapist does not cause change but merely enables it by providing conditions that foster the optimal functioning of the clients' inherent growth tendency. This perspective suggests that therapists need to surrender control of both process and content of sessions to their clients.

The type of intervention that these therapists identify as most helpful is that of reflection. They propose that reflections of feeling are the most articulate and precise form of empathic following response. In this type of response, while the therapist may reveal aspects of clients' experiences of which the latter may not have been previously conscious, that is not the therapist's primary intention. Rather, the therapist's primary intention is to share in the phenomenological and experiential world of the other and to understand it. Moreover these authors acknowledge that by reflecting certain aspects of clients' experiences the therapist may focus clients on some experiences rather than others. However, this is not the primary aim. Brodley (1990) contrasts the therapist's intentions in this approach with those in other experiential approaches; she suggests that to the extent that experiential therapists are more process directive they are more directive of client content so that the therapy is changed in some fundamental way. An essential difference between the form of client-centered therapy proposed by Brodley and others is the degree to which it emphasizes clients' agency within the session. In Brodley's form of client-centered therapy the emphasis is on clients' assuming as much responsibility for the direction and process of therapy as possible. This is in contrast to other forms of client-centered and experiential therapy where there is more shifting between clients as patients under the direction of their therapists and then as agents of their own experiences.

The focus in classical client-centered therapy is not so much on clients' interpersonal interactions but rather on clients' perceptions, feelings, and experience of others. The focus is more intrapsychic as opposed to interpersonal. Later developments in client-centered theory came to emphasize the importance of an interpersonal focus that would allow therapists more opportunity to be self-disclosing and revealing within the therapeutic encounter. Clients' growth in therapy was seen to be promoted by both increased understanding of their own intrapsychic processes as well as the interpersonal learning that occurred with their therapists.

## The Interpersonal Approach

The interpersonal focus grew out of Rogers's work with schizophrenics, encounter groups, and the wider social and political context (Lietaer, 1990; Zimring & Raskin, 1992; Rogers, 1970). Here the emphasis is on the role of genuineness, as the therapist adopts a more interpersonal focus within the therapeutic encounter. Rogers in his later years began to emphasize the therapist's role in the encounter as an important factor in the change process. Practitioners of this more interpersonal approach have also been influenced by the theory and practice of existential therapy, particularly the work of Yalom (1975, 1980). It was observed that while individual therapy promotes insight into oneself and the intrapsychic exploration of interpersonal problems, groups are useful in helping clients deal with dysfunctional relationship patterns (Lietaer, 1993). Work with groups made client-centered therapy more interactional, with therapists acting not only as alter egos to their clients but also as independent participants in the interaction who may at times express their feelings and observations about what is occurring between the participants (Lietaer, 1993). These writers within the client-centered tradition continue to emphasize the importance of the therapeutic relationship. An important task in both group and individual therapy is the construction and maintenance of a safe environment. Rogers attempted to do this by not steering the group in any particular direction and by listening as attentively as possible. However, Lietaer and Dierick (1996) suggest that client-centered group therapists need to be a little more directive of group process so as to clarify what is happening in the here and now and to maintain group cohesion. Some of the ways of working with groups, for example, being more directive and commenting on the therapeutic process, were also incorporated into work with individuals.

The focus on interpersonal processes gave added prominence to the notion of genuineness in the therapeutic relationship. In line with Rogers, Lietaer (1993) identifies genuineness as the most important of the three relationship conditions. He distinguished between two aspects of genuineness, an internal aspect and an external one.

The internal aspect of congruence refers to therapists' own internal experiencing with their clients, of which they need to be aware in therapy. Lietaer suggests that therapists need to be sufficiently mature and self-aware to be able to be nondefensive with their clients and open to the world of the other. This may be a challenge at times, as clients may make their therapists aware of aspects of themselves that they have not confronted before. To the extent that therapists are able to be in touch with their own experience they may be termed congruent.

The external aspect of congruence refers to the therapists' ability to reveal their experience to their clients. This is termed transparency. Lietaer cautions that therapists need to exercise transparency with responsibility. According to this criterion it is not necessary for therapists to share every aspect of their experience but only those that they feel would be facilitative of their clients' work. Transparency is always used in an empathic climate. The therapists' self-disclosure needs to flow out of deep involvement with the client. There are two guidelines for being transparent in the relationship. First, therapists should own their feelings using "I" messages as opposed to "you" messages. This is particularly important as therapists need to be careful not to sound evaluative or blaming of their clients (Lietaer, 1993; Watson & Greenberg, in press). Second, therapists need to be continually open to their clients' experiences and the impact of therapists' self-disclosures on them. Therapists should constantly check with their clients about the latters' experiences and use clients' experiential tracks as the touchstones in all interactions (Thorne, 1992). Another way that therapists can try to maintain the balance between congruence and empathy and clients' self-explorations is to keep self-disclosures brief and to end their responses with a focus on the clients' concerns (Thorne, 1992; Watson & Greenberg, 1995).

The interpersonal branch of client-centered therapy gives some credence to the psychological concept of transference. Lietaer (1993), like Gendlin, holds that as a function of interacting with other human beings—some of whom may have difficulties in their interpersonal relationships—there is a very high likelihood that therapists will experience what it is like to interact with their clients and to gain a fuller understanding of their clients' difficulties. However, client-centered therapists are not charged with the task of addressing the relationship difficulties as a means of facilitating change. Nor is their role to teach clients about patterns of interaction that arise from their own psychogenic histories (Lietaer, 1993; Watson & Greenberg, in press). Rather, these therapists believe that the relationship difficulties that emerge may evaporate to the extent that clients are exposed to a corrective emotional experience. If this occurs, the relationship difficulties may not need to be confronted directly in therapy. The exception to this occurs when the difficulties become chronic and focal so that they need to be addressed to facilitate the creation of a stronger and safer alliance between client and therapist as well as to assist clients in working through their interpersonal difficulties.

## The Relationship in Existential Therapy

As in Gestalt therapy, existential therapists believe that therapists need to be authentic in their relationship with their clients (May & Yalom, 1989). One of the most important concepts used by May and Yalom to characterize authenticity in the therapeutic relationship is that of presence. According to this view therapists must be fully present with their clients. This notion overlaps with the client-centered notion of congruence. However, in contrast to client-centered notions of the relationship, existential therapists believe that the client and therapist are interacting in a way that both "participate, and in which love and hate, trust and doubt, conflicts and dependence, come out and can be understood and assimilated" (May & Yalom, 1989, p. 269; Deurzen-Smith, 1988). These writers were concerned that the primary focus on the client in client-centered therapy might close off aspects of experience that require exploration. Thus existential therapists strive to be honest, open, and direct with their patients.

Existential therapists work to acquire clients' trust: while empathy is seen as vital to this process, it is not communicated with empathic reflections; rather, the emphasis is on a deep understanding of clients' difficulties without necessarily verbalizing or expressing this (Swildens, 1990). In the early stages of therapy existential therapists try to avoid confronting clients until the clients feel safe and courageous enough to engage in self-reflection. Existential therapists work hard to develop a climate of safety and security for their clients before they begin confronting clients with the responsibility for creating their life situations, and their avoidances of the givens of their existence that leave them feeling anxious and despairing. Later in therapy existential therapists assume a more equal position with their clients as they help their clients to examine and address their weaknesses and deficiencies. During this phase it is important for therapists to be supportive and to actively help their clients come up with alternatives to their current problems. The existential therapist might suggest alternatives, discuss options, consider the consequences of different courses of action, and give advice (Swildens, 1990).

As in more classical Gestalt approaches, and in interpersonal approaches to client-centered theory, existential therapists anticipate that clients will distort aspects of the therapeutic relationship based on previous experiences. The role of the existential therapist is to help the patient tease out reality from the distortions. Therapists assist with this from their own basis of self-knowledge and understanding of how others respond to them (May & Yalom, 1989). An important goal of existential therapy is to affirm the clients' experiences. Like client-centered practitioners, existential therapists realize the healing power for clients of being seen and accepted as they really are. It is assumed that this will have a positive impact on their relationships outside of therapy.

## The Relationship in Gestalt Therapy

Gestalt therapists have always seen the therapeutic relationship as an important source of new learning for their clients. This approach grew out of a disaffection with the psychoanalytic emphasis on the notion of transference and historical reconstruction. Like client-centered theorists, Gestalt theorists saw the relationship as involving real contact between the participants as well as the possibility that clients were projecting their prior experience onto their current relationship with their therapists. However, there was not a strong theory of relationship nor were there guidelines for the role of the relationship in practice, other than as a projection screen, or by contrast a source of genuine contact.

Initially Gestalt therapy was confrontational, operating from a view—drawn somewhat from its dynamic roots—of the importance of frustrating client manipulations. Clients were often viewed as manipulating the environment for support, rather than developing self-support. Over the years greater emphasis has been placed on respecting clients, providing them with support, validating them as authentic sources of experience, and relating to them less authoritatively. An important influence in this development has been Gestalt therapy work with people who are more fragile and suffer from personality disorders. With these people it became apparent that an empathic bond and a good working relationship with the therapist were important. In its early formulation, problems in the relationship between clients and therapists were thought to reflect projective, transferential processes. These were worked on not as interpersonal problems with the therapist but as projections that needed to be reowned. Clients were invited to put their therapists in an empty chair and dialogue with their imagined therapists. Therapists thus adopted a more experimentally oriented rather than a relational approach to therapy. While authenticity and genuineness were emphasized, there was little or no clarification of distinctions between therapeutic and nontherapeutic genuineness, and little attention was paid to establishing a relationship characterized by empathic listening and prizing, as in client-centered practice.

Recently a more interpersonal form or dialogic Gestalt therapy has replaced the classical approach in which the active experiment was the cornerstone of treatment. In this view, like its existential and client-centered counterparts, the therapeutic relationship is seen as a real, existential encounter between two people. This perspective is guided by Martin Buber's view of an I–Thou relationship, which emphasizes that encounters between individuals should be characterized by qualities of presence, inclusion, nonexploitativeness, authenticity, and commitment to dialogue (Jacobs, 1989; Yontef, 1991; Hycner & Jacobs, 1995). This more recent form of Gestalt therapy, rather than viewing relational problems as client projections, sees them as arising out of an interpersonal field (Wheeler, 1991; Yontef, 1991). Problems in the relationship between client and therapist are responded to supportively. Clients' growth is thought to be facilitated by the therapist working with the client to heal the ruptures that occur in the relationship. Thus Gestalt therapists focus on the present contacts between clients and therapists and attend to disruptions in these contacts. Therapists are highly aware of their own impact on clients momentary experience, focusing on disruptions in relational contact as both a source of discovery and an opportunity for new experience. Clients' awareness of patterns in their experiences and awareness of how they interrupt themselves, as well as the corrective experience of a helping dialogue, are all seen as curative.

As in client-centered therapy, the relationship is seen as an important vehicle for change in Gestalt therapy. However, there is less focus on the relationship and the avoidance of ruptures than in more classical client-centered approaches. In client-centered therapy the relationship is seen as both enabling and a primary source of change. It both facilitates deeper exploration and is internalized, thereby promoting self-empathy (Barrett-Lennard, 1997). In Gestalt therapy relational work that involves becoming aware of and working with the interruptions of contact is probably still seen as the predominate change process (Hycner & Jacobs, 1995), as opposed to a view that relational empathy and interpersonal confirmation provide a corrective emotional experience that helps repair developmental deficits.

## Experiential Therapy

In the experiential approaches (Gendlin, Greenberg, Mahrer, Rice, Lietaer, Leijssen, Sachse) therapists are seen as constantly needing to balance responsiveness with directiveness, as they continually assess whether to follow the clients' track or propose the use of more specific interventions like two-chair work or focusing. One way that process-experiential therapists attempt to balance these competing agendas is to give primacy to the clients' experience within the session. The clients remain the experts and final arbiters of their own experience within the session and in their lives more generally, and therefore any process directions or suggestions from therapists that may not fit are dropped in favor of clients' steering the process.

Experiential therapy sees the relational conditions as important in confirming and validating people. Not only are they confirmed as authentic sources of experience and understanding, but their experience is validated in the context of their current and historical realities. In addition, therapists constantly focus on the growing edge of clients' possibilities, strengths, and future goals, thereby confirming their capacity for growth. Growth is seen as emerging from both the interpersonal processes between clients and therapists as well as clients' reformulation of their own intrapsychic processes.

Experiential therapists emphasize the need to create a safe working environment for their clients (Elliott & Shapiro, 1992; Lietaer, 1992; Watson & Greenberg, 1994). It is important that clients and therapists have strong working alliances before they begin to engage in the more active Gestalt experiments and tasks. As in more classical client-centered approaches, process-experiential therapists establish trust and safety by responding to the live, poignant aspects of clients' narratives. This is done primarily with the use of empathic responses, using reflections, exploratory responses, evocative language, and metaphor to distill the special significance of events in clients' lives (Bohart, 1993; Greenberg & Elliott, 1997; Watson & Greenberg, 1998).

Process-experiential therapists differ from their more client-centered counterparts in that they use more questions and conjectures to explore and stimulate clients' inner experience, and pay more attention to specific client markers or statements that indicate that clients are experiencing particular cognitive–affective problems. These markers are then used by therapists to frame and focus clients' activities within the session. Therapists also engage in experiential teaching, helping clients become aware of the impact of specific types of internal processes, such as self-criticism, and they structure the sessions using tasks (Greenberg et al., 1993; Watson, 1996). Consequently process-experiential therapists must balance more directive responding with responsive attunement and careful tracking of their clients' experiences. If they are too directive they can lose touch with each client's focus of inquiry and risk rupturing the relationship, especially if they become overly controlling in the session (Watson, 1996; Watson & Greenberg, 1998). Sensitive attunement to clients in the session is all the more important, as ruptures in the alliance are often covert processes that are not discussed or even mentioned by them (Rennie, 1992; Watson & Greenberg, 1994). One way that process-experiential therapists attempt to stay in tune with their clients is to metacommunicate with them about the purpose and objective of certain interventions to determine whether clients see these as being congruent with their own expectations and goals in the session (Watson & Greenberg, 1995). Moreover clients are encouraged to voice dissent freely with their therapists so that a shared understanding can be negotiated. Therapists facilitate this by not acting as experts but merely as facilitators who suggest different tasks that clients may or may not want to try. Another way that therapists can sidestep the role of expert is to make suggestions and frame their understandings tentatively so that clients are encouraged to look to their own experience as a guide to the appropriateness of formulations, tasks, or reflections by their therapists.

Process-experiential therapy has attempted to provide a comprehensive theory of treatment by integrating Gestalt and client-centered approaches. It combines the relationship conditions of empathy, prizing, and congruence with more active interventions like empty-chair and two-chair work from Gestalt therapy, and focusing and evocative unfolding from Gendlin's and Rice's developments within client-centered therapy. In Gendlin's (1981, 1996) focusing approach to experiential therapy the relationship is seen as being of major importance. He sees listening as the second most important element, and focusing instructions as following on and being dependent on these. Everything done in therapy is seen as a product of interaction and as having an impact on the client's ongoing bodily sense. This is essentially a field or relational view of functioning rather than a purely intrapsychic view. Gendlin considers therapy as a real relationship between two people for the purpose of therapy in which the therapist is continually attempting to reach the struggling person within. In this approach the safety of the client supersedes all else, including theory, technique, or assessment. Although therapy may involve dealing with relational events such as covert difficulties or therapist internal reactions as a means of registering interactional problems, these are dealt with only as they arise, not as the primary focus of therapy. Other experiential therapists vary in the degree to which they emphasize the relationship versus tasks.

## THE FOCUS ON CLIENTS' EXPERIENCING IN THERAPY

We will now turn to the primary task in experiential approaches: clients' experiencing in therapy. Carl Rogers believed that people had within themselves the resources for self-understanding and the capacity to alter their behavior. He observed that an important change process in therapy seemed to be clients' movement from a rigid way of being in the world to a more fluid process in which they were in touch with their moment-to-moment inner experiencing. This led to the development of the experiential arm in client-centered therapy which emphasized the importance of clients' experiencing in therapy.

Rogers (1975) posited that change in therapy often resulted from a nonlinear process or shift as seen in focusing. He observed that "when a hitherto repressed feeling is fully and acceptantly experienced in awareness in the relationship, there is not only a definitely felt psychological shift, but a concomitant physiological change, as a new state of insight is achieved" (p. 210). The key to experiential therapy is the inward focusing of attention to articulate experience clearly. The therapeutic dialogue is distinguished by the inward direction of the clients' attention as they engage in an inner search, as opposed to the dialogue being like the social chitchat of a tea party.

## Focusing and the Phenomenological Perspective

Gendlin (1974) describes experiential therapy in these words: "The crux of experiential psychotherapy is the richer, fuller experiential process that occurs when one lets a felt sense form, when one lives and stays with that until the next step of speech or action emerges from that and when one then returns again to the level of the felt sense to take still further steps" (p. 239). Gendlin suggests that change or movement in therapy consists of the client's internal shift in experiencing as a result of accurately representing an internal felt sense. He conceptualizes experience as a process, and the occurrence of change depends on whether the ongoing living and experiencing process moves further and further as the inner sense is continually articulated. "The motor that powers psychotherapeutic change is a direct sensing into what is concretely felt (not emotions but an implicitly complex felt sense) and allowing that to form and to move" (Gendlin, 1974, p. 240). Gendlin (1974, 1981) developed the technique of focusing to assist clients to recognize and clarify their feelings. He stresses that clients need to turn their attention to their inner experience. Gendlin (1974) observes that within each individual there is a flow of experiencing to which that person can have recourse to discover the meaning of particular experiences for him-/herself. The main principle of the experiential method is to have people check whatever is said or done against their own concretely felt experiencing. People's experiencing was seen as full bodied and rich in detail, very immediate, intense, fluid, and capable of differentiation. An important aspect of experiencing is that it functions as an internal barometer against which one's representations of experience can be checked. Both Rogers and Gendlin distinguished feelings from emotions. The former are the result of the interaction of cognition and emotion. Feelings are the product of the symbolization of experience and reveal the cognitively felt meaings of one's experience, whereas emotions are the physical sensations or reactions that are a response to various environmental stimuli and reveal the pre-reflective import or significance that things have for one.

Even as he emphasized focusing and experiencing, Gendlin saw reflection as the primary tool of the client-centered and experiential therapist. He argued that it is through the use of reflection that therapists can check their understanding of their clients' experiences and stay in tune with what they are experiencing in the session. He suggested that there were two requirements necessary for a good reflection: first, the reflections should distill the essence of what clients are trying to say, or alternatively they should have a tentative, probing quality that stimulates clients' differentiation and exploration of their experiences; second, clients should be encouraged to check what their therapists say against an inner felt sense of experiencing. In this way experiencing acts like a barometer against which clients can check their symbolizations of their experience.

Gendlin's experiential model of therapy focuses on intrapersonal functioning. Therapeutic change and clients' growth is seen to emerge from their growing awareness of their experience and their symbolization of it in words. This process seems to transform clients' experiences so that they are able to move forward to encounter other aspects of themselves and the world. Thus Gendlin's focusing method emphasizes intrapsychic change processes within the client rather than interpersonal change processes within the therapeutic relationship as the important ingredient of change.

Mahrer (1989) has developed an experiential approach that differs from the other experiential approaches discussed here. His more radical line of experiential therapy sees no need for a relational component and focuses purely on promoting clients' experiencing in the session. Mahrer's concept of experiencing involves four essential aspects: (1) being in a moment of strong feeling; (2) welcoming the newly accessed way of being (or inner potential); (3) being experienced as the inner potential in an earlier life scene; and (4) prospectively translating this way of being into the world outside of therapy. He defines the essential common elements of different views of experiencing as a process of deeper exploration of a felt sense and the consequent opening up of a further internal felt sense leading to a cognitive/perceptual reorganization, an acceptance of one's inner potential and being, and behaving in accord with it. In addition experiencing involves encountering one's whole self and that of another in a process of meeting.

## The Constructivist/Information Processing Perspective

A number of other theorists within the person-centered tradition began to conceptualize clients' experiencing in terms of cognitive–affective information processing and meaning construction (Rice, 1974; Wexler, 1974; Zimring, 1974, 1990; Anderson, 1974; Toukmanian, 1992; Sachse, 1990). These theorists were influenced by Rogers's notion that human beings were active processors of information who actively constructed and organized their experience. In this view people are seen as active agents who create their own experience and are the recipients of it. Thus people discover the structure of their experience in the process of living it and feelings are generated in the process of organizing information (Greenberg et al., 1993; Wexler & Rice, 1974; Epstein, 1994).

This arm of client-centered theory sees cognitive processes as acting on and transforming information, the raw material of experience derived from both external and internal sources. The internal sources of information consist of sensory input from inner sources and stored information from long-term memory. External sources of information consist of the vast array of information which can be processed through the senses. It is in the process of organizing and making sense of this information that experience is generated and constructed. Thus experiencing is defined as the process of organizing and attending to the information from internal and external sources to make "sense" of the world. The information is organized in some way most commonly referred to as schemes (Rice, 1974; Wexler, 1974; Zimring, 1974; Toukmanian, 1994). Practice thus began to focus on helping clients to reorganize their schemes of themselves and the world.

Rice (1974) proposed that people have classes of experience which they may not have adequately processed. For example, clients may have felt so anxious in a particular situation that they were unable to process it. Alternatively, specific stimulus fields may be so wide or contain so much information that they are difficult to process. Either way, parts of the stimulus situation may be left out of clients' representations of their experience. Thus, the representations clients develop of events may not be accurate. Rice (1974) suggests that if one continues to encounter similar situations under such distorting conditions then a construction of these events is formulated that filters experience and guides behavior. These constructions are considered to be relatively enduring unless challenged by new information.

The goal of client-centered therapy, according to this view, is the differentiation and integration of meaning. Differentiation refers to the process of elaborating more specific facets of meaning. The therapist's function is to help clients to attend to information; to assist them with organizing information and integrating meaning across experience; and to evoke new facets of information. Rice (1974), like a number of other theorists (Butler, 1974; Gendlin, 1974), recognized the importance of heightening experience in order to symbolize it more accurately in awareness. Rice distinguished between the relationship factors that promoted clients' change processes in therapy and the task factors or specific techniques that therapists could use at different times to facilitate clients' experiencing within the session and assist in their information processing activities. The objective being to help clients access more information to induce changes in their faulty schemes and allow for improved functioning.

To facilitate access to new information Rice (1974) developed the technique of evocative reflection. With this technique the therapist attempts to rekindle clients' recollections of events so as to formulate successively more accurate accounts of their experience. Other techniques that were developed by client-centered therapists to heighten clients' access to their experiencing included the use of vivid language (Butler, 1974) and the use of metaphor. Later Toukmanian (1990, 1992), emphasizing the cognitive restructuring elements, extended the information processing function of the therapist by helping clients to actively differentiate the meaning of their experience and to reconstrue their experience by examining their memories and evaluations of events. Rainer Sachse (Chapter 13, this volume), working in a linguistic processing framework, developed a set of steps to access deeper levels of processing. The information processing perspective was to be pursued and furthered by Greenberg et al. (1993), as they attempted to locate experiential psychotherapy within current thinking on emotion and cognition.

## Existential Therapy

Existential therapy, like Gestalt therapy, grew out of psychoanalysis. Consequently in this approach people are seen as balancing and juggling conflicting conscious and unconscious forces. However, in existential therapy, the conflict that is at the core of human existence does not involve sexual and aggressive impulses; rather, it is between the individual and the givens of existence (May & Yalom, 1989; Tiryakian, 1962). The four basic concerns that define the human condition and with which everyone struggles include the concern with death, isolation, freedom, and meaninglessness. Existential therapists utilize a wide range of techniques in their practice, including interpretation, confrontation, advice, support, and empathy (Swildens, 1990). One of the primary objectives is to have clients to face the givens of existence and confront the attendant anxiety so that they can learn to live more authentically and responsibly in the moment.

The fundamental tasks clients perform in existential therapy are to explore and revise their SAWCS, the givens of existence, and their attendant anxiety (May & Yalom, 1989; Bugenthal & McBeath, 1995; Swildens, 1990). In order to revise their SAWCS clients need to articulate and represent their constructs of themselves and their world, and to reflect on and examine their own inner experiencing, emotions, goals, and apprehensions. Clients need to open themselves to change so as to formulate alternative constructions and perceptions of themselves and their world to develop more satisfying strategies for living (Bugenthal & McBeath, 1995). A primary task that clients engage in existential therapy is searching. This process is similar to unfolding or focusing (Gendlin, 1974) and is a way for clients to tap into processes that are not readily available to consciousness (Bugenthal & McBeath, 1995). Searching requires that clients be fully present to themselves during the psychotherapy hour. When present clients have an emotional investment, focused intention and are genuinely open to internal discovery.

Obstacles to searching and being present are termed resistances that can provide important information to both clients and therapists about the ways clients have learned to adapt and cope with life. It is important for both therapists and clients to understand and respect the latter's resistances so that they can be adapted to better serve the clients' life goals and tasks.

## Gestalt Therapy

Using the phenomenological method Gestalt therapists have long recognized the power of accessing experience in the here and now. They focus on the tasks of facilitating clients' awareness, experiencing, and contact with the external world. One of the central tenets of Gestalt therapy, like existential therapy, is to facilitate the individual in becoming more authentic. Stimulating experience to form vivid new awareness is the goal and is based on the notion that experience and action precede and are a necessary precursor to understanding. Gestalt therapists pay particular attention to what is occurring at the contact boundaries between self and others, and work to enhance clients' awareness of their own processes, needs, and wants. In doing this Gestalt therapists often focus on people's nonverbal behavior and their use of language. They may, for example, direct clients' attention to a sigh or a snarl on the lip, or ask clients to experiment with the effect on their experience of changing the word "it" into "I."

In this approach, increasing awareness by focusing on feelings, sensations, and motoric processes is the core process. Clients are encouraged to follow their awareness as it makes contact with or withdraws from the environment and figural experience in a disciplined manner. Awareness is followed as a continual process that changes moment by moment as a need is recognized, acted on, and satisfied, or as a goal is met or an interest followed. Gestalt therapy thus offers clients a means of exploring their manner of constructing reality in the moment that this is occurring. This is aimed at helping people become aware of their agency in constructing reality and in identifying and reworking any unfinished business that may have impeded contact with present reality.

The graded experiment was used as the major form of intervention. This experimental method involved setting up tasks in the session not so much to be completed as to promote discovery of intrapsychic processes. In the session experimental tasks like two-chair work and dream work were emphasized, but many other experiments were created in the moment to help clients intensify and embody their experiences. Creative experiments were created to meet the client's situation, such as asking the client to express resentment to an imagined other, to assert or disclose something intimate to the therapist, to curl up into a ball, to express a desire in order to make it more vivid, or to move freely and fluidly like water. The client's experience and expression were then analyzed for what prevented or interrupted completion of these experiments. The experimental method focused on bringing people's difficulties to the surface, and what interfered with task completion became the center of therapeutic attention. Therapists asked clients to become aware of and experience the interruptive processes that prevented feelings or needs from being expressed or acted upon. In this manner clients were able to gain insight into their own experience by discovery rather than interpretation. Thus clients enacted conflicts between parts of the self and had dialogues with others with whom they had unfinished business. In line with the idea that all parts of the dream are parts of the dreamer, clients were asked to identify with the different elements in their dreams and to set up dialogues between parts of the dream.

Creative use of imagery and experiment involved "Try this" followed by "What do you experience now?" This was referred to as behavioristic phenomenology in which observable behaviors were tried out in the here and now to generate experience which was then attended to and explored. In addition to the experiment, Gestalt therapists used a set of key questions designed to get at particular aspects of clients' functioning and promote creative adjustment to the environment. The experience-oriented questions were as follows: "What are you aware of?" "What do you experience?" "What do you need?" "What do you want or want to do?" Finally, at appropriate times, identity-related questions of the form "Who are you?" or "What do you want to be?" were also asked.

With more fragile clients who have not developed a strong sense of self or boundary between self and other, the development of awareness is more of a long-term objective. Promotion of experience and asking these clients such questions as "What do you feel?" or "Can you stay with this feeling?" would be pointless, as they have yet to develop an awareness of their internal world. With these clients the relationship is seen as the only therapeutic point of departure (Spagnola Lobb & Salonia, 1993). Thus a more relational form of work needs to be followed in which the process of contact with the therapist becomes the focus.

## Process-Experiential Therapy

In process-experiential therapy an important task is to bring emotions and their associated action tendencies into awareness. A process-experiential approach to therapy in addition pays great attention to the questions or problems clients pose about their experience as they explore their feelings. Client statements are viewed as markers that indicate aspects of experience that are currently troubling to clients and indicate that they are struggling to resolve certain experiences. For example, clients might find some of their reactions to be problematic or puzzling, or they might be in conflict about pursuing different courses of action, or they might express lingering and chronic bad feelings about a significant other, or express distress at having a cherished belief challenged, or be unclear and uncertain about how they are feeling. When these markers are heard and identified in therapy, therapists are able to differentially intervene in ways that can facilitate the resolution of these problems. For example, systematic evocative unfolding can be implemented to resolve a problematic reaction, chair work can be used at a conflict split or unfinished business, the creation of meaning task can be initiated when a cherished belief is challenged, or focusing can be applied at an unclear or absent felt sense.

Each of these techniques has as its primary objective the heightening of clients' inner experiences so that these can be symbolized more easily in awareness. Through the symbolic representation of their experience clients' needs, expectations, and characteristic ways of experiencing reality are revealed. Different interventions have been developed to help clients' resolve specific cognitive–affective problems and to heighten their access to their inner experience. Each intervention pursues particular types of exploration suited to specific types of problems and promotes different types of resolution. For example, systematic evocative unfolding facilitates clients' access to their memories of events and their emotional reactions through the use of vivid, concrete, and evocative language (Bucci, 1984; Watson & Rennie, 1994). To heighten clients' access to their experience, therapists ask clients to provide detailed and concrete descriptions of their external environment. These descriptions are then amplified by therapists with the use of vivid, imagistic language. This provides clients with the opportunity to represent external events more clearly and accurately and to access and attend to their own subjectively felt experience so as to represent it more fully in awareness. It serves to illuminate their patterns of responding as well as their personal styles of behavior that they may have developed from emotionally significant past experiences, thereby enabling clients to develop a new view of themselves.

Two-chair work helps clients to resolve self-critical internal dialogues. Self-critical introjects and self-statements are heightened in order to evoke an emotional response in the experiencing self. This emotional response is differentiated until a new adaptive emotional response to the critic emerges. When this precipitates a softening in the previously harsh critic, an integration of the previously opposing aspects of experience occurs. The unfinished business task tries to concretely evoke the presence of the other and his or her most salient characteristics to evoke an emotional reaction in the self which can then be symbolized in awareness. The previously unexpressed emotion is expressed, and the unmet need is mobilized. The promotion of dialogue with a significant other and the representation of the other's point of view often lead clients to change their view of the other and become more self-assertive. The significant other may be understood and possibly forgiven or may be held accountable for offenses committed. A variety of other tasks including focusing are used to facilitate exploration of different problem states (Greenberg et al., 1993).

It is important to evoke clients' emotional reactions to help them identify the impact of events, symbolize their reactions, and discover their needs and goals and the action tendencies inherent in their emotional reactions. This allows them to become aware of links between the external environment, their inner experience, and their behavior (Greenberg et al., 1993; Watson & Greenberg, 1996a, 1996b). Subsequently these links can be subjected to reflexive examination in the light of current goals, values, and environmental contingencies. Once the data from their emotional and rational systems has been integrated, clients are in the position to choose among alternative ways of acting to enhance their adaptation and growth and facilitate achievement of their life tasks and goals (Watson & Greenberg, 1996a).

Although process-experiential tasks are focused on intrapsychic processes, some of them indirectly facilitate interpersonal functioning. Systematic evocative unfolding is very useful in helping clients access the impact of external events and those aspects of their interpersonal transactions that can be particularly troublesome. Chair work is useful in teaching clients techniques of self-assertion and ways of negotiating with significant people in their lives. Moreover, to the extent that aspects of the therapeutic relationship are open to discussion, there is the possibility of clients becoming more congruent in their interpersonal transactions in the world at large. Specific types of relational events have been alluded to but not yet developed. Such events are as follows: dealing with alliance ruptures (Safran, Muran, & Samistag, 1994); promoting empathic understanding of misunderstanding (Rhodes, Geller, Elliott, & Greenberg, 1995); using therapists' experienced reactions as a source of dealing with client interpersonal patterns (Kiesler, 1982) and focusing on the positive tendencies of the inner struggling person to resolve therapist-experienced conflicts between genuineness and positive regard (Lietaer, 1993); and providing a basis for positive confrontations. In addition, the therapeutic relationship is seen as operating throughout the tasks, offering support and validation of emerging new experience. The relationship thus provides the interpersonal contact with confirmation, and empathy seen as essential in promoting self-empathy and growth.

## CONCLUSION

In this chapter we have examined the evolution of experiential praxis over the last 40 years. Specifically we have attempted to elaborate the differential emphasis by various proponents on the role of the relationship in promoting change and the role of specific experiential tasks to facilitate clients' access to their inner experience. In spite of the differential emphases within experiential approaches to therapy, it is to be hoped that future generations of experiential therapists will continue to see the value of both enhancing and maintaining the therapeutic relationship and of promoting clients' experiencing within the session. We believe that these two principles in conjunction with an appreciation of both intrapsychic and interpersonal components of functioning help define the essence of experiential psychotherapy.

# REFERENCES

Anderson, W. (1974). Personal growth and client-centered therapy: An information-processing view. In D. Wexler & L. Rice (Eds.), *Innovations in client-centered therapy*. New York: Wiley.

Barrett-Lennard, G. (1997). The recovery of empathy towards others and self. In A. Bohart & L. Greenberg (Eds.), *Empathy Reconsidered*. Washington, DC: APA Books.

Bohart, A. (1993). Experiencing: The Basis of Psychotherapy. *Journal of Psychotherapy Integration, 3*(1), 51–67.

Bozarth, J. (1990). The essence of person-centered therapy. In G. Lietaer, J. Rombauts, & R. Van Balen (Eds.), *Person-centered and experiential psychotherapy in the nineties*. Leuven, Belgium: Leuven University Press.

Brodley, B. (1990). Person-centered and experiential: Two different therapies. In G. Lietaer, J. Rombauts, & R. Van Balen (Eds.), *Person-centered and experiential psychotherapy in the nineties*. Leuven, Belgium: Leuven University Press.

Bucci, W. (1984). Linking words and things? Basic processes and individual variations. *Cognition, 17,* 137–153.

Bugenthal, J., & McBeath, B. (1995). Depth existential therapy: Evolution since World War II. In B. Bongar & L. Beutler (Eds.), *Comprehensive textbook of psychotherapy*. New York: Oxford University Press.

Butler, J. M. (1974). The iconic mode in psychotherapy. In D. A. Wexler & L. N. Rice (Eds.), *Innovations in client-centered therapy*. New York: Wiley.

Elliott, R., & Greenberg, L. S. (1993). Experiential therapy in practice: The process-experiential approach. In B. Bongar & L. Beutler (Eds.), *Comprehensive textbook of psychotherapy*. New York: Oxford University Press.

Elliott, R., & Shapiro, D. (1992). Client and therapist as analysts of significant events. In S. Toukmanian & D. L. Rennie (Eds.), *Psychotherapy process research: Paradigmatic and narrative approaches*. Newbury Park, CA: Sage.

Epstein, S. (1994). Integration of the cognitive and psychodynamic unconscious. *American Psychologist, 49*(8), 709–724.

Fagan, J. (1974). Personality theory and psychotherapy. *The Counseling Psychologist, 4*(4), 4–7.

Gendlin, E. (1964). A theory of personality change. In P. Worchel & D. Byrne (Eds.), *Personality change*. New York: Wiley.

Gendlin, E. T. (1974). Client-centered and experiential psychotherapy. In D. Wexler & L. N. Rice (Eds.), *Innovations in client-centered therapy*. New York: Wiley.

Gendlin, E. T. (1981). *Focusing*. New York: Bantam.

Gendlin, E. T. (1996). *Focusing-oriented psychotherapy: A manual of the experiential method*. New York: Guilford Press.

Greenberg, L. S., & Elliott, R. (1997). Varieties of empathic responding. In A. Bohart & L. Greenberg (Eds.), *Empathy reconsidered: New directions in psychotherapy*. Washington: APA Books.

Greenberg, L. S., Rice, L. N., & Elliott, R. (1993). *Facilitating emotional change: The moment-by-moment process*. New York: Guilford Press.

Greenberg, L. S., & Safran, J. D. (1987). *Emotion in psychotherapy: Affect, cognition, and the process of change*. New York: Guilford Press.

Hart, J. T. (1970). The development of client-centered therapy. In J. T. Hart &

T. M. Tomlinson (Eds.), *New directions in client-centered therapy*. Boston: Houghton Mifflin.

Heidegger, M. (1962). *Being and time* (J. Maquarne & E. S. Robinson, trans.). New York: Harper and Row. (Original work published 1949)

Hycner, R., & Jacobs, L. M. (1995). *The healing relationship in Gestalt therapy*. New York: Gestalt Journal Press.

Jacobs, L. M. (1989). Dialogue in Gestalt theory and therapy. *Gestalt Journal, 12*(1), 25–67.

Jaspers, K. (1963). *General psychopathology*. Chicago: University of Chicago Press.

Kiesler, D. (1982). Interpersonal theory for personality and psychotherapy. In J. C. Anchin & D. J. Kiesler (Eds.), *Handbook of interpersonal psychotherapy*. New York: Pergamon.

Klein, M. H., Mathieu-Coughlan, P., & Kiesler, D. J. (1986). The experiencing scales. In L. S. Greenberg & W. M. Pinsof (Eds.), *The psychotherapeutic process: A research handbook*. New York: Guilford Press.

Latner, J. (1992). The theory of Gestalt therapy. In E. C. Nevis (Ed.), *Gestalt therapy*. New York: Gardner Press.

Leijssen, M. (1990). On focusing and the necessary conditions of therapeutic personality change. In G. Lietaer, J. Rombauts, & R. Van Balen (Eds.), *Person-centered and experiential psychotherapy in the nineties*. Leuven, Belgium: Leuven University Press.

Leijssen, M. (1996). *Characteristics of a healing inner relationship*. Paper presented at the Third International Conference on Client-Centered and Experiential Therapy, Gmunden, Austria.

Lietaer, G. (1990). The person-centered approach after the Wisconsin Project: A personal view on its evolution. In G. Lietaer, J. Rombauts, & R. Van Balen (Eds.), *Person-centered and experiential psychotherapy in the nineties*. Leuven, Belgium: Leuven University Press.

Lietaer, G. (1992). Helping and hindering processes in client-centered/experiential psychotherapy: A content analysis of client and therapist post-session perceptions. In S. Toukmanian & D. L. Rennie (Eds.), *Psychotherapy process research: Paradigmatic and narrative approaches*. Newbury Park, CA: Sage.

Lietaer, G. (1993). Authenticity, congruence, and transparency. In D. Brazier (Ed.), *Beyond Carl Rogers: Towards a psychotherapy for the twenty-first century*. London: Constable.

Lietaer, G., & Dierick, P. (1996). Client-centered group psychotherapy in dialogue with other orientations: Commonality and specificity. In R. Hutterer, G. Pawlowsky, P. F. Schmid, & R. Stipsits (Eds.), *Client-centered and experiential psychotherapy: A paradigm in motion*. Frankfurt: Peter Lang.

Mahrer, A. R. (1989). *How to do experiential psychotherapy: A manual for practitioners*. Ottawa, Ontario, Canada: University of Ottawa Press.

May, R. (1969). *Love and will*. New York: Norton.

May, R., & Yalom, I. D. (1989). Existential psychotherapy. In R. Corsini & D. Wedding (Eds.), *Current psychotherapies*. Itasca, IL: Peacock.

Meador, B., & Rogers, C. (1979). Person-centered therapy. In R. Corsini (Ed.), *Current psychotherapies*. Itasca, IL: Peacock.

Mearns, D. (1994). *Developing person-centred counselling*. Newbury Park, CA: Sage.

Mearns, D., & Thorne, B. (1988). *Person-centred counselling in action*. Newbury Park, CA: Sage.

Melnick, J., & Nevis, S. (1992). Diagnosis: The struggle for a meaningful paradigm. In E. C. Nevis (Ed.), *Gestalt therapy*. New York: Gardner Press.

Mermin, D. (1974). Gestalt theory of emotion. *The Counseling Psychologist, 4*(4), 15–20.

Perls, F. (1969). *Ego, hunger and aggression*. New York: Random House.

Perls, F. (1973). *The Gestalt approach and eyewitness to therapy*. Palo Alto, CA: Science and Behavior Books.

Perls, L. (1976). New perspectives in Gestalt therapy. In W. L. Smith (Ed.), *The growing edge of Gestalt therapy*. Secaucus, NJ: Citadel Press.

Polster, E., & Polster, M. (1973). *Gestalt therapy integrated*. New York: Random House.

Raskin, N., & Rogers, C. R. (1989). Person-centered therapy. In R. Corsini & D. Wedding (Eds.), *Current psychotherapies*. Itasca, IL: Peacock.

Rennie, D. L. (1992). Qualitative analysis of the client's experience of psychotherapy: The unfolding of reflexivity. In S. Toukmanian and D. Rennie (Eds.), *Psychotherapy process research: Paradigmatic and narrative approaches*. Newbury Park, CA: Sage.

Rennie, D. L. (1993). Clients' deference in psychotherapy. *Journal of Counseling Psychology, 41*, 427–437.

Rennie, D. L. (1998). *Person-centered counseling: An experiential approach*. Newbury Park, CA: Sage.

Resnick, R. (1995). Gestalt therapy: Principles, prisms, and perspectives. *British Gestalt Journal, 1*, 3–13.

Rhodes, R., Geller, J., Elliott, R., & Greenberg, L. (1995, June). *Misunderstanding events*. Panel presentation at the meeting of the Society for Psychotherapy Research, Berkeley, CA.

Rice, L. N. (1974).The evocative function of the therapist. In D. Wexler & L. N. Rice (Eds.), *Innovations in clients-centered therapy*. New York: Wiley.

Rice, L. N. (1983). The relationship in client-centered therapy. In M. J. Lambert (Ed.), *Psychotherapy and patient relationships*. Homewood, Illinois: Dow-Jones Irwin.

Rice, L. N., & Greenberg, L. S. (1992). Humanistic approaches to psychotherapy. In D. K. Freedheim (Ed.), *History of psychotherapy: A century of change*. Washington, DC: American Psychological Association.

Rogers, C. R. (1942). *Counseling and psychotherapy*. Boston: Houghton Mifflin.

Rogers, C. (1951). *Person-centered therapy*. Boston: Houghton Mifflin.

Rogers, C. R. (1957).The necessary and sufficient conditions of therapeutic personality change. *Journal of Consulting Psychology, 21*, 97–103.

Rogers, C. R. (1959). A theory of therapy, personality, and interpersonal relationships, as developed in the client-centered framework. In S. Koch (Ed.), *Psychology a study of science*. New York: McGraw-Hill.

Rogers, C. R. (1959). *Client-centered therapy: Its current practice, implications, and theory*. Boston: Houghton Mifflin.

Rogers, C. R. (1961). *On becoming a person*. Boston: Houghton Mifflin.

Rogers, C. R. (1970). *Carl Rogers on encounter groups*. New York: Harper and Row.

Rogers, C. R. (1974). Empathic: An unappreciated way of being. *The Counseling Psychologist, 5*(2), 2–10.

Rogers, C. R. (1980). *A way of being*. Boston: Houghton Mifflin.

Sachse, R. (1990). The influence of therapist processing proposals on the explication process of the client. *Person Centered Review, 5,* 321–364.

Safran, J. D., Muran, C., & Samistag, P. (1994). Resolving therapeutic alliance ruptures: A task-analytic investigation. In A. O. Horvath & L. S. Greenberg (Eds.), *The working alliance: Theory, research and practice.* New York: Wiley.

Schneider, K. J., & May, R. (1995). *The psychology of existence: An integrative clinical perspective.* New York: McGraw-Hill.

Simkin, J. (1979). Gestalt therapy. In R. Corsini (Ed.), *Current psychotherapies.* Itasca, IL: Peacock.

Spagnola Lobb, M., & Salonia, G. (1993). What is the future in Gestalt therapy? *Studies in Gestalt Therapy: International Edition, 2,* 23–32.

Swildens, H. (1990). Client-centered psychotherapy for patients with borderline symptoms. In G. Lietaer, J. Rombauts, & R. Van Balen (Eds.), *Client-centered and experiential psychotherapy in the nineties.* Leuven, Belgium: Leuven University Press.

Taylor, C. (1975). *Human agency and language philosophical papers I.* Cambridge: Cambridge University Press.

Thorne, B. (1992). *Carl Rogers.* Newbury Park, CA: Sage.

Tiryakian, E. (1962). *Sociologism and existentialism.* Englewood Cliffs, NJ: Prentice-Hall.

Toukmanian, S. (1990). A schema-based information processing perspective on client change in experiential therapy. In G. Lietaer, J. Rombauts, & R. Van Balen (Eds.), *Client-centered and experiential psychotherapy in the nineties.* Leuven, Belgium: Leuven University Press.

Toukmanian, S. (1992). Studying clients' perceptual processes and their outcomes in psychotherapy. In S. Toukmanian & D. Rennie (Eds.), *Psychotherapy process research: Paradigmatic and narrative approaches.* Newbury Park, CA: Sage.

Vanaerschot, G. (1990). The process of empathy: Holding and letting go. In G. Lietaer, J. Rombauts, & R. Van Balen (Eds.), *Client-centered and experiential psychotherapy in the nineties.* Leuven, Belgium: Leuven University Press.

Van Balen, R. (1990). The therapeutic relationship according to Carl Rogers: Only a climate? a dialogue? or both? In G. Lietaer, J. Rombauts, & R. Van Balen (Eds.), *Client-centered and experiential psychotherapy in the nineties.* Leuven, Belgium: Leuven University Press.

Van Deurzen-Smith, E. (1988). *Existential counselling in practice.* London: Sage.

Watson, J. C. (1996). *An analysis of therapist interventions using the SASB model of interpersonal behavior in a good and poor outcome case in the experiential therapy of depression.* Paper presented at the annual meeting of the Society for Psychotherapy Research, Amelia Island, FL.

Watson, J. C., & Greenberg, L. S. (1994). The alliance in experiential therapy: Enacting the relationship conditions. In A. Horvath & L. S. Greenberg (Eds.), *The working alliance: Theory, research and practice.* New York: Wiley.

Watson, J. C., & Greenberg, L. S. (1995). Alliance ruptures and repairs in experiential therapy. *In Session: Psychotherapy in Practice, 1*(1), 19–32.

Watson, J. C., & Greenberg, L. S. (1996a). Emotion and cognition in experiential therapy: A dialectical-constructivist perspective. In H. Rosen & K. Kuelwein (Eds.), *Constructing realities: Meaning making perspectives for psychotherapists.* San Francisco: Jossey-Bass.

Watson, J. C. & Greenberg, L. S. (1996b). Pathways to change in the psychotherapy of depression: Relating process to session change and outcome. *Psychotherapy Research, 33*, 262–274.

Watson, J. C., & Greenberg, L. S. (1998). The alliance in short term experiential therapy. In J. Safran & C. Muran (Eds.), *The alliance in brief psychotherapy.* Washington, DC: APA Books.

Watson, J. C., & Rennie, D. (1994). A qualitative analysis of clients' reports of their subjective experience while exploring problematic reactions in therapy. *Journal of Counseling Psychology, 41*, 500–509.

Wexler, D. A., & Rice, L. N. (1974). *Innovations in client-centered therapy.* New York: Wiley.

Wheeler, G. (1991). *Gestalt reconsidered.* New York: Gardner Press.

Yalom, I. D. (1975). *The theory and practice of group psychotherapy.* New York: Basic Books.

Yalom, I. D. (1980). *Existential psychotherapy.* New York: Basic Books.

Yontef, G. M. (1991). *Awareness, dialogue and process: Essays on Gestalt therapy.* New York: Gestalt Journal Press.

Yontef, G. M. (1995). Gestalt therapy. In A. S. Gurman & S. B. Messer (Eds.), *Essential psychotherapies: Theory and practice.* New York: Guilford Press.

Yontef, G. M., & Simkin, J. S. (1989). Gestalt therapy. In R. Corsini & D. Wedding (Eds.), *Current psychotherapies.* Itasca, IL: Peacock.

Zimring, F. M. (1974). Theory and practice in client-centered therapy. In D. A. Wexler & L. N. Rice (Eds.), *Innovations in client-centered therapy.* New York: Wiley, 117–137.

Zimring, F. M. (1990). Cognitive processes as a cause of psychotherapeutic change: Self-initiated processes. In G. Lietaer, J. Rombauts, & R. Van Balen (Eds.), *Person-centered and experiential psychotherapy in the nineties.* Leuven, Belgium: Leuven University Press.

Zimring, F. M., & Raskin, N. J. (1992). Carl Rogers and client/person centered therapy. In D. K. Freedlehm, H. J. Freudenberger, J. W. Kessler, S. B. Messer, D. R. Peterson, H. H. Strupp, & P. L. Wachtel (Eds.), *History of psychotherapy: A century of change.* Washington, DC: APA Books.

Zinker, J. (1977). *Creative process in Gestalt therapy.* New York: Brunner/Mazel.

# 2

*****

# The Theory of Experience-Centered Therapies

## Leslie S. Greenberg
## Richard Van Balen

*A theory of functioning* in the experience centered therapies, has tended to follow on the heels of a more developed theory of practice. In this chapter we offer a review and revision of the experiential theory of human functioning to reflect developments in practice. The theory of client-centered, existential, and Gestalt therapies and their more recent developments will be reviewed as the basis of the theory guiding current experiential/phenomenological approaches. We will follow the review with a theoretical synthesis and revision that we believe more closely fits the current practice of experiential therapy. In this synthesis, theoretical concerns with the notion of the actualizing tendency and with the concepts of denial and the possibility of direct access to experience are addressed. A theory of experiential construction is proposed to help clarify these issues.

## BASIC ASSUMPTIONS

The basic assumptions underlying experiential approaches are that human beings are aware, experiencing organisms who function holistically to organize their experience into coherent forms (Perls, Hefferline, & Goodman, 1951; Rogers, 1951; Gendlin, 1962; Mahrer, 1978, 1983, 1986, 1996; May, 1958, 1960, 1981; Yalom, 1975, 1980, 1989). People are therefore viewed as purposive, meaning-creating, symbolizing agents whose subjective experience is an essential aspect of their humanness (Frankl, 1959, 1968). In addition to the emphasis on subjective awareness and experience, in these phenomenological approaches the operation of an integrative, formative tendency, oriented toward survival, growth, and the creation of meaning, has governed an experiential view of functioning. Behavior is seen as the goal-directed attempt of people to satisfy their needs as experienced in the field as perceived (Rogers, 1951; Perls et al., 1951), and consistency with the self-concept has been seen as a determining factor regulating behavior.

A general principle that has united all experientially/phenomenologically oriented theorists is that people are wiser than their intellects alone. In an experiencing organism consciousness is seen as being at the peak of a pyramid of nonconscious organismic functioning. Of central importance is that tacit functioning is an important guide to conscious experience, is fundamentally adaptive, and is potentially available to awareness. Internal experience is seen as being potentially most available to awareness when the internal deployment of attention is supported by the interpersonal field. Interpersonal safety and support are viewed as key elements in promoting an increase in the amount of attention available for self-awareness and self-exploration. In addition, experiments in directed awareness are seen as helping both to focus attention on inchoate experience and to intensify its vividness.

The self is central in explaining human functioning. Although theorists differed in their views of the nature of the self, all were self theorists. Rogers, who developed the most systematic self theory, equated the self with the self-concept. Gestalt theory equated the self with the integrated whole and the agent of growth. Existentialists viewed self as a quality of existence. All, however, adopted the idea of an active integrating self as a guiding construct.

The person was viewed as a complex system, operating in a field in which greater awareness of more aspects of experience—of self and the environment—promoted integration and adaptive engagement with the environment. We will argue that within this tradition the major view of the self, although sometimes implicit, has been one of the self as a dialectically operating dynamic system (Thelen & Smith, 1994; Pascual-Leone, 1987, 1990a, 1990b, 1998), in which healthy functioning results when as many parts as possible are integrated in awareness. In this view it is the integration of ever-developing facets of experience, including polar aspects (Perls, 1969; Mahrer, 1986) as well as different levels and types of experience (Rogers, 1961; Greenberg & Safran, 1987), that is seen as central in healthy functioning.

## CLASSICAL THEORY

The major theoretical influences on current experiential therapy come from Rogers's (1951, 1959) statement of client-centered therapy, Gendlin's (1962, 1964, 1973, 1974, 1996) development of this approach into a focusing view, and Perls and his collaborators' (1951) views of Gestalt therapy (see also Perls, 1969). In addition the contribution of existential theory (May, 1960;

Yalom, 1980) and Mahrer's (1983, 1996) experiential view will be touched on when they add a unique perspective.

Both client-centered and Gestalt therapy moved from earlier structural theories to later, more process-oriented views of functioning. The structural and process views are discussed below.

## Client-Centered Structural Theory

Two major structural constructs were used to explain functioning, self-concept and organismic experience.

### *Self-Concept*

Self-concept or self-structure was an important construct in client-centered theory. For Rogers (1959) it is an organized *conceptual* Gestalt consisting of the individual's perceptions of self and self in relation to others, together with the *values* attached to these perceptions. The self-concept is not always in awareness but always is available to awareness. It is a changing process but at any moment it is a fixed entity. My self-concept is thus the view I have of myself plus my evaluation of that view. A person may, for example, perceive her-/himself as a good student, of superior intelligence, and as loving her/his parents and value these positively as well as seeing her-/himself as unattractive to the opposite sex and as competitive, and view these negatively.

Attitudes toward self were seen as important determiners of behavior and, although needs were also seen as important determiners of behavior, the particular way a need was satisfied was to *select a behavior to be consistent* with a self-concept (notice the dialectical interaction between elements). In this view difficulty in maintaining consistency between strong needs and self-concept caused distress and resulted in defensive maneuvers in an attempt to keep perception of behavior consistent with one's self view. This led to maladjustment.

### *Organismic Experience*

Experience is "anything observed or lived through, an actual living through of an event, ... individuals reaction to events, feelings" (*Webster's New World Dictionary*, 1979, p. 645). Experience, according to Rogers (1959), is all that is going on within the organism that is potentially available to awareness. To experience means to receive the impact of sensory or physiological events happening in the moment. Experiencing according to Gendlin (1964) is the process of concrete bodily feeling. This constitutes the basic matter of psychological phenomena. Experience is thus a datum; it is what happens as we live.

## Gestalt Structural Theory

Gestalt theory has a variety of different structural models. One, identical to client-centered theory, is that there is a conflict between an image (self-concept in client-centered theory) that the person is trying to actualize and what in Gestalt is called the self-actualizing tendency (organismic experience and actualizing tendency in client-centered theory). In the Gestalt view the process of introjection is crucial in forming the "shoulds" by which people try to manipulate the self to behave and experience in accord with the dictates of one's image. One of Perls's major breaks away from Freudian theory involved the rejection in normal development of the necessity of identification and introjection processes to form a superego, in favor of organismic wisdom as the guide to socialization. A "top dog" based on introjected "shoulds" was seen as being at the basis of the dysfunction of self-manipulation. The top dog was seen as evoking its opposite, the underdog, which opposed the self-coercion of the top dog.

A more formal structural theory was offered in Perls et al. (1951). In this, three aspects are conceived of as necessary to explain the functioning of the self, which was seen as the totality: the id, the ego, and the personality. Personality was seen as the structured aspect of functioning, like a self-concept or a social role, that had become habituated. It was viewed as the source of an inauthentic, false self. The ego was seen as an agent that variedly identified with, or alienated, aspects of id functioning. The id was seen as the spontaneous, organismic, preverbal level of experiencing. In addition a core set of interruptive mechanisms were posited. These were seen as producing poor awareness and disturbances of contact, as preventing the ego's identification with emerging experience as well as preventing contact between emerging id experience and the environment. The original mechanisms discussed were introjection, projection, and retroflection.

In Gestalt theory the person was also viewed as being constituted by various parts and as functioning by the integration of polarities. In essence a modular theory of self was postulated in which there existed different parts of the person that needed to be integrated. A further semistructural view was also offered by Perls (1969) in a theory of the layers of neurosis. Here five layers were posited: The synthetic layers made up of a *phony*, social-role layer, and a *phobic*, avoidant layer; this is followed by the *impasse* (or stuck) layer and the *implosive* layer in which action was turned inward; if these layers were all traversed the person reached an authentic, *explosive* layer, involving the healthy expression of anger, sadness, joy, or orgasm.

There are a number of problems with the above structural models. First, a self-concept, especially in Rogers's model, is given a governing role in a manner that does not match the spontaneous or automatic process nature by which much experience and behavior occur. Much of our conduct is free of reflection or conscious concern. Our views of how we should be, and our concepts of ourselves, as important as they are, do not appear to regulate all our behavior. Life has more complexity, depth, passion, and pain than can be described by struggles to be consistent and to maintain an image. In addition the source of the self-concept is most fundamentally others' views of the self. This fails to explain the complexities of personal organization that result from such sources as loss, trauma, neglect, human emotionality, and lived experience.

## Motivational Theory in Client-Centered and Gestalt Theory

Both client-centered and Gestalt posited a holistic actualizing tendency. Rogers's notion of an actualizing tendency developed from an initial view of a growth and development tendency into its later definition as the "inherent tendency of the organism to develop all its capacities in ways which serve to maintain or enhance the organism" (Rogers, 1959, p. 196). The latter view added the idea of the actualizing of all capacities to the notion of the adaptive function of a growth and development tendency. The actualizing tendency view was highly important in that it offered a nonhomeostatic view of functioning. The person was not guided by deficiencies but was proactive.

Perls started with the Gestalt psychology view of people as active organizers of their world with a tendency toward closure or completion of experience. This was offered as an alternative to views of people as determined either by their history or by the environment. Rather organismic regulation was seen as central. This view developed in the 1960s into one of a self-actualizing tendency, described metaphorically as that tendency by which an acorn develops into an oak tree. Perls in this period tended to shy away from systematic theorizing and, continuing to describe this tendency in a metaphoric vein, he often said that an elephant needs to grow up to be an elephant and an eagle needs to grow up to be an eagle, and that neither should attempt to grow up to be the other. Although human development was not seen by either Rogers or Perls as the unfolding of a genetic blueprint, their views have often been criticized on this account, and Perls's metaphors are clearly open to this interpretation. Rather than a view of a genetic blueprint that was actualized, theirs was a commitment to a view that there was some inherent organizing tendency that led infants to learn to walk and to develop, led humankind to learn to maintain themselves and to use tools, and led people to develop verbal concepts, strive for meaningful interpersonal contact, and for a sense of personal mastery.

In addition it was the holistic nature of this formative tendency that was emphasized over any specific drives or needs. All theorists drew on Goldstein's (1939) observation and conceptualization of an actualizing tendency to describe the holistic human tendency to organize capacities so as to optimally cope. Maslow (1954, 1968, 1971) subsequently defined the actualizing tendency in terms of a hierarchy of needs, moving from needs at the lower biological survival level to those at the higher "being" level. Perls, however, rejected these levels and adopted a more dynamic principle that stated that the most dominant need in the situation emerged to organize the field. All the theorists also emphasized the tendencies of people to thrust toward autonomy from external control, a view that fitted the autonomy-oriented view of health of the times. Perls, for example, stressed that maturation involved moving from environmental support to self-support. Rogers, however, strongly emphasized the prosocial nature of the actualizing tendency. People, according to Rogers, when guided by this tendency, were trustworthy, reliable, and constructive. Here both Perls and the existentialists differed somewhat from Rogers, placing greater emphasis on the importance of the integration of polarities over any inherent tendency toward goodness.

Rogers posited the development of *a need for positive regard* in addition to the actualizing tendency. This was seen as a persistent and pervasive need that is universally present in all human beings. This was a basic motive that was added to the actualizing tendency, or was seen as a major aspect of it. In Rogers's view this need rapidly transformed into a need for positive *self-regard* and promoted the subsequent development of conditions of worth that satisfied the need for love, primarily from caretakers. Thus in order for Rogers's theory to be coherent, a second regulatory principle, the need for positive regard, came into existence in addition to the actualizing tendency.

Together with the actualizing tendency Rogers proposed the existence of an *organismic valuing process*. This involved a regulatory or feedback mechanism that evaluated experience against a criterion set by the actualizing tendency to ensure that behavior would meet its need. This valuing process was thus the ultimate governor of functioning. How this tendency set the criterion and how the valuing process operated, however, remained somewhat of a mystery.

Perls, on the other hand, saw needs as central to functioning, and he offered a homeostatic model of organismic regulation in which the most dominant need emerged in relation to the situation and health involved acting on the environment to meet that need. He distanced himself from Maslow's hierarchy of basic needs, holding that there were thousands of psychological needs. The process by which the most dominant need emerged remained unclear, however. Examples of the most dominant need emerging in nature were given in place of an explanation of any mechanism—examples such as when a thirsty buck's need for survival from the imminent danger of being attacked by a lion overrides its survival need for water and leads to it fleeing the water hole. This was a field theory of motivation in which the need was not purely innate but emerged out of an organism–environment interaction. One sees this, for example, when one's loneliness and need for contact is sensed most acutely on seeing others being close, or when sexual desire is as much stimulated by the presence of an exciting other as by an internal drive.

Choice has been emphasized as a key motivational process by existential theorists, who along with Perls proposed that awareness leads to choice. Increased awareness was seen as enhancing need regulation, and choice was seen as key in determining the means whereby a need was met. Although Rogers valued self-determination and choice, his theory tended to put the actualizing tendency and the organismic valuing process in the driver's seat more than did the other traditions, which placed greater emphasis on awareness plus choice as guiding principles.

The notion of an actualizing tendency and its operation has been an ongoing source of difficulty and misunderstanding in this tradition. The nature and scientific basis of the actualizing tendency, as well as the relationship between this tendency and self-determination and choice, have long been a focus of discussion and critique. In addition, how organismic regulation operates remains a mystery. These problems will be further discussed in the section "A Synthesis: Experiential Construction," later in this chapter.

## Theory of Dysfunction

Dysfunction according to Rogers occurred due to *incongruence between self-concept and experience*. A state of incongruence exists when the self-concept differs from the actual experience of the organism. Thus if I see myself as loving but feel angry and vengeful, I am incongruent. Organismic experience that is consistent with both the organismic valuing process and conditions of worth can be accurately perceived and symbolized. However, experiences that contradict conditions of worth would, if accurately perceived and assimilated, frustrate the need for positive self-regard. Rather, these are selectively perceived distorted or denied to awareness to make them consistent with self-worth. Thus begins people's basic estrangement from themselves. A person can no longer live as a whole integrated person. We now have people divided within themselves.

Threat or anxiety occurs if accurately symbolized experience violates the consistency of the self-concept. This leaves a person vulnerable. Anxiety is thus the response of the organism when a discrepancy between self-concept and experience threatens to enter awareness and to cause a disruption of the self-concept. However, in response to strong needs, behavior inconsistent with the self-concept does occur. In such instance the person often disowns the experience or behavior as not "me."

This view is summarized in Figure 2.1, in which the subception of incongruence between a self-concept, guided by a self-actualizing tendency, and organismic experience, guided by an actualizing tendency, leads to either healthy acceptance, or immediate distortion or denial of experience or fragmentation of the self-concept.

Health, according to Gestalt theory, in a similar fashion to Rogers, involved the owning of emerging experience, whereas dysfunction involved the automatic *disowning or alienation of this experience*. A variety of interruptive mechanisms including introjections, projections, and retroflections were seen as preventing need satisfaction. Other phenomena such as conflict be-

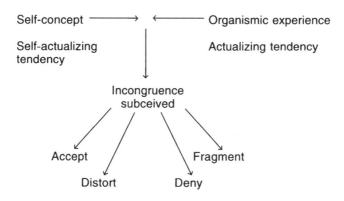

FIGURE 2.1. Incongruence model.

tween polarities, habits, unfinished business, avoidance, and catastrophizing were also seen as important processes that produced dysfunction. Some confusion also existed between different views of dysfunction and change. One view, reflecting a psychoanalytic influence, held that awareness or discovery of previously unaware contents was curative, implying that hidden contents were pathogenic. Pathology in this view resulted from the inability to integrate one's representations and reactions to certain experiences into one's existing self-organization. In another view the unacceptable is dealt with not by expelling it from consciousness (repression) but by failing to experience it as one's own (disowning). Therapy thus needed to promote reowning a fuller experiencing of what one was talking about, and possibly already knew, rather than making the unconscious conscious. In addition what is important in this view is that what is disowned is not itself pathogenic. Rather, it is the healthy or the traumatic that is disowned. Dysfunction occurs because of the disowning of healthy growth-oriented resources and needs or because of the avoidance of pain. It is the owning and reprocessing of experience to assimilate it into existing meaning structures, as opposed to consciousness of repressed contents, that is the key change process in an experiential view. This is an essential difference from classical psychoanalytic views in which it is motivated efforts for indirect gratification of infantile or immoral needs that is denied to awareness. In existential theory, similar to the Gestalt view, dysfunction was seen as resulting from lack of authenticity, alienation from experience, and the resultant lack of meaning.

In yet another view it was more awareness of the *process* of identification and alienation of experience that was the road to health. Awareness of functioning was seen as providing people with the option to choose if and when to own experience (Perls et al., 1951). Therapy then was seen as offering experiments of deliberate awareness to promote the experience of people as active agents in their experience, so that they began to experience that "It is me who is thinking, feeling, or doing this" (Perls et al., 1951, p. 238). This process view of dysfunction was focused on awareness of interruptions rather than on reowning interrupted experience. Awareness of how one functioned was seen as leading to choice, and it was the regaining of this capacity that was the road to health.

One of the problems with all the theories, however, was the tendency to posit one universal mechanism to explain all psychological distress. All dysfunction fell under one common principle, be it incongruence, denial, disowning, lack of awareness, or loss of meaning. Any singular ("global") view of dysfunction is, however, unable to explain all problems. Problems stemming from such diverse phenomena as lack of self-esteem, attachment disorders, childhood maltreatment, and dysfunctional family interactions, as well as such heterogeneous conditions as depression, panic, addiction, and obsessive–compulsive, borderline, and other personality disorders, cannot all be explained by one major dynamic. In addition the dominant incongruence or disowning view suggests that experience is denied or disclaimed, and this assumes that experience exists fully formed, outside of awareness or ownership. This creates the problem of explaining both how experience is kept unaware or disclaimed and exactly how the dysfunctional processes of denial or disowning are undone. Process theories arose as an answer to this latter problem.

# PROCESS THEORY

## Process Theory in Client-Centered Therapy

### Rogers's Model

In his process conception, Rogers (1958) offered a conceptualization of health that saw change not as occurring as an evolution from stability through change to a new level of stability but rather as involving a transition from stability to flux, from rigidity to flow, and from structure to process. In optimal functioning, experience, in this view, loses its structure-bound quality and becomes freely flowing. No longer is it the self-concept that mediates the organism's actions and experience, and no longer is it denied contents that are pathogenic.

No longer was there a self-concept that admitted or disallowed certain feeling, but only an experiencing subject. The self and experiencing now coincided: "the self at that moment is the feeling" (Rogers, 1961, p. 147). Successful therapy would lead to functioning in a process manner of moment-by-moment symbolization of experience. Functioning by means of a self-concept would be dysfunctional. The theory basically shifted from a structural to a process conception of functioning that was more constructivist in nature.

## Gendlin's Model

In his theory of experiencing, Gendlin (1962, 1964, 1974) more fully articulated a process-oriented view and clearly moved away from denial views. He started from the premise that people are experiencing beings and stressed the interactional character of all naturally occurring forms of life. The absence of important forms of interactions, interactions that carry processes forward, were seen as the major cause of disturbance of spontaneous organismic process, or what he referred to as a bodily way of being-in-the-world. Gendlin argued that optimal self-process was indicated by an ever-increasing degree of using experiencing as a referent in which felt meanings *interact* with verbal symbols to produce an explicit meaning. Felt meanings are tacit form of knowing based on a bodily sense or a perception of an event (Merleau-Ponty, 1962). They are implicitly felt but not explicitly known. In this view both implicit and explicit meanings are in awareness. Implicit meanings just are not fully formed or fully processed, and they need to be further processed and developed, or in Gendlin's terms, carried forward and completed by symbolization. Explicit meanings are not already *in* the implicit meaning. Rather, we complete and form them when we explicate. Implicit meaning are full of implications and "may have countless organized aspects, but this does not mean that they are conceptually formed, explicit, and hidden" (Gendlin, 1964, p. 140). They are thus clearly preconceptual: "Only when interaction with verbal symbols (or events) actually occurs, is the process actually carried forward and the explicit meaning formed" (Gendlin, 1964, p. 141). According to Gendlin, experiencing is thus essentially an interaction between feeling and symbols just as bodily life is an interaction between body and environment.

Gendlin (1973) proposed a totally unified bodily process. He referred to a layered structure consisting of four levels: (a) the physiological body; (b) the interactions with the physical environment (behavior in the sense of moving etc.); (c) the interaction with others (interpersonal relationships); and (d) the ability to symbolize and, as part thereof, a person's reflection on his or her own experiencing process. These four dimensions can be compared with the four levels in existentialism: *Welt*, *Umwelt*, *Mitwelt*, and *Eigenwelt*.

Important here is that each higher level of functioning adds something to the functioning of the previous ones (Van Balen, 1996). This means that the human body is influenced in its functioning by all four levels, which makes the body a "verbal" body. The most influential dimension in the total functioning is the fourth one—the symbolic level. This also means that, when the process unfolds in an optimal way, these four dimensions function together as a whole and that symbolization, whether in words or in behavior, is the fruit of a complex but harmonic total process.

The carrying forward of each level of interaction, viewed separately, is a function of the completion of a sufficient variety of interactions at that level

(Gendlin, 1973; Van Balen, 1996). An impoverishment at each of the inter-action levels may result either from limited opportunities for adequate inter-action (as, e.g., in a caged animal) or from the absence of or incompleteness of the unfolding of one's own interaction responses (as, e.g., in the lethargy of extended television viewing). When the process of interaction is blocked, the internal interruption or block has to be overcome and the process of unfolding reinstated. Thus, the tears never wept have to be wept first, or the pent-up rage must first be expressed, before an evolution at that level can take place.

For human beings symbolization at the fourth level of the experiencing process, letting a real "felt sense" emerge in symbolized form and reflecting on it, immediately alters the process course at the three other levels. Thus symbolizing that one feels appreciation or resentment toward another per-son alters one's interactional stance toward the other, one's tendency to move toward or away from the other, and one's internal sensations. And it is this "living further," as Gendlin calls it, that allows people to intervene in their own history. Living further allows them to realize themselves as co-construc-tors of their own experience, instead of remaining the product of heredity and history. This is viewed as a means of coming to an authentic way of life. Existential theory (Frankl, 1959, 1968; May, 1981; Yalom, 1980, 1989) adds further perspectives on the nature of an authentic life, highlighting the impor-tance of both meaning and the future. It also identifies the types of issues, such as freedom, death, and aloneness, that we face in living authentically.

According to Gendlin (1964, 1973), conceptual rather than experien-tially based living results in "structure-bound" functioning and this produces dysfunction. "Structure-bound" functioning at the fourth level means that conscious symbolizing activity has been channeled solely toward conceptual end products (words, signs, etc.) and away from the concrete experiencing process. In this mode of functioning the implicit experiencing process is miss-ing. One's conscious experience is just a frozen whole that will not give up its structure to yield something new or engage in a next step. Thus one is stuck, for example, in a view of oneself as bad or the world as cruel. One has forgotten—or never really learned—to pay explicit attention to one's under-lying experiencing process. Indeed, reflection then becomes "thinking about" instead of "thinking and living from within." One continues to look for a solution by using what one knows rather than reaching for "the more"—what one can, but does not yet, explicitly know. Thus therapy is a process of trying to gain access to the not yet known where one tries to get at what is the "more" in "it," where "it" is the implicit sense. The key to this accessing consists in attention to one's own experiencing process, using experiencing "as a referent," and letting oneself and one's meanings be shaped by a real "felt sense" and then reflecting on this meaning.

This view makes it clear that the essence of change is not simply the admission of denied feelings to awareness but the quality of the process of symbolization. Indeed, it is the source of the symbolization and whether or not it is rigid and frozen or fluid and richly differentiated that is important. The difference with earlier views is immediately clear. For Rogers and Perls in the structural models the accent was on unhindered admittance of experiential data to awareness. Incorrect conscious conceptualizations were caused by a ban on material entering awareness—essentially a denial or distortion process. In healthy functioning the organismic process, as such, was viewed as entering awareness unhindered as a preformed whole.

The opposite is the case in the process view. The so-called admission of feelings that happens in therapy is replaced by a form of "living further," or construction, a completion of the interactive process. It is only by crowning an experience by symbolization that one makes experiential knowledge ultimately one's own. One therefore continually creates as well as discovers who one is (Greenberg et al., 1993). Adequate symbolization is thus the basis of healthy self-functioning.

Awareness and symbolization in this view is also the specifically human level of functioning. Humans are symbolic creatures, and it is this level of functioning that forms the bridge between the original, innate organization and culture. Meaning is not only created out of experience, but experience is created out of the meaning reached. As in all interactions, this is a two-way street. A smoothly functioning fourth level of symbolic bodily interaction is a constant source of reciprocal action between knowledge and experience. These levels are thus continuously tested out against one another and adjusted. This form of interaction allows not only knowledge processing but also a kind of bodily digestion of this knowledge, which then, when later experienced and symbolized again, has acquired an idiosyncratic personal quality and is thus no longer identical to that which was attained previously.

Thus Gendlin offers a sophisticated process conception of functioning in which the implications for practice involve facilitation of the process of focusing on a bodily felt referent, both by experiential responding that points to the implicit felt sense and by explicit processing instructions that facilitate focusing on the bodily felt sense. These forms of intervention are designed to unblock a stuck process of interaction and to explicate the implications of one's felt sense rather than to admit something new to awareness or change a self-concept. In this view the causes of dysfunction or the means of blocking of the process are, however, still not very clearly specified. Gendlin's model emphasizes a description of healthy functioning and its promotion, but the mechanisms of dysfunction are somewhat less clear.

## Process Theory in Gestalt Therapy

### Perls and Goodman's Model

Gestalt therapy began, under that name, with a field theory of human functioning. Although Frederick S. Perls had come from a psychoanalytic background, he strove toward an alternate conceptualization that came to fruition with the influence of Laura Perls in his work with Paul Goodman. These theorists proposed a self as process model.

This theory in essence made two proposals: first, that the self is the *synthesizing agent*, the artist of life, who creates contact at the organism–environment boundary; and, second and somewhat different, that the *self is contact* with the environment, and that it comes into being at the moment of contact. Contact is defined as the person's given experience of the world at any moment. Contact is a key term and refers both to an orienting, perceptual aspect, the forming of meaningful wholes of experience and personal meaning, and to an active, motoric aspect, a behavioral action on the environment to satisfy a need.

According to the first view, the self creates aware solutions to problems that arise at the contact boundary. Thus to solve the problem of rising out of bed in the morning the self organizes one to move by imaging projects that lie ahead, thereby propelling one toward the day. According to the second view, when there is full contact there is full self, and when there is little contact there is little self. Thus the self comes into existence in the experience, and I "am" my experience. Self, according to this second, more radical process view, therefore swells and fades. The self in a Gestalt view is thus not a concept, an object, or a structure but rather a function and/or a process, the creator of contact and withdrawal, and the process of coming into being. It is the system of contacts making contact in the organism–environment field and is "flexibly various" (Perls et al., 1951, p. 235). It is both the process and the everchanging product of a dynamic synthesis of many elements.

Within this process view Paul Goodman's contribution to Gestalt was essentially to offer a relational approach to the view of self. First, as stated above, the self was seen as a source, or organizer, of agency in the behavioral field. This clearly emphasized the *organizing, constructive capacities* of the person as the essential function and defining activity of the processes called "self." This organizing process was, however, located not within, as a drive, nor without, as a conditioner, but was seen as occurring at the boundary between the organism and the environment (Perls et al., 1951; Wheeler, 1991, 1995). The self was thus removed from the "inner individual" and seen as a field process. Self was the meeting point of internal and external achieved by a process of dynamic synthesis of all elements of the field.

In line with interpersonal theory (Sullivan, 1950, 1953) the organism was seen as being born into a preexisting field. Awareness was the capacity to respond to changes in the field. Contact with otherness, a sense of difference, was the most basic characteristic of experience. Discrimination, or attention to difference, is thus crucial in the creation of experience. An evershifting boundary was seen as a forming a "me" and a "not me" by this process of attending and discriminating. The primary datum of awareness was a felt difference, an experience of "me" and "you," of self and other. Being self-aware involved awareness, while I'm doing something, that I am doing it. In this view in order to survive and grow people had to be aware of both the inner world of desire and the outer world of people and things (Wheeler, 1991, 1995). In experiential or phenomenological terms life then consists of relating inner and outer, of integrating the world of wishes and fears with the world of resources and dangers. Life is thus the ongoing process of need satisfaction in an interpersonal environment, and it involves continuous contact and negotiation with other people who are engaged in the same process.

Self, in process terms, is thus the *activity of the integration of inner and outer* (Perls et al., 1951; Wheeler, 1991; Yontef, 1993). The self thus is on the surface, not somewhere deep inside, and it forms continually, *at the everchanging boundary*, between the organism and the environment, in order to fulfill needs, solve problems, and deal with obstacles. The self as function integrates the whole field of experience into coherent, usable wholes of understanding, meaning, and action. My self, as process, is "my experience." This is similar to Rogers's view that the self at any moment is one's feeling.

This process/field view of self was later represented in the basic model of functioning represented in the Gestalt Experience Cycle (Polster & Polster, 1973; Zinker, 1977). In this view, as shown in Figure 2.2, a dominant need emerges at the contact boundary from the organism's interaction with the environment. This emergence of a need is seen as a field event, not as an internal drive. In this process the person, in a need-facilitating context, attends to and becomes aware of the need (say, for comfort), and then proceeds through the stages of the mobilization of excitement (feeling a desire for contact) to the stage of action in the world (say, reaching out or asking for a hug) to a final stage of contact and completion (in which the hug is

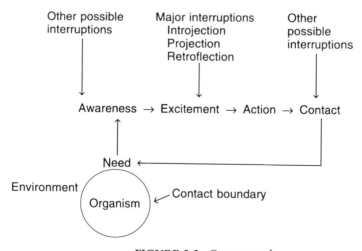

FIGURE 2.2. Contact cycle.

truly sensed and enjoyed) and the need is met. Need satisfaction allows attention once again to be paid to the next emerging need, and a repeat of the cycle occurs. Various interruptions can be experienced that prevent completion, interruptions such as thinking one should be strong or that others will see one as weak. This cycle is offered as a description of the process of living. People who live according to this natural rhythm are flexible, clear, and effective (Polster & Polster, 1973). When the need cycle is interrupted, a situation results in which people remember and return to the unmet needs and the unresolved feelings, seeking to finish the unfinished (Zeigarnik, 1927; Mazur, 1996). Therapy involves awareness of contact interruptions and promotion of need satisfaction.

Gestalt therapy's process/functional view of the self as the formation of figures against backgrounds and Gendlin's process views of symbolizing implicit experience, as important as they are, are both somewhat incompatible with the notion of a person having a structural core and a sense of continuity. The problem with a purely process, "no-self" view is that we often do feel that we are, in many ways, the same person we always were, and this makes ideas about the constancy of the self ring true phenomenologically (Yontef, 1993). This presents a problem for a purely process view that claims to be phenomenologically based. The necessity for a structural construct of some sort or some other process arises if one wishes to explain our sense of continuity (cf. Varela, Rosch, & Thompson, 1991). It appears that even in endorsing functional/process views of the self, the recognition of some enduring structural aspect has still been maintained as necessary in understanding human functioning, both in Gestalt and client-centered theories. Thus notions of self-concept, structure boundness, and character are all still used albeit often as the dysfunction-producing aspect. Conceptualization of different aspects of self, as both subject and process ("I") and object and structure ("me"), are probably all necessary in devising an adequate self theory. The notion of identity is hard to dispose of, as we all have the experience of sameness (Riceur, 1992) as well as of being in process.

## A SYNTHESIS: EXPERIENTIAL CONSTRUCTION

Integrating and developing experiential theory in line with modern views on emotion, constructive cognition, and the operation of dynamic systems, a dialectical constructivist model of experiential therapy has recently been proposed (Greenberg et al., 1993; Greenberg & Pascual Leone, 1995, 1997; Pascual-Leone, 1991, 1998; Watson & Greenberg, 1997). In this view a person is seen as a symbolizing, meaning-creating being who acts as a dynamic system constantly synthesizing information from many levels of processing and from both internal and external sources into a conscious experience. Three major levels of processing—innate sensory motor, emotional schematic memory, and conceptual level processing—are identified (Greenberg & Safran, 1987, 1989; Greenberg et al., 1993). In addition people are seen as organizing experience into emotion-based schemes[1] that then play a central role in functioning and the creation of meaning.

This view of the dynamic construction of experience and meaning supports a form of practice in which emotions play an important role and both the therapeutic relationship and therapeutic work on specific problems are seen as aiding change. Change is viewed as occurring by the co-construction of new meaning in a dialogue between the client and therapist in which the therapist plays an active role in confirming the client's emotional experience and in helping the client synthesize an identity based on strengths and possibilities.

In this view integration or synthesis of emotion schemes and levels of processing to create new meaning becomes the operative process, and a principle of *coherence* can be viewed as supplementing the principle of congruence or consistency in explaining healthy functioning. Thus it is not simply that "I" become aware of my "feelings," or that my self-concept and experience are consistent, but that I form a coherent sense of myself as, say, angry or sad—a form that successfully organizes aspects of experience together into a coherent whole that is viable in a given situation. In this view, aspects of experience as well as levels of processing are coordinated to fit together in an affiliative relationship with each other, integrated into a coherent whole that makes sense and is identified as a part of one's self-organization. This view helps overcome the problem, in both language and thought, of presuming the operation of any preexisting hidden content or meaning that comes to awareness or is accepted into a self-concept. Rather, there is an ongoing process of synthesizing levels of processing and modules of experience in a complex internal field. Each module of experience is itself a developing self-organizing system which has its own voice, and all aspects exist in states of dialectic tension with each other. Reowning is seen as the integration of varied aspects of experience into coherent forms. This involves awareness and meaning creation as well as identification with disclaimed action tendencies.

In this dialectical view the emphasis is on the person as an *active agent*, constantly organizing or configuring (see Bohart, 1993, 1995; Mahoney, 1995) experience and reality into meaningful wholes. Both discovery of elements of experience and creation of new meaning operate in tandem, neither process being privileged over the other (Greenberg et al., 1993). In addition both emerging internal experience and interpersonal validation are seen as active ingredients in the process of change.

In accord with Gendlin, symbol and referent are viewed as interacting to carry meaning forward, and newly symbolized experience is organized in different ways to construct new views. Attending to and discovery of preconceptual elements of experience influence the process of meaning construction. People are then viewed as constantly striving toward making sense of their preconceptual experience by symbolizing it, explaining it, and putting it into narrative form. New experiential elements can come from many sources, both from within and sometimes from without, to influence constructions. Preconceptual tacit meaning carries implications and acts to constrain but does not determine meaning. Rather, it is synthesized with conceptual, explicit meaning to form explanations constrained by experiencing (Greenberg & Pascual-Leone, 1995).

In this process the self is seen as that human agency which acts to become aware of and creatively fulfill needs and resolve problems that arise for the person in his or her interactions with the environment. Awareness of ways in which one functions that interfere with forming needs thus can become an important therapeutic focus. Need emergence is seen as a field event rather than as an inner drive and emerges by the self synthesizing internal and external elements into coherent forms. Needs and goals along with meaning are thus as much created as discovered. The inability to identify and form needs, and thereby a clear, coherent sense of self, is seen as leading to a weakened self-organization lacking in coherence and vitality.

This experiential, constructivist view is designed to address a number of issues in the existing models. These are (1) the nature and role of the self and self-concept; (2) the nature of experience, and the role of the actualizing tendency and self determination; (3) the problem of process and flux versus structure and sameness; and (4) the source of dysfunction.

## The Self and the Self-Concept

Here the term "self" refers not to an entity but to the tacit level of organization that acts as the integrating agent of experience that separates what is me from what is not me. The self operates as a dynamic system organizing the elements of experience into a coherent whole and works by a process of dynamic/dialectical synthesis (Pascual-Leone, 1987, 1990a, 1990b; Thelen & Smith, 1994; Smith & Thelen, 1993). In this view, the self can be seen as involving a community of voices constantly in dialogue (Elliott & Greenberg, in press; Hermans, Kempen, & van Loon, 1992). In this dialogical self there is no central or hierarchical control, but all elements add weight in an ongoing synthesis process in which the resulting self-organization, a momentary state such as feeling shy or being assertive, is the result of the synthesis. Conscious control is but one aspect that can influence the synthesis process and is always itself influenced by tacit knowing processes in a never-ending circular process of mutual influence. In line with Stern (1985) we see the self as being dynamically synthesized into possessing a sense of coherence, agency, continuity, and affectivity. One's sense of self is thus an emergent sense synthesized from more basic elements of experience of which the affectively toned sensorimotor experiences of infancy are reference points for the ordering of much later experience and for one's developing sense of self. Emotion is thus seen as the "glue" of the identity formation process.

In a dialectical constructive view of experiential theory the self-concept, our view of ourselves, is replaced by the notion of the narrative construction of an identity—the story we tell to understand and explain our lives. Rather than this being a structure, a concept of the self, it is the ongoing process by which a person *makes sense of experience* and explains his or her actions (Guidano, 1987, 1991). This involves a conscious conceptual process influenced by learning, by values, and by a variety of different cognitive and evaluative processes involved in the creation of meaning. Rather than possessing a fixed self-concept, people operate by a set of tacit organizing processes by which they actively evaluate and reflect on their experience and create stories or views of who they and others are, and how and why things happened (Watson & Greenberg, 1997; Greenberg & Pascual-Leone, 1995).

The self in our view operates by means of a dynamic relationship between tacit emotional experience and explicit conceptual knowing (cf. Guidano, 1987, 1991). Our deeper structures or emotion schemes are constantly apprehending reality and producing complex internal responses that are being tacitly synthesized to produce a sense of internal complexity. This acts as a felt sense that is constantly being organized by a conscious, more focused style of analytical reasoning and formed into self-views and plans of action. We are thus dialectical experiencers constantly synthesizing many levels of information to form two streams of consciousness, one tacit and one explicit, and finally synthesizing these two streams into unified conscious experience. Many levels and modules of experience are thus synthesized in our continual efforts to make sense of our experience.

## Experience, Actualizing, and Self-Determination

The experiential therapies, although emphasizing the bodily felt nature of experience, have been silent on how this bodily felt basis of experiencing is created; taking a phenomenological perspective, they have treated experiencing as the given datum. It just happens. We have suggested, rather, that experiencing can be understood as the synthesized product of a variety of sensorimotor responses and emotion schemes, tinged with conceptual memories, all activated in a situation (Greenberg et al., 1993). In this view the coordination of collections of neurons (schemes) that have been coactivated (evoked by the same releasers) and are cofunctional (can be comfortably applied together) produces a complex internal field (Greenberg & Pascual-Leone, 1995, 1997; Pascual-Leone, 1987, 1989, 1990a, 1990b, 1991). This field provides one with a sense of internal complexity to which one can refer and in which at any moment much more is contained than any explicit rendition could capture.

Imagine, for example, telling the story to a friend of an occurrence the previous evening, one of standing in line for a movie, then turning around and suddenly seeing someone whom you either wished desperately to avoid or whom you were amorously longing to meet. Depending on which occurred, you might be able to speak at length from two entirely different senses of internal complexity generated in the moment by complex tacit synthesis. You could talk about how you felt in this moment and how you felt about it, drawing on all kinds of different images and explicating complex felt meanings and their implications. All these tacit meanings occurred in the field of internal complexity but were not necessarily processed consciously in the moment, as you greeted the other person.

It is important to note that this bodily felt sense of internal complexity is *not only multidetermined* by many modalities and modes of processing, such as auditory, visual, kinesthetic, emotional, and semantic, *but is also overdetermined*; that is, the resultant is produced by as many determinant causes as there are compatible processes that might jointly inform the performance. Experience is thus produced by more than one set of causes, even if a partial set of all the determinants found therein would suffice to produce the same result. In this view conscious experience is overdetermined in the sense that many schemes or aspects are coordinated in its production (Pascual-Leone, 1989, 1990a, 1990b; Greenberg & Pascual-Leone, 1995). A subset of these schemes might often suffice to produce the same result. Thus as many authentic performance/meanings may be generated as there are semantically distinct schemes synthesized in one's internal field, overdetermining the performance. An experience thus means both "this" and "this," even though the two determinants may differ and either could have sufficed to produce the result. Explanation of why one feels or does something is thus not a simple rational or linearly causal process. We experience things for many reasons, all of which converge to overdetermine the final state. Conscious meaning then occurs by the symbolization of aspects of internal complexity into symbols that create distinctions in experience. These symbols in turn can be further organized by reflection to generate new felt meanings (Watson & Greenberg, 1997; Greenberg & Pascual-Leone, 1997).

Tacit decentralized control in a synthesis system of this nature makes it always possible to perceive more than we currently experience and to experience more than we currently attend to. New sets of tacit experience are always available to be explicated in consciousness. Experiencing is thus a tacit level of meaning generated by a dynamic synthesis of sensory, schematic, and conceptual levels of processing that integrate by a type of summation of related or mutual elements into a totality—a Gestalt with figural and background aspects.

In relation to the actualizing tendency we suggest that it is the biologically adaptive emotion system that provides the scientific basis for the actualizing tendency and the associated organismic valuing process. The actualizing tendency, as posited by the original theorists, actually contains at least three major aspects: first, the formative aspect, the process that integrates all aspects into coherent forms; second, an adaptive or directional aspect that works to maintain and enhance the organism; third, the notion of actualization of potential, the process of becoming who one "truly is" or becoming "all that one can become."

Preferring a more biologically based view of this tendency, Greenberg et al. (1993) see it as a growth and development tendency oriented toward increased complexity via exploration, and differentiation and integration of functioning, that results in greater adaptive flexibility. The aim is to be viable in a given environment rather than to actualize potential or become all one can be. The actualizing-of-potential view is based more on a set of values than on a biological tendency. We support a view that incorporates the first two aspects of the actualizing tendency, the holistic and the adaptive exploratory/assertive aspects, without including the third actualization-of-potential aspect. In our view the idea of becoming "who one truly is" is one of the paradoxes that resulted from the structural and actualizing of potential points of view. A structural view allows for a denied "true self" hidden under a false self. An actualizing-of-potential view assumes that such a potential exists. This thinking promoted a view of therapy as involving helping people to change to be who they truly are. Rather, in the dynamic system view being proposed, we are always being ourselves, with different self-organizations emerging at different moments as syntheses of elements. In this view certain self-organizations, such as self-accepting ones, are far more harmonious than others, such as self-coercive or avoidant organizations. Thus it is the functioning of the self that is important—functioning in such a way that our internal relations are affiliative or harmonious, rather than that some preexisting content is accepted.

In addition, in our view self-actualization is highly interpersonal. It results not only by means of the self-organization of some type of biological tendency but also through confirming dialogue with another person. In an I–Thou dialogue (Buber, 1958, 1965) each person is made present by the other. The therapist is seen as *contacting and confirming* the other by focusing on particular aspects of the client's functioning. First, there is a continual focus by the therapist on the client's subjective experience, confirming the person as an authentic source of experience. Second, there is a selective focus on that which is emotionally adaptive and growthful and on the person's exploratory, assertive tendencies and strengths. It is the therapist's focus on clients' subjective experience, on their exploratory, assertive tendencies, and on their strengths that helps guide growth and development.

People in our view are often struggling and confused. Both "good" and "bad" inclinations do exist as possibilities. Therapy is the co-constructive dialogue in which both the therapist and client struggle to discern and confirm the client's health-promoting tendencies and possibilities, thereby adding to their strength in the synthesis (Friedman, 1972, 1985; Van Balen, 1990; Watson & Greenberg, 1995). Growth thus truly emerges from the "in-between," from the two working together in a collaborative alliance toward the client's survival and enhancement, and to the confirmation of life. The therapist's ability to see and focus on possibilities in the client's experience and help construct the implications of experience is an important element in promoting the client's directional tendency.

Experience is rich with not yet articulated implications. New meanings always can be created from a person's field of internal complexity. Thus becoming oneself is really the unfolding of the implications of internal experience. This involves discovering some of the constituents and organizing them into coherent wholes in a growth-promoting interaction with another. The growth tendency is thus seen as being guided (1) *from within*, by an emotion system that operates by evaluating situations in relation to one's well-being (Frijda, 1986; Lazarus, 1991a, 1991b; Greenberg & Safran, 1987; Greenberg et al., 1993; Greenberg & Paivio, 1997), and (2) *from without*, by the other, who sees, focuses on, and confirms the tendency to grow. The multiple internal and external elements are dialectically synthesized into a holistic response. Thus growth occurs in an interpersonal field. The growth tendency is a biological tendency that develops and is strengthened by being focused on, symbolized, and confirmed in a dialogue.

The operation of the biosocial nature of this process is well demonstrated in a "visual cliff" experiment with toddlers and their mothers (Sroufe, 1996). The toddlers, who would not normally venture out onto a visual cliff when referencing their own reactions alone, were clearly affected by the facial expression of their mothers on the other side of the cliff. If, as the hesitant infants explored the cliff, the mothers facially expressed joy, the infants proceeded over it toward their mothers, whereas if the mothers facially expressed fear, the infants rapidly moved back from the cliff. The toddlers thus integrated internal and external cues to guide action. It is the operation of this biological–interpersonal synthesizing system that, in effect, results in adaptive growth and development. Supported by another, this biosocial tendency has goals of adaptation and viability more than actualization of inherent potential.

Experiencing, however, as well as resulting from an integration of inner and outer influences, needs to be explained in terms of its internal processes of generation. In this view, initially inwired biologically adaptive affective processes that provide basic action tendencies and expressions, such as fear responses to a looming shadow, joy to a facial configuration, and anger at restraint, become more organized as the child develops. In fact, Scherer (1984) has suggested that emotional responses are generated by a series of preconscious evaluative checks that move progressively from evaluation of the more basic and inherent dimensions of an event, such as novelty, pleasantness, and goal/need significance, to the more complex and socially referenced dimensions, such as one's potential to cope with the event, and the norm and self-concept compatibility of the event. Thus the generation of a simple discrete emotion such as anger or joy is itself a complex synthesis of a variety of differentially complex tacit evaluations. As a child's cognitive capacities develop, the child, in addition to generating its basic emotional responses, represents to itself not only its own emotional reactions to situations but also the evoking situation and beliefs about its own and others responses. They become more and more differentiated, and, with the child's development of conceptual capacities, they come to incorporate more learned and inferred rules and beliefs. Emotion-based schemes that integrate inner with outer, as well as sensory memorial and cognitive elements, are thus formed and serve as the basic units of psychological functioning (Greenberg & Paivio, 1997; Greenberg et al., 1993; Pascual-Leone, 1991).

When emotion schemes are evoked they do not act singly but produce emotional experience via a dynamic synthesis process in which all evoked schemes are synthesized in an internal field to form, out of the evoked elements, the most coordinated, coherent unity possible. This referent, when attended to, is available to consciousness as current preconceptual experience and can be symbolized explicitly in conscious awareness. The process of symbolization which is an aspect of the synthesis creates a conscious meaning that both influences experience and is influenced by it. Symbolized experience is further open to reflective processing and is used in reasoning about and explaining the person's circumstances (Watson & Rennie, 1994).

Symbolization and reflective processing therefore serve to both organize and reorganize meaning (Watson & Greenberg, 1997). Both of these mental processes are guided and constrained by what is activated in the field of internal complexity. They do not however *represent* it, in the sense of forming a copy; rather, they *organize* it to create meaning grounded in experience (Bohart, 1995). In addition, once experience is symbolized, in awareness reason is brought to bear on experience to plan and produce action. Thus emotional experience informs reasoned action. In this process emotion signals what is of concern to us and then we figure out what to do to get our needs met. Cognition in this way is seen as predominantly serving affective goals (Greenberg & Paivio, 1997; Pascual-Leone, 1991).

In this view, in line with the existentialists, conscious choice and will are seen as the final arbiters of action. Existence precedes essence, and we ultimately choose who we are to become. We therefore can choose to attend to and integrate our emotional experience, or we can choose to attempt other more alienated ways of living. Choice and will are governed by attentional allocation, and it is this element in the construction process over which we all have some control. By directing our attention in particular ways to particular facets of experience we can influence our experience. Although this is not a simple process, nor one which can easily be controlled rationally, attentional allocation is the component of the synthesis process over which, even if it be by the "heave of our will" (James, 1890/1950), we have some control. Affect, however, always exerts a more powerful influence on attentional resources and allocation than does reason. Therapy therefore needs to focus attention on emotional experience rather than purely concern itself with the content of cognition and cognitive control.

## Process and Structure

In terms of the process–structure dichotomy in self theory, we recognize that although life is a constant process of creation in each moment, there is also stability in who we are. The stability in our view comes not from an overarching self-concept but from the *structure* and *function* of the building blocks—our emotion schemes—and from the construction of narrative identities. First, schemes carry our learned connections between situations, experiences, and responses, thus accounting for some of the regularity in behavior. Second, more functionally, the same or similar schemes are often coactivated and are integrated in similar ways, according to their ability to cofunction, thereby producing similar experience and performance. Third, conscious explanations of experience and events account further for some of the regularity. We repeatedly construct the same stories.

Moments of similar experience therefore often result from a process of repeatedly synthesizing similar elements in similar ways and repeatedly making sense of them in the same way. Thus we may often get annoyed or feel worried in similar situations. These similar ways of functioning and constructing meaning reflect what can be thought of as core organizing principles (Guidano, 1991). These principles exist, then, not as contents of consciousness as such, nor as explicit beliefs, but as generalized rules of operation—rules of the way evoked material is tacitly synthesized and the way we put things together and make sense of our experience. The coordination and summation of those elements that fit result in the construction of similar states.[2]

## Dysfunction

Dysfunction in this constructive experiencing process occurs not through one singular mechanism alone, such as incongruence (Rogers, 1951), interruptions of contact (Perls et al., 1951), or a blocking of the meaning creation process (Gendlin, 1964). Rather, we believe dysfunction arises via many possible routes.

At the most global level we see the inability to integrate aspects of functioning into coherent, harmonious internal relations as a major source of dysfunction. Thus it is problems in self-organization that are seen as producing dysfunction. This view incorporates both Rogers's and Perls's views of incongruence and integration as well as Mahrer's view of the importance of affiliation between operating potentials. Conflict in this view occurs between different self-organizations, between different voices, not between conscious and unconscious or moral and immoral; and disowning, in effect, is a process of the construction of one possible self-organization and thereby the exclusion of another. Denial and disowning are viewed as problems in the synthesizing and self-organizing functions of the self.

At another level, in line with Gendlin, Perls, and Rogers, we see the inability to symbolize bodily felt constituents of experience in awareness, or symbolizing them in restricted or rigid ways, as another central source of dysfunction. Thus one may not be aware or able to make sense of the increasing tension in one's body as resentment, or be unable to symbolize as resentment the constituents of experience that support that construction. This leaves one confused and disoriented. A third major source of dysfunction involves the activation by minimal cues of core maladaptive emotion schemes. This leads either to the experience of painful emotions or a maladaptive weak/bad sense of self (Greenberg & Paivio, 1997). The operation of this process implies that not all basic internal experience is an adaptive guide, and that in addition to the benefits of becoming aware of the basic constituents of experience, basic experience itself sometimes requires therapeutic change. For example, in posttraumatic stress syndrome the emotion system often signals an alarm when no danger is present. Similarly abuse or poor attachment histories can lead to maladaptive experience of, or mistrust of, interpersonal closeness, or a desire for relational experiences that are not in one's best interest.

The above three general processes of dysfunction are supplemented by the operation of a large variety of more specific cognitive–affective processing difficulties that arise in therapy and provide opportunities for therapeutic interventions best suited for these states. The occurrence of different specific states helps explain different types of dysfunction (Rice & Greenberg, 1984). We have described a variety of specific problems as sources of particular types of experiential difficulties (Greenberg et al., 1993). Examples are problematic reactions, in which one's current view of an experience and one's reaction don't fit; self-evaluative splits, in which one part of the self negatively evaluates another; unfinished business, involving unresolved emotional memories; and statements of vulnerability involving a fragile sense of self. All involve different types of schematic processing problems. Each state requires different interventions designed to deal with the specific cognitive–affective processing problems. This offers a differential view of dysfunction in which current determinants and maintainers of disorders are identified by a form of process diagnosis in which therapists identify markers of in-session opportunities for implementing specific types of interventions and change processes.

Thus, specific problems in living, such as depression, might be seen as predominantly involving some of the above general processes, say, an inability to symbolize, and the evocation of maladaptive schemes. Each person's depression, in addition, may be seen as involving more specific processing difficulties, for example, people with self-critical depressions manifest lots of self-evaluative splits in therapy, whereas people with dependence depressions present a lot of unfinished business with significant others (Greenberg & Watson, 1998).

## CONCLUSION

People in this view are thus dynamic systems attempting to maintain the coherence of their organizing processes by continuous synthesis and restructuring. The person grows toward greater and greater complexity and coherence by constantly assimilating her or his own experience, integrating incongruities and polarities. Growth is inherently dialectical. This view does not privilege an internal process of feeling over the meaning-creating processes of symbolization and reflection, nor does it privilege internal experience over contact with others. Rather, it sees a dialectical synthesis of all elements, emotion and cognition, internal and external, biological and social, as the crucial act in the creation of meaning. It is thus itself a synthesis of phenomenological, constructivist, and relational/field theory views.

An important point is that in symbolization of experience, making the implicit explicit is not a process of representation but rather a process of construction, always limited and not complete. Not all tacit information is used in any construction. Thus we can always explore for what more there is, reconfigure, and see it in a new way. Explicit knowledge needs to adequately fit, make sense of, and integrate elements into a coherent meaningful whole. Once we make a conscious model of our experience, this acts as an identity or becomes our representation of ourselves. We then reflect on this, and this creates new experience. We have many views of our self and are constantly revising them. Thus we do not *have* a self-concept or even a self but are constantly forming both. We are engaged in an ongoing process of creating coherence and unity. In each moment we are the expression of one of many possible selves.

Dysfunction does not always result from a conflict between experiencing and a self-concept based on introjected conditions of worth. Rather, we integrate different aspects of experience and different levels of processing; we synthesize bodily felt experiencing and conceptual meaning. The later may include convictions and conditions of worth but is not totally dominated by them. Dysfunction occurs via different general and specific types of processing problems that undermine sound meaning creation. In addition, we reject any notion of a vitalistic tendency in which a genetic blueprint is actualized for the person to become who he/she "truly is." Rather, we envisage an interpersonally facilitated exploratory/assertive growth tendency that is oriented toward contact with the environment, attachment to others, and increased complexity, coherence, and adaptive flexibility.

Therapy, in turn, involves focusing on this adaptive capacity, confirming it, as well as promoting different types of exploratory processing to facilitate different types of problem resolution. In addition, therapy promotes awareness of blocks and interruptions of the person's strengths and exploratory/assertive problem-solving capacities so that awareness becomes fluid rather than fixed on reworking of unfinished situations. In therapy one thus provides a relational environment that will help strengthen the adaptive self, will create process-enhancing interactions that will not interfere with or block healthy self-organizing processes, and will recognize the client as expert on his or her own experience. Additionally one focuses on evoking maladaptive schemes in therapy in order to make them accessible to new experience and uses different active methods of facilitating the resolution of different specific processing difficulties, again always recognizing clients as having privileged access to their experience and as having the ability and the right to choose their own direction (Greenberg et al., 1993). Therapy is thus both exploratory, focusing on strengthening the self, and problem focused, oriented toward the resolution of specific emotional concerns.

The problem of the origins of the wisdom of the body, or the scientific basis of the organismic valuing process, is solved by realizing that emotion is a basic biologically adaptive system that serves an organizing function in human experience and operates by evaluating situations in relation to our well-being. The formative tendency is viewed as working by means of a dynamic systems process of the dialectical coordination of many elements to form the most inclusive coherent synthesis of activated elements. It works through the medium of both a basic biologically adaptive emotion system and the human symbolic capacity and drive to make sense of things, in the service of goals to survive and to maintain and enhance the self. Thus the organism is always producing a directional tendency informed by all its learning, experience, and interaction.

Further, human beings live and grow in the context of relationships and function by attention being allocated to some aspect of the organism/environment field. Attention operates under the control of emotion, interest, reason, conscious effort, and the salience of environmental stimuli. Attending leads to the creation of emotional meaning that organizes the person for action. At the point of symbolization, reasoning, aided by imagination, invents possible solutions and guides action. Goals, and plans for their attainment, are reflected on and evaluated, and the person decides on a course of action. Action on the chosen alternative then follows. This process involves emotion, reason, choice, and above all an ongoing process of dynamic synthesis of many elements including feelings, memories, beliefs, values, things learned, anticipations, all constantly being integrated as the self reorganizes itself to meet the challenges of the environment.

## NOTES

1. The term "scheme" is used rather than "schema" following Pascual-Leone (1987) and Piaget (1969) to emphasize the scheme as action-oriented experience producing structure rather than cognitive representational experience.

2. The synthesis process thus produces particular patterns or states that represent the stable enduring areas or attractors of dynamic system functioning (Van Geert, 1994). Our identity, character structure, or even cognitive styles are the result of the "attractiveness" of particular states. This view of the origins of order is in line with views of modern complexity theorists where order is seen as emerging out of chaos by the coordination of dynamic processes into stable states (Lewin, 1994).

Change and creative adjustment is, however, always imminent by the incorporation of new elements that will influence the totality, bumping the system out of stable states, thereby precipitating new configurations of experience. Thus we can readily shift from worrying obsessively to focusing on novelty, or from being organized as vulnerable to being organized as angry to being organized as sad. Each style or state represents a stable state in a dynamic process. Change here involves changing the probability of emergence of specific states or styles rather than change in these states or styles themselves.

## REFERENCES

Bohart, A. (1993). Experiencing: The basis of psychotherapy. *Journal of Psychotherapy Integration, 3*, 51–68.

Bohart, A. (1995). Configuration and constructivism from an experiential perspective. *Journal of Constructivist Psychology, 8*(4), 317–326.

Buber, M. (1958). *I and thou.* New York: Scribner's.

Buber, M. (1965). *The knowledge of man.* New York: Harper Torchbook.

Elliott, R., & Greenberg, L. S. (in press). Multiple voices in process-experential therapy: Dialogue between aspects of the self. *Journal of Psychotherapy Integration.*

Frankl, V. E. (1959). *Man's search for meaning: An introduction to logotherapy.* New York: Simon & Schuster.

Frankl, V. E. (1968). *Psychotherapy and existentialism: Selected papers on logotherapy.* New York: Washington Square Press.

Friedman, M. (1972). Dialogue and the unique in humanistic psychology. *Journal of Humanistic Psychology, 12*(2), 7–22.

Friedman, M. (1985). *The healing dialogue in psychotherapy.* New York: Aronson.

Frijda, N. H. (1986). *The emotions.* Cambridge, UK: Cambridge University Press.

Gendlin, E. T. (1962). *Experiencing and the reaction of meaning.* New York: Free Press of Glencoe.

Gendlin, E. T. (1964). A theory of personality change. In P. Worchel & D. Byrne (Eds.), *Personality change.* New York: Wiley.

Gendlin, E. T. (1973). Experiential psychotherapy. In R. Corsini (Ed.), *Current psychotherapies.* Itasca, IL: Peacock.

Gendlin, E. T. (1974). Client-centered and experiential psychotherapy. In D. A. Wexler & L. N. Rice (Eds.), *Innovations in client-centered therapy.* New York: Wiley.

Gendlin, E. T. (1996). *Focusing-oriented psychotherapy: A manual of the experiential method.* New York: Guilford Press.

Goldstein, K. (1939). *The organism.* New York: American Book.

Greenberg, L. S., & Paivio, S. C. (1997). *Working with emotions in psychotherapy.* New York: Guilford Press.

Greenberg, L. S., & Pascual-Leone, J. (1995). A dialectical constructivist approach to experiential change. In R. Neimeyer & M. Mahoney (Eds.), *Constructivism in psychotherapy.* Washington, DC: APA Press.

Greenberg, L. S., & Pascual-Leone, J. (1997). Emotion in the creation of personal meaning. In M. Power & C. Brewin (Eds.), *Transformation of meaning.* London: Wiley.

Greenberg, L. S., Rice, L. N., & Elliott, R. (1993). *Facilitating emotional change: The moment-by-moment process.* New York: Guilford Press.

Greenberg, L. S., & Safran, J. D. (1987). *Emotion in psychotherapy: Affect, cognition, and the process of change.* New York: Guilford Press.

Greenberg, L. S., & Safran, J. (1989). Emotion in psychotherapy. *American Psychologist, 44,* 19–29.

Greenberg, L. S., & Watson, J. (1998). Experiential therapy of depression: Differential effects of client-centered relationship conditions and process experiential interventions. *Psychotherapy Research, 8,* 210–224.

Guidano, V. (1991). *The self in process.* New York: Guilford Press.

Guidano, V. (1987). *Complexity of the self.* New York: Guilford Press.

Hermans, H., Kempen, H., & van Loon, J. (1992). The dialogical self: Beyond individualism and rationalism. *American Psychologist, 47,* 23–33.

James, W. (1890). *The principles of psychology.* New York: Holt. (Reprinted, New York: Dover, 1950)

Kaplan, M., & Kaplan, M. (1987). *Psychotherapy, 24*(15), 245–253.

Lazarus, R. S. (1991a). Cognition and motivation in emotion. *American Psychologist, 46,* 352–367.

Lazarus, R. S. (1991b). Progress on a cognitive–emotional–relational theory of emotion. *American Psychologist, 46,* 819–834.

Lewin, R. (1994). *Complexity.* New York: Macmillan.

Mahoney, M. (1995). *Human change process.* New York: Basic Books.

Mahrer, A. R. (1978). *Experiencing: A humanistic theory of psychology and psychiatry.* New York: Brunner/Mazel.

Mahrer, A. R. (1983). *Experiential psychotherapy: Basic practices.* New York: Brunner/Mazel.

Mahrer, A. R. (1986). *Therapeutic experiencing: The process of change.* New York: Norton.

Mahrer, A. R. (1996). *The complete guide to experiential psychotherapy.* New York: Wiley.

Maslow, A. H. (1954). Motivation and personality. New York: Harper.

Maslow, A. H. (1968). *Toward a psychology of being.* New York: Van Nostrand.

Maslow, A. H. (1971). *The farther reaches of human nature.* New York: Viking Press.

May, R. (1958). Contributions of existential psychotherapy. In R. May, E. Angel, & F. Ellenberger (Eds.), *Existence: A new dimension in psychiatry and psychology.* New York: Basic Books.

May, R. (Ed.). (1960). *Existential psychology.* New York: Random House.

May, R. (1981). *Freedom and destiny.* New York: Norton.

Mazur, E. (1996). The Zeigarnik effect and the concept of unfinished business in Gestalt therapy. *British Gestalt Journal, 5*(1), 18–23.

Merleau-Ponty, M. (1962). *The phenomenology of perception* (C. Smith, Trans.). London: Routledge & Kegan Paul.

Pascual-Leone, J. (1987). Organismic processes for neo-Piagetian theories: A dialectical causal account of cognitive development. *International Journal of Psychology, 22,* 531–570. Also in A. Demetriou (Ed.), *The neo-Piagetian theories of cognitive development: Towards an integration.* Amsterdam: North-Holland.

Pascual-Leone, J. (1989). An organismic process model of Witkin's field-dependence–independence. In T. Globerson & T. Zelniker (Eds.), *Cognitive style and cognitive development.* Norwood, NJ: Ablex.

Pascual-Leone, J. (1990a). An essay on wisdom: Toward organismic processes that make it possible. In R. J. Sternberg (Ed.), *Wisdom: Its nature, origins, and development.* New York: Cambridge University Press.

Pascual-Leone, J. (1990b). Reflections on life-span intelligence, consciousness and ego development. In C. Alexander & E. Langer (Eds.), *Higher stages of human development: Perspectives on adult growth.* New York: Oxford University Press.

Pascual-Leone, J. (1991). Emotions, development and psychotherapy: A dialectical constructivist perspective. In J. D. Safran & L. S. Greenberg (Eds.), *Emotion, psychotherapy, and change.* New York: Guilford Press.

Pascual-Leone, J., & Irwin, R. (1998). Abstraction, the will, the self and modes of learning in adulthood. In M. Smith & T. Pourchot (Eds.), *Adult learning and development: Perspectives from educational psychology.* Mahwah, NJ: Erlbaum.

Perls, F. S. (1969). *Gestalt therapy verbatim.* Lafayette, CA: Real People Press.

Perls, F. S., Hefferline, R., & Goodman, P. (1951). *Gestalt therapy: Excitement and growth in the human personality.* New York: Dell.

Piaget, J. (1969). *The mechanisms of perception.* London: Routledge & Kegan Paul.

Polster, I., & Polster, M. (1973). *Gestalt therapy integrated.* New York: Brune-Mazel.

Rice, L. N., & Greenberg, L. S. (1984). *Patterns of change: An intensive analysis of psychotherapeutic process.* New York: Guilford Press.

Riceur, P. (1992). *Oneself as another.* Chicago: University of Chicago Press.

Rogers, C. R. (1951). *Client-centered therapy.* Boston: Houghton Mifflin.

Rogers, C. R. (1958). A process conception of psychotherapy. *American Psychologist, 13,* 142–149.

Rogers, C. R. (1959). A theory of therapy, personality, and interpersonal relationships as developed in the client-centered framework. In S. Koch (Ed.), *Psychology: A study of a science* (Vol. 3). New York: McGraw-Hill.

Rogers, C. R. (1961). *On becoming a person.* Boston: Houghton Mifflin.

Scherer, K. R. (1984). On the nature and function of emotion: A component process approach. In K. R. Scherer & P. Ekman (Eds.), *Approaches to emotion.* Hillsdale, NJ: Erlbaum.

Smith, L. B., & Thelen, E. (Eds.). (1993). *A dynamic systems approach to development: Applications.* Cambridge, MA: MIT Press.

Sroufe, L. A. (1996). *Emotional development: The organization of emotional life in the early years.* New York: Cambridge University Press.

Stern, D. N. (1985). *The interpersonal world of the infant: A view from psychoanalysis and developmental psychology.* New York: Basic Books.

Sullivan, H. S. (1950). The illusion of personal individuality. *Psychiatry, 13,* 317–332.

Sullivan, H. S. (1953). *The interpersonal theory of psychiatry.* New York: Norton.

Thelen, E., & Smith, L. B. (1994). *A dynamic systems approach to the development of cognition and action.* Cambridge, MA: MIT Press.

Van Balen, R. (1990). The therapeutic relationship according to Carl Rogers: Only a climate? a dialogue? or both? In G. Lietaer, J. Rombauts, & R. Van Balen (Eds.), *Client-centered and experiential psychotherapy in the nineties.* Leuven, Belgium: Leuven University Press.

Van Balen, R. (1996). Theory of personality change: A comparison of Rogers. In R. Hutterer, G. Pawlowsky, P. Schmid, & R. Stipsits (Eds.), *Client-centered and experiential psychotherapy: A paradigm in motion.* Frankfurt am Main: Lang.

Van Geert, P. (1994). *Dynamic systems of development: Change between complexity and chaos.* Hertfordshire, UK: Harvester Wheatsheaf.

Varela, F. J., Rosch, E., & Thompson, E. (1991). *The embodied mind: Cognitive science and human experience.* Cambridge, MA: MIT Press.

Watson, J. C., & Greenberg, L. S. (1995). Alliance ruptures and repairs in experiential therapy. *In Session: Psychotherapy in Practice, 1*(1), 19–32.

Watson, J. C., & Greenberg, L. S. (1997). Emotion and cognition in experiential therapy: A dialectical-constructivist position. In H. Rosen & K. Kuelwein (Eds.), *Constructing realities: Meaning making perspectives for psychotherapists.* San Francisco: Jossey-Bass.

Watson, J. C., & Rennie, D. (1994). Qualitative analysis of clients' subjective experience of significant moments during the exploration of problematic reactions. *Journal of Counseling Psychology, 41,* 500–509.

*Webster's new world dictionary.* (1979). Toronto: Nelson, Foster & Scott.

Wheeler, G. (1991). *Gestalt reconsidered.* New York: Gardner Press.

Wheeler, G. (1995). Shame in two paradigms of therapy. *British Gestalt Journal, 4*(2), 76–85.

Yalom, I. D. (1975). *The theory and practice of group psychotherapy* (2nd ed.). New York: Basic Books.

Yalom, I. D. (1980). *Existential psychotherapy.* New York: Basic Books.

Yalom, I. D. (1989). *Love's executioner and other tales of psychotherapy.* New York: Basic Books.

Yontef, G. M. (1993). *Awareness, dialogue and process: Essays on Gestalt therapy.* Highland, NY: Gestalt Journal Press.

Yontef, G. M. (1995). Gestalt therapy. In A. S. Gurman & S. B. Messer (Eds.), *Essential psychotherapies: Theory and practice.* New York: Guilford Press.

Zeigarnik, B. (1927). Das Behalten erledigter und unerledigter Handlungen. *Psychologie Forschung, 9,* 1–85.

Zinker, J. (1977). *Creative process in Gestalt therapy.* New York: Brunner/Mazel.

# II

\*\*\*\*\*

# FOUNDATIONAL PROCESSES

# 3

*****

# Empathic
## *A POSTMODERN WAY OF BEING?*

Jeanne C. Watson
Rhonda Goldman
Greet Vanaerschot

*Empathy is a basic* client-centered process that is complex and multi-faceted. While it simultaneously forges an alliance and builds therapists' relationships with their clients, it also serves to deconstruct clients' realities and subjective worldviews. In this chapter we will define empathy as it is known and practiced within the experiential tradition. We will examine its function in humanistic psychotherapies and discuss its value as a potent change mechanism in psychotherapy. Then we will look at various types of empathy that have been identified by experiential therapists before discussing the various cues that therapists use to assist them in communicating empathically with their clients.

Carl R. Rogers was at pains to distinguish empathy from identification. He defined empathy as the ability "to perceive the internal frame of reference of another with accuracy and with the emotional components and meanings which pertain thereto as if one were the person without ever losing the as if condition" (1959, pp. 210–211). While identification reflects a fusion of perspective and feeling with another so that one totally shares the other's perspective, empathy implies a more distant perspective—one that is infused with cognitive understanding of the other's phenomenological world and frame of reference. To some degree empathy is at the basis of all successful communication between peoples. However, the degree and scope of empathy varies with the nature of the relationship and the purposes to which it is ultimately applied. To communicate successfully with another person one must understand not only what they are saying but how they are feeling, what their intentions are, albeit in a limited way, and what they require of you in the process. This is illustrated quite well in a cartoon that depicts a chieftain of a South Sea island urging his tribes people to hide their high-tech gadgets, including televisions and stereos, because the anthropologists have arrived. The chieftain obviously not only understood the anthropologists' objectives, intentions, and what they required of him and his people but empathized sufficiently not to disappoint them.

One of Rogers's primary intentions in psychotherapy was to facilitate clients' self-directed change processes. He realized that empathy was a potent way of having clients actively explore and resolve the problematic issues in their lives that brought them into therapy. Rogers proposed that empathic responding would enable therapists to immerse themselves in the world of another, to swim in it and come to understand what was significant and what it feels like to be the other. To do this therapists need to become involved in the therapeutic relationship as a real other, offering their own presence as one who is meeting, trusting in, and confirming that which is most basic in the individual's experience at any given moment. Therapists are encouraged to stop being observers and evaluators of their clients behavior and to bracket their own values and preconceptions of the world. Rogers described it in these words: "Empathy is a process. . . . [It] involves being very sensitive moment to moment to the changing felt meanings which flow in the other person. . . . [It] means temporarily living in his/her life, moving about in it delicately without making judgments, sensing meanings of which he or she is scarcely aware" (1975, p. 1833). From this perspective therapists may be viewed as anthropologists, trying to discover the other from the inside out. By walking as a companion, offering themselves and trying to live in the other's world albeit temporarily and only through discourse, therapists can help clients unleash their potential to heal or help themselves. A number of theorists suggest that unconditional regard and empathy are opposite sides of the same coin—one cannot be empathic without being unconditionally prizing (Bozarth, 1997; Keil, 1996; Lietaer, 1993). Moreover, an important yardstick for determining how empathic one is being is to check the extent of one's unconditional regard for the client. If that is low, it is likely that one is not being as empathic as one might be in the situaton (Keil, 1996).

Empathy has a number of very important functions in experiential therapy. First, it provides clients with an affirming therapist presence that facilitates the development of a safe working environment and helps to forge and maintain a good working alliance. Second, empathic responding models a way of being for clients that may facilitate their developing better ways of regulating their affect and of soothing themselves. By being empathic, therapists can model nurturing, affirming ways of being with clients that the latter may internalize. Empathic responding also helps clients access more adaptive emotions that may not be in awareness. Third, empathic responses are important change mechanisms in their own right, as they help clients to deconstruct and reorganize their worldviews consisting of their experiences, histories, assumptions, values, needs, and behaviors. Empathy can be communicated both by one's attitude (nonverbal behaviors), and by specific empathic responses for example, empathic affirmations, empathic conjecture among others.

## EMPATHY IN THE SERVICE OF THE RELATIONSHIP

Rogers (1965, 1975) saw empathy as vital to providing clients with an optimal environment in which change could be effected. Rogers suggested that restricted and maladjusted experiencing can only be reduced and altered when people are in safe environments. In such safe, unthreatening contexts people may be able to examine the threatening aspects of their experience and replace their introjected value systems with their own organismic valuing process, which is open to information from a variety of sources and leaves individuals free to behave and experience in more open and comprehensive ways (Watson & Greenberg, 1998). The objective in client-centered and experiential therapies is to provide a safe climate in which people can once again access those parts of themselves that they have distorted or denied to awareness so as to allow greater congruency in functioning and to devise more satisfying ways of being (Rogers, 1965; Vanaerschot, 1993, 1997). Rogers believed that people were capable of changing their conditions of worth and altering their self-concept if they were exposed to nurturing, nonevaluative environments where they could safely acknowledge organismic experiences that were at odds with their self-concept (Vanaerschot, 1990, 1993; Watson & Greenberg, 1998).

The therapeutic relationship has long been recognized as an important component of change in psychotherapy, and much effort continues to be expended to determine the components of a good working alliance (Horvath & Greenberg, 1994; Henry, Schacht, & Strupp, 1986; King, Mallinckrodt, & Coble, 1996; Safran, Muran, & Samistag, 1994; Elliott, 1985; Lietaer, 1990). The provision of empathy by the therapist is viewed as essential to the development and maintenance of the therapeutic alliance by numerous authors (Bohart & Greenberg, 1997; Safran et al., 1994; Rhodes, Hill, Thompson, & Elliott, 1994). It is essential that clients feel safe with their therapists if they are to engage productively in the work of therapy. Safety refers to the affective components of the relationship and clients' experiences of their interactions with their therapists. A review of the research literature shows that clients value feeling accepted, prized, understood, supported, and affirmed by their therapists. Elliott (1985, 1990) and Lietaer (1992) have observed that clients who did well in therapy reported that their therapists' warmth, interest, involvement, support, empathy, respect, patience, and understanding were helpful to them. It is highly likely that these factors are highly related to therapists' empathic responsiveness to their clients. In contrast, when clients feel criticized, belittled, controlled, or neglected by their therapist they are unlikely to do well at the end of therapy. Thus empirical evidence would seem to confirm Rogers's view that the provision of an empathic climate is important to clients' well-being and progress in therapy (Rogers, 1975; Vanaerschot, 1993).

Experiential therapists work to create strong alliances with their clients. This means working toward establishing agreement on the tasks and goals of therapy and developing a bond. The bond is seen as developing out of two important processes: first, it stems from clients feeling understood by and trusting of their therapists; second, the bond is fed by clients' sense of hope that grows out of their perception that they are working with their therapists in a manner that will lead to the resolution of their problems. Thus empathic responses serve three main functions in terms of building the alliance: (a) they convey understanding of clients' subjective perceptions of the world; (b) they help clients articulate and symbolize their own sense and manner of constructing their problems; and (c) they help clients and therapists formulate the goals and tasks of therapy.

There are a number of important consequences for the relationship or alliance that follow from clients feeling safe in therapy. One of the most important is that they feel free to self-disclose. This has been referred to as the meta-task of therapy and is the primary vehicle by which clients and therapists come to know and understand clients' experiences of their worlds (Watson & Greenberg, 1994, 1995). It is through self-disclosure that clients are able to engage in self-examination, deconstruction, and reorganization of their experience.

A second important function of empathy for the relationship is that it mitigates the power imbalance so that clients learn to assume responsibility for their own process and find the solutions to their problems. They learn to feel trusted and respected by their therapists and to see the other as a companion who can facilitate certain experiences and tasks but not necessarily as the expert with the answers or solutions to their problems. A fundamental tenet of humanistic approaches to psychotherapy is the maintenance of as equitable a power balance as possible, given that each participant has a very unique role within the therapeutic encounter. This is especially important for those groups who may feel disempowered by various life circumstances that prevent them from realizing their potential.

Third, empathy helps therapists perceive and understand their clients' goals and helps guide their choice of tasks in order to facilitate their realization. A recent study that looked at differences between good-outcome and bad-outcome cases in client-centered and process-experiential therapy determined that while all clients felt that they had a good bond with their therapists, those clients who felt that there was agreement with their therapists on the goals and tasks early on in therapy did better at the end of therapy (Weerasekera, Linder, Greenberg, & Watson, 1998). Thus agreement on the goals and tasks of therapy may be crucial to good outcome. One way of insuring that there is a match between clients and therapists is for the latter to be empathic to their clients' objectives and know how to match their techniques with their clients' goals. This is also true in client-centered therapies, where there is less emphasis on techniques. In client-centered therapy an important component of successful therapies may be therapists' abilities to focus clients and help them track relevant experiential questions (Klein, Mathieu-Coughlan, & Kiesler, 1986; Gendlin, 1981, 1996). One way this can be accomplished is if therapists are empathically attuned to that which is emotionally and experientially significant for their clients.

Fourth, empathy has been found to be essential to alert therapists to the presence of ruptures and to help heal them when they occur in the therapeutic alliance (Safran et al., 1994; Rhodes & Hill, 1994). Together with congruence, therapists' abilities to hear and respond empathically to clients' negative feelings about them as therapists or their therapeutic endeavors seems to be the most important ingredient for maintaining and strengthening the alliance over time, and in preventing early termination and poor outcomes. Given the importance of the therapeutic alliance in facilitating change, few would question the usefulness of empathy in ensuring its development and maintenance. However, the question still remains: How is empathy curative?

## EMPATHY IN THE SERVICE OF THE SELF

While numerous authors acknowledge that empathy is useful in building the therapeutic relationship and creating conditions of safety, many still see it as a means to an end or as producing the necessary preparatory groundwork to ensure the successful seeding of their specific therapeutic operations, for example, interpretations (Kohut, 1977) or challenges to clients' views of reality (Linehan, 1997). According to these theorists the provision of empathic responding is fundamentally relational: it is an effective way to make clients feel safe within the therapeutic encounter; it helps them feel understood and cared for by their therapists; and it serves to validate clients' subjective realities, their perceptions, and feelings. However, empathic responding does more than merely assist the development of the relationship. Some of the important processes that it facilitates are the development of awareness and self-soothing behaviors and the containment of overwhelming emotions.

### Developing Awareness

As stated earlier an important function of empathy is to help clients access those aspects of their experience that are outside of awareness. Rogers saw empathic responding as a way in which therapists could provide their clients with fresh canvases on which to paint (i.e., express) their perceptions and subjective experiences of reality without worrying about the judgments of others. The primary aim is to create conditions of safety and lowered threat and to validate clients' perceptions and organismic experience so that they can begin to formulate new views of themselves and reorganize their self-structures (Lietaer, 1992; Rogers, 1975; Thorne, 1992; Bozarth, 1990; Brodley, 1990). Emotional processing is an important component of healing. Emotions have important adaptive qualities that guide and direct people toward accessing and thus meeting fundamental needs and goals. When information from one's emotional processing is not accurately articulated in awareness, the orienting function of the adaptive system is defeated. Empathy helps people become aware of their emotions.

## Self-Soothing and Containing Experiences

Another important consequence of providing an empathic, safe environment is that therapists model ways that clients can learn to be with themselves that might not be part of their current repertoire. Clients learn what it means to be validated, to feel nurtured, and to feel accepted (Rogers, 1965, 1967; Barrett-Lennard, 1997; Vanaerschot, 1990). This is particularly important for clients who have grown up in critical and rejecting environments and who may not have developed positive nurturing introjects from others. These clients may lack the ability to soothe themselves and may seek other more self-destructive ways of managing and containing their emotions. The objective of empathic responding for these clients is to help them acknowledge their feelings and to know that their feelings are received in a respectful and caring environment. As clients begin to talk about their feelings and represent what is happening to them, they are able to use their cognitive abilities to gain a new perspective on events and their behavior (Kennedy-Moore & Watson, in press). Symbolically representing experience and reflexively examining it are ways of containing overwhelming feelings that can help to strengthen clients' coping abilities as they acquire distance from them by talking about them as opposed to acting them out. Ideally clients will come to learn to be more responsively attuned to their own needs and to protect and nurture themselves independently of their therapists. In this way empathy serves to strengthen clients' sense of self. Clients become more self-assertive as they acknowledge and respect their own feelings, gain confidence as they voice them, and begin to see ways of acting congruently that are more satisfying and acceptable.

## EMPATHY IN THE SERVICE OF DECONSTRUCTION

To understand how empathy functions to deconstruct people's worldviews it is important to grasp how Rogers saw healthy functioning. Healthy functioning is characterized by an openness to experience and a state of congruence. Lietaer (1993) defines this as a way of being that is characterized by flexibility, openness, and the ability to hold concepts of the real and ideal self tentatively so that they can be accessible and receptive to new information and experience and subject to change if necessary. Thus it is not a state of harmony but rather a sophisticated level of cognitive–affective development rather like Piaget's level of formal operations with respect to interpersonal and intrapersonal knowledge. According to this perspective, perceptions are accurate and open to corroboration or disconfirmation depending on the evidence at hand. If people are functioning optimally, experiences are seen as limited and differentiated, they are accurately located in space and time, and dominated by facts which can be evaluated in multiple ways. Moreover at this level of functioning people are aware of different levels of abstraction and are able to test inferences and abstractions against reality (Meador & Rogers, 1979; Rogers, 1959). Thus well-adjusted people are able to experience in a comprehensive and thorough manner, thereby leaving open the possibility of synthesizing different aspects of experiencing into an organized whole that is satisfying to them and consistent with their current values, desires, needs, and demands of their environment.

In addition to these more cognitive activities, the fully functioning person trusts his or her feelings, which are viewed as the integration of emotions together with their cognitively felt meanings (Bohart & Tallman, 1997; Rice, 1974; Rogers, 1965; Toukmanian, 1993). According to this view people are not dominated by their feelings, but rather the information obtained from their feelings is available to awareness to be integrated with information from other sources and used as a guide in determining future actions. Rogers defined mature behavior as the ability to perceive in a comprehensive and thorough manner, be nondefensive, accept responsibility for one's behavior, accept responsibility for being differentiated from others, make evaluations in accord with the information from the senses and organismic valuing, accept others as unique, and prize oneself and others (Meador & Rogers, 1979; Rogers, 1959). In a nutshell Rogers saw healthy functioning as fluid, malleable, and evolving (Watson & Greenberg, 1998).

While Rogers (1975) emphasized that empathy was an attitude, he also distinguished between empathy as it is experienced covertly by the therapist and empathy as it is communicated to the client. Thus it is not enough to merely feel empathic toward one's clients; one has to be able to demonstrate one's understanding of their experience and world in order for them to feel understood and further facilitate their change process. In examining how empathy interacts with clients' own cognitive and self-reflective abilities, our focus will be on empathic responding or communicated empathy and its role in psychotherapy.

An important function for Rogers of empathically responding to clients was that it enabled them to get in touch with aspects of experience that were previously outside of awareness. However, the view of empathy that high-lights its role as facilitating the relationship does not sufficiently highlight that it is a way of facilitating clients' self-reflection in therapy.

It is human beings' capacity to determine, evaluate, and reflect on the significance of things for themselves that sets them apart from other animals. Self-reflective agents are people with a sense of themselves and their lives, which they can evaluate and about which they can make choices (Taylor, 1990). An important way for clients to become aware of themselves and their lives is by articulating their sense of situations and the import or significance of events. This information is provided by feelings. Once clients are aware of their subjective response to events they are able to apprehend their action tendencies and subject these to strong evaluation in the light of their needs, goals, values, and standards (Watson, 1996; Watson & Rennie, 1994). This process is facilitated in experiential therapy by therapists empathically re-sponding to their clients' feelings so as to help them acquire a better sense of those feelings and the impact and import of different situations for them. An important effect of helping and closely tracking clients' feelings is that they function as an undercurrent or the thread that leads therapists to the clients' core experiences that require further processing.

Empathic responding holds up a mirror to clients of what they are feel-ing and experiencing so that they can see it more clearly and consider it freshly. Through empathic responding and mirroring, experiential therapists help clients to articulate and reflect upon their own subjective perceptions of the world and constructions of reality. Therapists validate and explore clients' appraisals, affects, needs, and action tendencies in relation to situations that occur in everyday life, as well as the assumptive frameworks from which they operate. Thus therapists help clients access adaptive emotions so that they can better orient themselves in the world in order to meet their needs and goals; they also help clients to freely and effectively examine and reevaluate their values and objectives so as to construct alternative worldviews and ways of being. This in turn leads to greater self-acceptance and the formation of new views of self that allow people different modes of operating in interper-sonal relationships. By empathically responding to their clients' subjective experience, therapists help to give it form which objectifies and clarifies it for clients so that they can look at it in a new way and evaluate their actions, feelings, and values to create alternative ways of being in the world that are more personally satisfying (Watson & Rennie, 1994; Watson & Greenberg, 1996).

Empathic responding helps clients to deconstruct their subjective frame-works. Experiential therapists respect clients autonomy and ability to judge their own behavior and to begin to see the links between various environ-mental stimuli and their feelings and actions. Rogers saw clients as being primarily responsible for seeing the discrepancies and incongruities between various aspects of their behavior, feelings, and goals. However, it is likely that as therapists struggle to truly grasp their clients' worlds, incongruencies and discrepancies may be highlighted (Keil, 1996). Noting incongruencies in clients' narratives is performed very differently in experiential therapies than in other modalities. In many approaches therapists assume the need to comment on and dispute clients' views of reality and perhaps even step out and judge what their clients are saying, or offer interpretations of their clients' unconscious motivations. In these cases therapists are asserting some objective reality to which they have privileged access, whereas in experiential therapies it is almost by accident that the discrepancies emerge. Moreover, it is only in the service of understanding that the therapist may comment on them; it is the client who judges and ultimately determines whether they are valid, accurate, or worthwhile.

In an empathic approach, as therapists reflect the impact of different events and try to represent their clients' views tentatively, implicit in their elaboration of their clients' worlds is that this is a subjective view of reality and that there might be other views of the same landscape. Moreover as clients try to articulate and symbolize their experience for the other it becomes clearer and better defined, and as therapists struggle to understand and apprehend their clients' realities they help to uncover clients' assumptions, leaving these open to questioning and reevaluation by the latter. Empathy at its most highly developed level brings knowledge that is at the periphery into focus (Beech & Brazier, 1995; Rogers, 1975; Truax, 1961; Neville, 1995). In this way it serves to deconstruct clients' dominant views of their experiences and reality and bring that which has been marginalized and silenced to center stage. As such, it is quite revolutionary and empowering for clients. As therapists work with clients to deconstruct their realities, the latter learn that knowledge is relative—and that there are an infinite number of other ways of knowing and being.

An example from a therapeutic transaction will help to illustrate this aspect of empathic responding. A client who was struggling to differentiate herself from a severely disturbed mother whom she had cared for from an early age was exploring how trapped she felt and unable to venture out on her own. This is how she described it:

CLIENT: I am so caught I feel as if I am suffocating, yet moving out is out of the question.

THERAPIST: So somehow for you even though you feel the life being snuffed out of you it is just too difficult to leave.

CLIENT: Yes . . . but when I hear you say it out loud it hits home . . . I can see more clearly how damaging it really is . . . I never properly considered how damaging it is to me and yet to abandon her seems so cruel. I feel that I would be punished . . . struck down. It's as if I do not deserve to live unless I can save her, it's just too too selfish.

THERAPIST: So somehow taking care of yourself and saving yourself seems too selfish and that is just somehow unacceptable?

CLIENT: Yes . . . but I want to be free and have a life of my own like other people. I just don't know quite how to achieve that.

Here the therapist is responding each time in a tentative, probing voice. It can be observed that while she empathically reflects her client's experience she implicitly heightens the impact of that experience and keeps it in the foreground using imagery like "snuffed out." In this way the therapist is also implicitly questioning and focusing the client on her belief that it would be too difficult to leave. It is the client who ultimately evaluates the impact of that experience and later determines that there has to be a better balance in her life so that she does not forfeit all to the care of her parent. This is achieved by the therapist attending closely to the client's experience of being in the world and holding it up for closer scrutiny by means of empathic reflections. Therapists can respond empathically to their clients by using numerous different techniques, including empathic reflections, empathic conjectures, empathic evocation, and empathic exploration, focusing, empty-chair work, systematic evocative unfolding, and two-chair work (Greenberg, Rice, & Elliott, 1993).

## TYPES OF EMPATHIC RESPONSES

How do we convey empathy? A number of different types of empathic responses including empathic understanding, empathic affirmation, empathic evocation, empathic exploration, and empathic conjecture have been identified (Greenberg et al., 1993; Greenberg & Elliott, 1997). Each of these serve a slightly different function in experiential therapy.

### Empathic Understanding Responses

These are simple reflections that are intended to communicate understanding of clients' experiences. They may also be symbolic representations of clients' implicit experiences that they themselves have not quite stated fully. These responses begin to fill out the canvas on which clients' life experiences will be drawn. Thus they also begin to help clients see aspects of their experience freshly and in new ways. The following is an example of an empathic understanding response to a client who was grieving the loss of a brother:

CLIENT: It's like all my life I've just been . . . been brave and warding off the confusion and fear and the distress all the way along, all the way along.

THERAPIST: So there's never been time to allow yourself to feel the fear and confusion, you always had to keep going.

CLIENT: And then . . . and then Bobbie was the light you know, it's like when I was a little kid Bobbie was that.

THERAPIST: He was the lighthouse in the storm, your guide.

Here the therapist is working with the client to symbolize the role her brother played in her life. They are giving the clients's experience more form and color so that it can be better understood and the impact of the loss can be processed.

## Empathic Affirmation Responses

These responses are meant to affirm and corroborate a client's sense of self and situation. They convey a sense that the therapist is right beside the client and sees and understands how good or bad things seem to be right now. At these moments therapists are not pushing clients to explore their experience but are rather standing together with them confronting it as it truly is. For example:

CLIENT: I feel so trapped and without resources now. (*beginning to sob*) I don't know what I will do. . . . It feels so . . . so hopeless.

THERAPIST: It feels so painful right now as if there is no way out.

Here the therapist acknowledges and shares the client's bleak view; however, by locating it in the present she is implying that it may be of limited duration and that things might change.

## Empathic Evocation

With these responses therapists are trying to concretely evoke and heighten clients' experiences of events so that their impact and significance become clear. By heightening clients' access to their inner experiences therapists can help clients to better differentiate their emotional reactions and obtain clearer views of their situations. To do this therapists try to use fresh, connotative language that will throw clients' experiences into sharp relief (Rice, 1974). For example:

CLIENT: Looking at that situation was so hard. It took me by surprise—it's really, really fresh and unresolved, uhhmm—it's not that it was difficult or painful . . . those words don't fit, but it was that it was so intense that it just was overwhelming.

THERAPIST: So its like sort of a tidal wave hit you.

CLIENT: Yes, exactly . . . it just hit me and was so overpowering. It seems so devastating that I don't know where to start.

The therapists use of an evocative metaphor has helped to distill the clients' experience and put her in touch with its impact in a more differentiated and intense way.

## Empathic Exploration

These types of responses have a probing tentative quality to help clients explore the peripheries and margins of their experience. These responses are attempts to have clients go further into the tunnel of their experience, to unpack and illuminate aspects of it of which they are unaware and that might give them a somewhat different view. It is in this way that therapists help to reveal what is unspoken and assumed by clients.

Greenberg et al. (1993) do not distinguish between different types of empathic exploration responses, yet it seems that these responses can be used to have clients examine their assumptions, their feelings, and their evaluations of events. Often therapists will pose these reflections with a somewhat questioning tone; for example, a therapist may attempt to empathically explore and open up a client's evaluation of a particular situation by saying, "So you think this is the end of the relationship?" Alternatively a therapist may probe the client's feelings about a particular situation so as to help clients to differentiate their feelings more precisely to arrive at a clearer understanding of the impact of different events and their unique meaning to the client. For example, a therapist who was trying to have her client describe the pain she was feeling at the loss of a significant relationship said, "I don't know, you just feel very raw inside almost like you have been wounded . . . ?" Another therapist was trying to help her client develop an alternative model of a marriage partnership. The woman was having difficulty expressing disagreement with her husband on some important issues, as she believed that it was her place to support her husband and follow his lead irrespective of the consequences to herself. Her therapist focused on this belief with an empathic reflection saying, "So somehow you feel you have no right to express yourself, you have to just go along."

With empathic exploration responses therapists focus clients' attention on specific aspects of their experience and in particular their feelings, evaluations, and assumptions. This enables clients to reflect on their evaluations and assumptions and the aspects of their experience that might be contributing to their current view and appraisal. Moreover, this enables them to reexamine their perspectives and assumptions before determining how they wish to act. Alternatively, therapists may state their reflections so as to have the client attend to some of the more salient aspects of their environment. For example, "I'm not sure, but there just seems to be something in his tone of voice or expression that you find withering." Here clients are being asked to go beyond that which they have represented and to peer into other corners of their experience to see if something has been missed, or could be rendered more fully, and to reevaluate and confirm their perspective and construction of reality.

## Empathic Conjecture

These responses are attempts by the therapist to tease out the implicit meanings of what the client is saying. Here the therapist is attentive to the nuances of the clients' experience. Usually this requires that therapists be attentive and highly sensitive to the language their clients are using as well as their nonverbal behaviors as they try to amplify and develop what the client is saying. Empathic conjectures require therapists to be aware of and sensitive to the whole of their clients' experiences, as often the conjectures flow out of a deep understanding of clients' life contexts. While the information offered by the conjectures may be based on a hunch or a guess, it is still very much from within clients' frames of reference. Therapists do not impose their own framework, but rather like good jazz musicians they synergistically develop a melody with their clients of what it is like to experience the world as they do (Bohart & Tallman, 1997).

Empathic conjecture is when therapists try to distill the personal meaning of events for their clients. For example, a client was puzzled by her reaction to a production of Henrik Ibsen's *A Doll's House*. After she left the theater, while walking up Broadway she found herself sobbing without understanding why. She began to explore the event with her therapist: "I was so struck by Nora's performance, she gave such a contemporary interpretation. I never realized fully before how difficult it was for her to decide to leave. I guess the play is about secrets. . . . You know she realizes at the end that she is married to a stranger and that she has been her father's daughter and then her husband's wife but never truly herself. So that in some sense her existence had been inauthentic." As the client speaks the therapist feels that the material is charged for the client: although she is focusing on the play it seems emotionally significant to her. In an attempt to distill its personal meaning the therapist tries to articulate something about Nora's plight that somehow may be relevant to the client:

THERAPIST: So there is something about her not being true to herself . . . a sense of betrayal . . . I'm not sure that she sold herself short that somehow disturbs you, left you feeling sad?

CLIENT: Yes, I think after I left I felt somehow regret that I was not in New York producing plays of that caliber. It had once been a dream of mine.

THERAPIST: So somehow you feel that you have betrayed a dream, sold yourself short.

The communication of empathy is not restricted to the types of responses just described. However, these types of responses focus therapists' attention on what their clients are saying and help them to follow their clients as opposed to becoming more distant and evaluative. Empathy can be communicated in numerous other ways in experiential therapy. Watson and Greenberg (1994) suggest that empathy can also be enacted in the therapeutic encounter with more task-focused interventions like focusing, two-chair work, systematic evocative unfolding, and empty-chair work. Experiential therapists are sensitively attuned to the questions and issues that clients are trying to resolve in therapy. Once these questions or markers have been identified or observed by therapists they can demonstrate empathic understanding of their clients' objectives by suggesting ways that might work to achieve their ends. Experiential therapists try to expand clients' options in therapy to help them engage in those activities that might be most productive to resolve the problems that they have brought in. Thus to suggest to someone that they engage in two-chair work to help them resolve a conflict is a little like offering a thirsty person water. It clearly indicates that you have heard the client's need and are sufficiently attentive and sympathetic to help him or her meet it. In suggesting various therapeutic tasks therapists, if they have correctly understood their clients, can communicate their understanding of the core of clients' problems. Thus often they are able to demonstrate that they are attending to the centrality of their clients' messages. This is recognized as an important component of empathy by numerous scholars (Bohart & Tallman, 1997; Elliott, 1982).

The potential difficulty with suggesting tasks and moving out of a more reflective mode of responding even temporarily is that therapists can become caught up in their own agenda, which may cloud their vision of their clients' positions. Consequently experiential therapists need to be more sensitively attuned when implementing more directive interventions so as not to lose sight of their clients and their concerns. Moreover less experienced therapists may be so entranced with the technology that they do not see the efficacy and the special role that empathy plays in helping clients to resolve their problems. The directive techniques are embedded in empathic responding as therapists and clients try to symbolize and express the latter's experiences and to co-construct the latter's reality. Direction without empathy would not only be potentially damaging to the relationship, possibly contributing to the development of power struggles and a sense for clients of being ignored and invalidated, but it would undermine the important goal of having clients become sufficiently differentiated and autonomous so as to assume responsibility for their own functioning in different contexts. Moreover, it would be difficult for clients to learn to soothe themselves and to be more nurturing of their own needs if their therapists were not sensitively attuned.

## FACILITATING THERAPISTS' EMPATHY

Experiential therapy is both a set of skills that can be learned through instruction and modeling and an art that requires a careful balance between both (1) *leading clients* through emotional exploration and (2) *following clients* to help them symbolize experience as well as tolerate affect. While we have identified and described various types of empathic responses, it is difficult to specify which types of empathic responses are best at different times. Clearly the art of experiential therapy is one of achieving a fine balance between leading and following, knowing when clients need a gentle nudge or when they need to be nurtured and bathed in compassion. There are some guidelines, however.

In looking at how therapists can become empathic, a distinction needs to be made between processes internal to the therapist and more observable client processes. Vanaerschot (1990, 1997) emphasizes empathic listening by the therapist, whereas others emphasize specific client behaviors that alert therapists to salient, poignant, and central aspects of their clients' experiences (Rice, 1974; Greenberg et al., 1993; Klein et al., 1986). By empathic listening Vanaerschot (1993) is referring to the therapists' experiencing process while listening to their clients. She suggests that therapists act as surrogate experiencers for their clients and come to experience in a very real, visceral way what their clients are experiencing. She describes an empathic-resonance process whereby the clients description of their experience elicits a bodily felt sense in the therapist. It is this bodily felt sense that provides the therapist with the data that enables him/her to symbolize clients' experiences, which can then be confirmed and subjected to revision. According to this view it is important for therapists to take the time to determine how their clients' narratives, particularly their description of events, is impacting on them so that a felt sense can form. In addition, therapists need to be congruent about their own experiences so that they can take note of them and use them productively in the session. When listening empathically therapists must be open to the experience of another so that it can be tasted and absorbed. Rice (1974) cautions that therapists need to suspend their own value frameworks and must be careful not to reach for closure too quickly. A high tolerance for ambiguity is demanded of a truly empathic therapist. However, as stated earlier, it is not enough to only listen empathically; empathy must also be communicated to the client.

Therapists bring a number of cognitive–affective capacities to their ability to be empathic; the most important of these, as noted by Rogers (1975), is imagination. The stories and experiences that clients share activate our imaginations and allow us to formulate a sense of their landscape. This is often fueled by therapists' tacit knowledge developed from their life experience, clinical wisdom, literature they have read, and their accumulated general understanding of the world and its diversity. However, it is not limited to their personal experience but can transcend it. By actively imagining clients' experiences, therapists can begin to infer what it is like to be them. Through this process therapists can ask themselves what they might feel in response to what their clients have told them. This provides them with a clue to their clients' subjective states and may form the basis for empathic exploration of their clients' inner experiences. It is in this way that therapists can make process distinctions between clients' expression of core emotions and other secondary and instrumental emotions (Greenberg & Elliott, 1997). For example one client was talking about how angry she was at her sister. The therapist had suggested they do an empty-chair task to further the client's processing of the negative experience. After she asked the client to describe her sister in the empty chair, the therapist was aware that the figure that emerged was that of a helpless, pathetic waif. It struck the therapist that the clients' more core affective reaction might actually be sadness at her sister's plight and that the expression of anger came from a sense of frustration at seeing her sister so hurt and damaged. When the therapist tentatively reflected that the client's description of her sister was very pathetic and asked her if she felt sad, the client immediately burst into tears and began to explore her own sense of hopelessness with respect to her sister's situation.

Empathic responses that attempt to access clients' primary or core feelings and bypass secondary emotions do not invalidate clients' experiences but rather are tentative attempts to go beyond such responses to help clients access more primary and adaptive emotional responses. The backdrop of all empathic responding is a tentative, exploratory attitude that implies a process of discovery during which the therapist is holding up the flashlight on ongoing momentary experience, observing, conjecturing, and feeding back their perceptions of their clients' world. However, ultimately and unequivocally clients are the experts of their own experience.

Another guideline to help therapists decide how to intervene differentially is when they feel that clients' problems or particular emotional states are fuzzy and unclear; or if therapists are unsure of their clients' needs, then empathic exploration can be used to differentiate clients' emotional reactions. Alternatively, to obtain a clearer sense of clients' situations, therapists might use evocative unfolding responses to help clients describe their situations more clearly and graphically. At times, if therapists are aware that clients are exploring new or "uncharted" territory and that they are feeling fragile and vulnerable, therapists may use empathic affirmation responses to actively support their clients, helping them to hold onto and tolerate their newly felt experiences.

By attending to certain aspects of clients' experiences therapists can become more responsively attuned to their clients. It is important not to package or merely parrot back to clients what they have told you just moments before. Somehow therapists need to be able to hear what is most significant or central in their clients' stories. There are a number of ways that client-centered therapists have learned to attend to the critical, poignant aspects of clients' narratives. While many of these measures were initially developed for research purposes, they resulted from fine-grained analyses and descriptions of clients' processes and can serve a useful purpose for both novice and experienced clinicians who would like to develop a third ear for listening to their clients' narratives. These scales have a variety of different ways of identifying how close clients are to their experience in the session. This can be very useful, as an important aspect of empathy is not only understanding but knowing how to respond to clients. After all, this is what empathic attunement is really about.

One way responsiveness to clients can be enhanced is if therapists are alert to the possible meanings inherent in different client vocal qualities. Rice, Koke, Greenberg, and Wagstaff (1979) developed the clients' vocal quality scale. This identified four different types of client vocal quality that can be used to alert therapists to clients' internal resources and involvement with their experience. The four categories of voice were focused, emotional, externalizing, and limited. (1) *Focused voice* indicates that a client is symbolizing experience in new and fresh ways. At these junctures clients have turned their attention inward and are trying to capture the fine nuances of their feelings to render them in words. (2) *Emotional voice* indicates that clients are experiencing their feelings in the moment, so their narrative is interrupted by signs of anger or pain, for example, crying. (3) *Externalizing voice* has a rehearsed, practiced quality and seems to indicate that clients are distant from their experience. It is not live, vivid, or fresh in the moment. (4) *Limited vocal quality* indicates that clients are also distant from their experience. In this way it is similar to an externalizing voice except that clients with limited voice seem fragile and as if they are walking on eggs. In contrast, an externalizing voice is robust and clients appear quite resilient.

Another way therapists can be attentive to clients' distance from their experiences is with the experiencing scale (Klein et al., 1986). The experiencing scale differentiates the content of clients' narratives into seven categories. At lower levels of the scale clients are seen to be focused outward and not in touch with their own inner referents or their own experience. At level 4, clients begin to use their own inner experience as an anchor for the events in their lives. They are more aware of their impact on them. At level 5, clients' narratives shift as they pose an experiential question about why or for what reason they function in specific ways. This is a very important task in experiential therapy—that of turning inward and beginning to explore why one operates as one does. If clients are able to successfully track and explore their experiential question, they are likely to gain an altered perspective of their problems or reach some satisfactory resolution identified as level 6. At level 7, clients' experiencing is fluid, not fixed: it is constantly evolving in the moment and open to reconstruction as new information becomes available.

Clients' use of focused voice and/or the posing of an experiential question alerts therapists to the need for empathic conjecture and exploration as together they work to give the clients' experience more clarity. The goal at these times is to work with clients to construct a fresh view of their problems. Similarly when clients show emotional vocal quality therapists are alerted to the problematic, painful, and difficult aspects of clients' experiences that need to be focused on and reflected so that clients can reprocess them. At times like this empathic affirmation or possibly an empty-chair task might be appropriate ways to communicate empathic understanding of clients' experiences. In contrast, when clients are showing an externalizing vocal quality or are at lower ends of the experiencing scale and are not making any reference to their inner experiences, therapists need to be more evocative in their responding in order to heighten clients' experiencing in the session and to help them access it. When clients' vocal quality is external it is often difficult to develop an inside feel for their world, as their accounts seem glib and packaged so that the impact of events is not as clearly differentiated. With limited vocal quality therapists may need to be especially gentle in their dealings with their clients, as this may indicate that the client does not have the psychological resources to adequately deal with their problematic experiences.

In addition to using clients' vocal quality as a guide to what is significant for them and to choose between different ways of responding empathically, therapists can attend to the content of clients' narratives. Most notably clients use of language can alert therapists to significant events or aspects of experience that might be useful to focus on in the session. The use of vivid, unusual, or idiosyncratic language by clients can indicate aspects of experience that are particularly noteworthy and worth exploring.

In this chapter we have defined empathy as an attitude, a type of listening, and a way of responding that shows that therapists are actively and sensitively attuned to their clients. As Bohart and Greenberg (1997) concluded in their recent review of different approaches to empathy, it is a complex process involving a variety of intentions, functions, and behaviors, rather than a singular entity. We have suggested that empathy is more than a way to build and maintain a positive therapeutic alliance, for in addition it helps to gently and carefully deconstruct clients' worldviews so as to subject them to careful scrutiny and reflection. Finally different types of empathic responses were identified and illustrated, and ways for therapists to develop greater attunement with their clients' experiences were discussed. Empathy is the foundation of all interactions between human beings and the cornerstone of experiential therapists' practice.

## REFERENCES

Barrett-Lennard, G. T. (1997). The recovery of empathy towards others and self. In A. Bohart & L. S. Greenberg (Eds.), *Empathy reconsidered: New directions in psychotherapy*. Washington, DC: APA Books.

Beech, C., & Brazier, D. (1995). Empathy for a real world. In R. Hutterer, G. Pawlowsky, P. Schmid, & R. Stipsits (Eds.), *Client-centered and experiential therapy: A paradigm in motion*. Vienna: Lang.

Bohart, A., & Greenberg, L. S. (Eds.). (1997). *Empathy reconsidered: New directions in psychotherapy*. Washington, DC: APA Books.

Bohart, A., & Tallman, K. (1997). Empathy and the active client: An integrative cognitive–experiential approach. In A. Bohart & L. Greenberg (Eds.), *Empathy reconsidered: New directions in psychotherapy*. Washington, DC: APA Books.

Bozarth, J. (1990). The essence of person-centered therapy. In G. Lietaer, J. Rombauts, & R. Van Balen (Eds.), *Client-centered and experiential psychotherapy in the nineties*. Leuven, Belgium: Leuven University Press.

Bozarth, J. (1997). Empathy from the framework of client-centered theory and the Rogerian hypothesis. In A. Bohart & L. Greenberg (Eds.), *Empathy reconsidered: New directions in psychotherapy*. Washington, DC: APA Books.

Brodley, B. (1990). Client-centered and experiential: Two different therapies. In G. Lietaer, J. Rombauts, & R. Van Balen (Eds.), *Client-centered and experiential psychotherapy in the nineties*. Leuven, Belgium: Leuven University Press.

Elliott, R., Filipovick, H., Hargack, L., Gaynor, J., Renischiessel, C., & Zapaolka, J. K. (1982). Measuring response empathy: The development of a multicomponent rating scale. *Journal of Counseling Psychology, 29,* 379–387.

Elliott, R. (1985). Helpful and non-helpful events in brief counseling interviews. An empirical taxonomy. *Journal of Counseling Psychology, 32*(3), 307–322.

Elliott, R. (1990). The impact of experiential therapy on depression. The first ten cases. In G. Lietaer, J. Rombauts, & R. Van Balen (Eds.), *Client-centered and experiential psychotherapy in the nineties*. Leuven, Belgium: Leuven University Press.

Gendlin, E. T. (1974). Client-centered and experiential psychotherapy. In D. Wexler & L. N. Rice (Eds.), *Innovations in client-centered therapy*. New York: Wiley.

Gendlin, E. T. (1981). *Focusing*. New York: Bantam.

Gendlin, E. T. (1996). *Focusing-oriented psychotherapy: A manual of the experiential method*. New York: Guilford Press.

Greenberg, L. S., & Elliott, R. (1997). Varieties of empathic responding. In A. Bohart & L. Greenberg (Eds.), *Empathy reconsidered: New directions in psychotherapy*. Washiington, DC: APA Books.

Greenberg, L. S., Rice, L. N. & Elliott, R. (1993). *Facilitating emotional change: The moment-by-moment process*. New York: Guilford Press.

Greenberg, L. S., & Safran, J. D. (1987). *Emotion in psychotherapy: Affect, cognition and the process of change*. New York: Guilford Press.

Henry, W. P., Schacht, T. E., & Strupp, H. H. (1986). Structural analysis of social behaviour: Application to a study of interpersonal process in differential psychotherapeutic outcome. *Journal of Consulting and Clinical Psychology, 54,* 27–31.

Horvath, A. O., & Greenberg, L. S. (1994). *The working alliance: Theory, research, and practice*. New York: Wiley.

Keil, W. (1996). Hermeneutic empathy in client-centered therapy. In U. Esser, H. Pabst, & G. Speierer (Eds.), *The power of the person-centered approach: New challenges, perspectives, answers*. Köln: GwG.

Kennedy-Moore, E., & Watson, J. C. (in press). *Emotional expression*. New York: Guilford Press.

King, J. L., Mallinckrodt, B., & Coble, H. (1996). Family dysfunction, emotional awareness, and client attachment to therapist. In D. M. Kivlighan, Jr., & B. Mallinckrodt (Chairs), *Interpersonal problems in the psychotherapy relationship: Manifestation, resolution, and outcome*. Symposium conducted at the annual meeting of the American Psychological Association, Toronto, Ontario, Canada.

Klein, M. H., Mathieu-Coughlan, P., & Kiesler, D. J. (1986). The experiencing scales. In L. S. Greenberg & W. M. Pinsof (Eds.), *The psychotherapeutic process: A research handbook.* New York: Guilford Press.

Lane, & Schwartz (1987). Levels of emotional awareness: A cognitive–developmental theory and its application to psychopathology. *American Journal of Psychiatry, 144*(3), 133–143.

Lietaer, G. (1990). The client-centered approach after the Wisconsin Project: A personal view on its evolution. In G. Lietaer, J. Rombauts, & R. Van Balen (Eds.), *Client-centered and experiential psychotherapy in the nineties.* Leuven, Belgium: Leuven University Press.

Lietaer, G. (1992). Helping and hindering processes in client-centered/experiential psychotherapy: A content analysis of client and therapist post-session perceptions. In S. Toukmanian & D. Rennie (Eds.), *Psychotherapy process research: Paradigmatic and narrative approaches.* Newbury Park, CA: Sage.

Lietaer, G. (1993). Authenticity, congruence, and transparency. In D. Brazier (Ed.), *Beyond Carl Rogers: Towards a psychotherapy for the twenty-first century.* London: Constable.

Linehan, M. (1997). Empathy in cognitive-behavioural therapy. In A. Bohart & L. S. Greenberg (Eds.), *Empathy reconsidered: New directions in psychotherapy.* Washington, DC: APA Books.

Meador, B., & Rogers, C. (1979). Person-centered therapy. In R. Corsini (Ed.), *Current psychotherapies.* Itasca, IL: Peacock.

Neville, B. (1995). Five kinds of empathy. In R. Hutterer, G. Pawlowsky, P. Schmid, & R. Stipsits (Eds.), *Client-centered and experiential therapy: A paradigm in motion.* Vienna: Lang.

Rhodes, R., Hill, C., Thompson, B. J., & Elliott, R. (1994). Client retrospective recall of resolved and unresolved misunderstanding events. *Journal of Counseling Psychology, 41,* 473–483.

Rice, L. N. (1974).The evocative function of the therapist. In D. Wexler & L. N. Rice (Eds.), *Innovations in clients-centered therapy.* New York: Wiley.

Rice, L. N., Koke, C., Greenberg, L. S., & Wagstaff, A. (1979). *Manual for client vocal quality,* vol. 1. Toronto: Counseling and Development Centre, York University, North York, Ontario, Canada.

Rogers, C. R. (1951). The necessary and sufficient conditions of therapeutic personality change. *Journal of Consulting Psychology, 21,* 97–103.

Rogers, C. R. (1959). A theory of therapy, personality, and interpersonal relationships, as developed in the client-centered framework. In S. Koch (Ed.). *Psychology: A study of science.* New York: McGraw-Hill.

Rogers, C. R. (1961). *On becoming a person.* Boston: Houghton Mifflin.

Rogers, C. R. (1965). *Client-centered therapy: Its current practice, implications, and theory.* Boston: Houghton Mifflin.

Rogers, C. R. (1975). Empathic: An unappreciated way of being. *The Counseling Psychologist, 5*(2), 2–10.

Safran, J. D., Muran, C., & Samistag, P. (1994). Resolving therapeutic alliance ruptures: A task-analytic investigation. In A. O. Horvath & L. S. Greenberg (Eds.), *The working alliance: Theory, research, and practice.* New York: Wiley.

Taylor, C. (1990). *Human agency and language.* New York: Cambridge University Press.

Thorne, B. (1992). *Carl Rogers.* Newbury Park, CA: Sage.

Toukmanian, S. (1990). A schema-based information processing perspective on client change in experiential therapy. In G. Lietaer, J. Rombauts, & R. Van Balen. (Eds.), *Client-centered and experiential psychotherapy in the nineties.* Leuven, Belgium: Leuven University Press.

Toukmanian, S. (1992). Studying the clients' perceptual processes and their outcomes in psychotherapy. In S. Toukmanian & D. Rennie (Eds.), *Psychotherapy process research: Paradigmatic and narrative approaches.* Newbury Park, CA: Sage.

Truax, C. (1961). A scale for the measurement of accurate empathy. Psychiatric Institute Bulletin (Wisconsin), *1,* 12.

Vanaerschot, G. (1990). The process of empathy: Holding and letting go. In G. Lietaer, J. Rombauts, & R. Van Balen (Eds.), *Client-centered and experiential psychotherapy in the nineties.* Leuven, Belgium: Leuven University Press.

Vanaerschot, G. (1993). Empathy as releasing several microprocesses in the client. In D. Brazier (Ed.), *Beyond Carl Rogers: Towards a psychotherapy for the twenty-first century.* London: Constable.

Vanaerschot, G. (1997). Empathic resonance as a source of experience-enhancing interventions. In A. Bohart & L. Greenberg (Eds.), *Empathy reconsidered: New directions in psychotherapy.* Washington, DC: APA Books.

Watson, J. C. (1996). An examination of clients' cognitive-affective processes during the exploration of problematic reactions. *Journal of Consulting and Clinical Psychology, 63,* 459–464.

Watson, J. C., & Greenberg, L. S. (1994). The alliance in experiential therapy: Enacting the relationship conditions. In A. Horvath & L. Greenberg (Eds.), *The working alliance: Theory, research and practice.* New York: Wiley

Watson, J. C., & Greenberg, L. S. (1995). Alliance ruptures and repairs in experiential therapy. *In Session: Psychotherapy in Practice, 1*(1), 19–32.

Watson, J. C., & Greenberg, L. S. (1996). Emotion and cognition in experiential therapy: A dialectical–constructionist perspective. In H. Rosen & K. Kuelwein (Eds.), *Constructing realities: Meaning-making perspectives for psychotherapists.* San Francisco: Jossey-Bass.

Watson, J. C., & Greenberg, L. S. (1998). The therapeutic alliance in experiential psychotherapy. In J. D. Safran & S. Muran (Eds.), *The therapeutic alliance in brief psychotherapy.* Washington, DC: APA Books.

Watson, J. C., & Rennie, D. (1994). A qualitative analysis of clients' reports of their subjective experience while exploring problematic reactions in therapy. *Journal of Counseling Psychology, 41,* 500-509.

Weeresekera, P., Linder, B., Greenberg, L. S., & Watson, J. C. (1998). Manuscript in preparation.

# 4

✳✳✳✳✳

# Dialogic Gestalt Therapy

## Gary Yontef

*There has been a growing* trend in the last two decades for state-of-the-art practice of Gestalt therapy to be guided by a more explicated and consistent understanding of three cornerstones of its integrated theoretical framework: field theory, phenomenology, and dialogue. Field theory provides a way of thinking, phenomenology offers a way of defining and working with awareness, and dialogue delineates the necessary relationship between therapist and patient. Together they form the foundation of the whole that is Gestalt therapy.

This trend returns to and enhances the basic principles of Gestalt therapy and moves away from the "California model" that popularized Gestalt therapy from the mid-1960s through the mid-1970s. From the first Gestalt therapy publication, *Ego, Hunger and Aggression* (Perls, 1942/1992), there has been a serious intent to create a system of theory and practice that melds creative use of active phenomenological techniques with a therapeutic relationship based on the model of existential dialogue and that moves from a static perspective of history and structure to one that centers on here-and-now process.

The widespread attention received in the popularization phase by dramatic, cathartic, effective techniques, anti-intellectualism, and interpersonal confrontation diverted attention from more solid Gestalt therapy practice and overshadowed the theoretical basis of Gestalt therapy (Yontef, 1995). Solid practice and theory of Gestalt therapy was not only concerned with techniques but more importantly with relationship; not only focused on here-and-now process but also studied individual structure (e.g., diagnosis) and history; not only the individual but also the social/cultural context; not only focused on feelings but also on cognitive processes and philosophy (Perls, Hefferline, & Goodman, 1951/1994; Yontef, 1993, 1995). This illustrates a principle of Gestalt field theory: integration of polarities. In Gestalt therapy field theory dichotomies are considered artificial dualisms that are based on partial understanding. A more holistic understanding is sought in which the dualisms are unified into natural polarities, for example, yin and yang (Perls, 1942/1992).

State-of-the-art practice of Gestalt therapy has been guided by the cornerstone principles discussed above. Knowledge gleaned from this practice has led not only to clarification and refinement of the principles and their application but an integration of the principles with each other. Experience has led to an increasing emphasis on the importance of the therapist understanding, respecting, and orienting to what the patient actually experiences. This is a form of intimate contact and requires a softer, more accepting, more peaceful way of relating than encounter-group-like confrontation. In the balance between clinical frustration and support, support is now considered more important and necessary than was previously believed (Yontef, 1997a, 1997b).

Gestalt therapy has been associated with a focus on process as it unfolds one moment at a time, especially micro-focusing on the observed behavior and emotions of the patient at each moment, making interventions that actively focus and intensify awareness and behavior and often lead to cathartic release. The empty-chair and the two-chair experiments, sometimes combined with nonverbal expression of affect, were probably the best known of such techniques. But the list of experiments of active focusing that are used in Gestalt therapy is infinite. A patient biting her or his lip might be asked to bite harder or say something biting. A patient saying everything is fine and tapping fingers might be asked to tap harder, sometimes leading to pounding gestures that bring previously underground resentment into awareness and expression.

But the experiments are means of phenomenological exploration and not attempts at cathartic release or behavioral training (Yontef, 1995). Not only are a very wide variety of interventions used, but therapists are invited to be creative about finding or creating other techniques that apply the principles and fit the moment. Gestalt therapy has been called "permission to be creative" (Zinker, 1977, p. 3ff).

For example, an experiment was created in working with Amy, a 35-year-old woman who frequently focuses on her difficulty in establishing intimate contact with men but has no idea what she does that interrupts connection. In sessions she looks away whenever there is excitement or increased intensity of contact between us or between her and other group members. Focusing here and now on her averting her eyes is an experiment that helps her experience what she does out of the consulting room much more effectively than abstract discussion.

## CONCEPTIONS AND MISCONCEPTIONS

One style of Gestalt therapy, incorrectly identified by some as the essence of Gestalt therapy, is limited to what is immediately observable and the recognized context narrowed to only include the immediate therapeutic moment. In this approach to Gestalt therapy, attention to structure—what in field theoretical terms is considered to be repetitive processes, or to what phenomenologists refer to as invariants—was eschewed in favor of living in the here and now (based on the Principle of Contemporaneity; Lewin, 1936, 1951). This involved relating to the individual at each unique moment. A corollary of this style seems to be an attitude that a therapist's understanding does not have to include considerations of diagnosis, history, personality type, and culture.

Inferring Gestalt therapy theory and methodology from observations of demonstrations of the California model, rather than investigating the ordinary practice or theory of Gestalt therapy, led many to erroneously assume that the essence of Gestalt therapy is "Gestalt therapy techniques" and that catharsis and breaking down defenses were the aim of the techniques. Unfortunately, when cliches such as "there is nothing but the here and now" were loosely bandied about, or techniques were demonstrated without theoretical explication, practitioners were left with a misleading impression of naïveté, of simplistic contemporaneity, and the understanding that techniques could be responsibly or effectively used without considerations of relationship and overall methodology and philosophy. At the level of practice, good Gestalt therapists have always centered on what the clinical situation called for and have not adhered to this simplistic view.

Gestalt therapy theory is actually more inclusive, flexible, and clinically astute than its myth and very supportive of creative variation from dogma. The conception of the now is part of complex issues of time and space in field theory and phenomenology, which is far from simplistic or naive (Yontef, 1993). This has been more clearly explicated in the last decade and a half.

For example, it is now clearly held that contemporaneous awareness can support any awareness, even if not physically observed in the room by the therapist at a moment in a session, and that the background can be as broad as the sophistication of the therapist and the patient allows. The exploratory lens alternates between a narrow micro-focus and a wide focus as clinically needed. Although the act of experiencing takes place contemporaneously, the reference of the experience can be past, present, or future—in the room or anywhere in the universe. The perceived "now" can be as narrow as a fraction of a second or as wide as a lifetime. The focus and the width of what is currently perceived of as "now" changes with each moment. It is also true that there are repetitions or invariants, for instance, character structure, that must be included in an insightful awareness of contemporaneous functioning or effective or safe practice of psychotherapy.

The therapist must be present-centered with the patient, but his or her map must be broader than a moment. Larger gestalten are essential to here-and-now work, just as the conception of the larger picture must be validated or invalidated in the phenomenological micro-focused work of the moment. The long-term needs of the patient may well develop from supporting what emerges at each moment as advocated by Gestalt therapy theory, but how this is done in terms of relationship, technique, and focus must vary according to personality pattern, strengths, weaknesses, and so forth, and this is often not clear enough without consulting an understanding of larger gestalten to make sense out of what is happening in the therapy hour.

## Example 1: Bob

In this example, simple attention by Bob to his present experience allowed a meaningful story to evolve and a relationship to develop, gradually broadening his present experience by including awareness of previously unaware affect and processes of avoidance.

Bob, a well-dressed, middle-aged man, was referred by his wife's therapist because "he needs something for himself." He had been a solid and reliable support while his wife was going through the aftermath of her mother's death and her own successful recovery from cancer. A very articulate professional man, he told his wife's story very clearly. However, questions such as "What are you experiencing right now?" were answered only with talk about aspects of his wife's travail without giving any attention to his own feelings. My noting this lack of naming any of his own feelings was shrugged off. He did confirm that he subjectively felt the tension I observed (fidgeting, compression in his fingers, tight breathing, a voice that was huskier than his natural voice).

In his second session I continued to share my understanding of what Bob was experiencing (empathic attunement), asked about his actual experience, and disclosed my observations. His spontaneous stream of consciousness provided sufficient emotional focus that I did not suggest any active focusing experiments other than asking what he felt at the moment. During that session he came to realize and acknowledge that he knew his thoughts but was usually out of touch with his feelings. In the third session tears showed in his eyes as he talked of his sleepless nights caring for his wife, how he loved her, and the pain he felt when he recognized her pain. I was touched, which showed on my face, and while no explicit mention was made of this, he appeared to notice, and his experience of his own sorrow deepened. After he cried and wiped his eyes, I asked, "What do you experience now?" He said he felt relieved and noticed his tension had left. For the first time in our work he was not fidgeting, his knuckles were not white, his voice was more natural.

While during most of the first three sessions Bob talked about his story, the point of phenomenological focus and maximal contact between us were the moments of here-and-now, present-centeredness. He felt his grief, he felt relief, he learned something about his awareness process, and was affected by our engagement—he was the center of someone's caring rather than his being the caretaker and problem solver.

## Example 2: Tom

In this example, the therapist's attention to a broader field was needed before the patient could begin either to tell his story or focus on his immediate affective experience. Later, here-and-now focusing led to intensive exploration of childhood abuse.

Tom was also a middle aged man referred by his wife's therapist. While a straightforward here-and-now focus on affect and armoring worked well with Bob, the same was not true of Tom. Bob was oversocialized, talked of the important events in his life, functioned well in his career, had a satisfying and stable marriage, and showed no signs of serious character pathology. Tom, on the other hand, chatted amiably about psychological processes in his life, but without meaningful focus on either story or here-and-now process. Gentle efforts to clarify story, current experience, or what he wanted from therapy were not successful in the first session. He canceled his second appointment at the last minute. I wondered about alcohol or drug abuse. Subsequent interactions with the patient and the referring therapist revealed that Tom was an alcoholic whose wife considered him abusive and threatened divorce if he did not get therapy.

Good therapy with Tom required some awareness by the therapist of events outside the therapy hour that Tom avoided bringing into the hour. This started with working on his resentment about being pressured into therapy and his denial of there being any problem. Work eventually included extensive work on his background of being abused as a child by an alcoholic father. While the work was experiential, the background of his life had to be carefully explored. As this background was discussed, the patient began to recognize the depth of his emotional baggage from his childhood. Real progress started when he connected his immediate experience in the therapy hour, especially his reaction to the therapist, with his emotional history.

## Summary

While current Gestalt therapy practice focuses on what is being experienced here and now, it is also guided by understanding historical and characterological background factors. These background factors help organize the current field. It is the relationship of what is in immediate awareness and these background factors that makes meaning of what is happening in the therapy hour. This relationship of figure and ground is the gestalt that illuminates what therapy with this person requires, the patient's needs and strengths, what sequencing and timing is optimal for maximum effect with this patient, also enabling the therapist to be aware of particular dangers in therapy with this specific patient. Thus experience at one time and place is made meaningful by the context of background experience, that is, repetitive, ongoing experiences and patterns occurring in the world prior to and outside of the consulting hour. This is illustrated by work with Margaret, in Example 3, below.

Full awareness—and a therapeutic methodology to reach that capacity—requires a blend of the fluidity of here-and-now process (fast-moving process) and the predictability of invariant structure (slow-moving process). In the fluidity of narrow focusing in the present, both the felt experience of the patient and the structural aspects are clarified. On the other hand, present experience is clarified by the information about structure/invariants that funnels into present-centered exploration. It is only when the therapist integrates this information that intensive experiential work can be safe, sophisticated, relevant, and effective.

## CONTACT AND THE DIALOGIC RELATIONSHIP

The first goal in dialogic Gestalt therapy is to "meet" the patient existentially, to "start where the patient is" and then make contact on as empathic a basis as circumstances allow. From that point all purposes and design are jointly constructed by patient and therapist. The therapist's prime directive is to contact the patient rather than "fix" or move the patient.

Contact, a crucial concept in Gestalt therapy, refers to "what one is in touch with." Interpersonal contact is seen as being in contact with self and other. Contact is one of the characteristics of awareness; that is, one cannot be aware without being in contact with something. However, contact can occur without awareness, for example, worrying about something without being aware that one is doing so. Another example: a person making a vehement defense of the righteousness of his behavior may actually be in touch with shame and guilt without being fully conscious of it. In this case the emotional energy of the shame and guilt is not allowed to become figural, hence it is relegated to background status. In such a situation the person does not sense or feel the shame and guilt in focal awareness, but nevertheless the shame and guilt energize the behavior. The person is in contact with shame and guilt and aware of something else. In Gestalt therapy these contact and awareness process are explored phenomenologically—the therapist does not tell the patient what he or she "really feels" (interpretation).

Dialogue is a special form of contact in which people are in touch with each other and share what they experience *without aiming for an outcome*, each appreciating the other as a separate source of experience and worthiness, both saying what they mean and meaning what they say. In dialogic contact the meeting is not an instrumental action done in order to reach some other goal, but rather contact with the other person is an end in and of itself. In a dialogic relationship this contact continues over time.

Much is said in modern Gestalt therapy about dialogue being the basis of good therapy (Hycner, 1985; Hycner & Jacobs, 1995; Jacobs, 1989; Yontef, 1993) and training/supervision (Yontef, 1997a, 1997b). It is recognized that "dialogue" in therapy is a modification of the fully mutual "I–Thou" referred to by Martin Buber. In therapy the attitude is retained, but the dialogue is modified to honor the task and context of therapy.

Dialogue in therapy has the following characteristics:

1. *Inclusion.* The therapist simultaneously swings as fully as possible into an approximation of what the patient experiences while maintaining his/her own experience. This brings together fully sensing the patient's phenomenology as if one were the patient while maintaining full awareness of self as a different person who cannot feel exactly what the other feels.

2. *Confirmation.* In practicing inclusion the therapist makes the patient's existential existence real by imagining it, making it a shared experience. This confirms the patient by accepting both what is and what could be (potential for growth).

3. *Presence of therapist.* The dialogic therapist relates to the patient with open, authentic, and disclosing presence—with discrimination about context, the demands of the therapy situation, the patient's strength and state, and ethical limitations. In my opinion, inclusion, confirmation, and presence work in the therapeutic relationship only when the therapist feels and shows genuine warmth, tenderness, kindness, respect, and caring.

4. *Commitment to dialogue.* The dialogic therapist surrenders to what emerges between the patient and therapist and to the process of the dialectical formation of new wholes. This differs from the therapist moving the patient to some vision of health and is antithetical to the nonhorizontal viewpoint of only the patient changing and the therapist staying the same. In good dialogic therapy, the therapist's own phenomenology is influenced and changed by the interaction. This is especially important when there is disagreement between therapist and patient, for example, when the patient is critical of or disappointed with the therapist.

## THE PARADOXICAL THEORY OF CHANGE: AWARENESS THROUGH DIALOGUE

The paradox of the paradoxical theory of change is that the more one tries to be who one is not, the more one stays the same (Beisser, 1970). Healing is making whole; trying to be who one is not sets up internal conflict and not wholeness. Real growth is knowing and identifying with one's self. The more one claims who one is, the more one can grow; on the other hand, the more one disclaims change and tries to stay the same, the less one grows—and even withers and declines as the world around changes. People are not static but always in transition. At each moment a new figure is always emerging. People grow by identifying with this emerging figure.

The paradoxical theory of change presents the answer to an apparent dilemma: How can therapy be dialogic? Therapy is supposed to help patients improve in some way. Does this not mean moving toward a goal? Goals are something to aim for, but a dialogic relationship is defined as not aiming. Can therapy proceed without goals? How can therapy be dialogic?

The development of a sense of self as being worthy of love and respect, a sense of self that is cohesive, accurate, and self-accepting, is developed in interaction from early childhood on. It is not developed internally separate from the relational events that support and define the self (Perls et al., 1951/ 1994). In Gestalt therapy theory, the sense of self is relational. There is no "I," no person, no sense of self, isolated from the interhuman environment. When a child's emerging figures are met by disinterest or attack, a shame system rather than one of identifying with self is likely (Yontef, 1993, 1996; Lee & Wheeler, 1996).

The Gestalt therapy attitude is that an accurate and loving sense of self can be developed in psychotherapy and that this depends on the quality of contact and relationship and also the potency and pertinence of the awareness work. The dialogic relationship provides the matrix of a relationship with someone who is respected and that accurately understands, respects, and cares about the patient. Nonverbal factors such as tone of voice, intonation, and demeanor are very powerful in this regard. When the factors of relationship and technique are synchronized, phenomenological awareness work enables a person to have and identify with an accurate sense of self and others.

The phenomenological attitude supports self-identification by accepting the validity of the patient's subjective experience. Clarification of self and other, identification with self, and acceptance of other is supported in Gestalt therapy by the phenomenological method and dialogic relating. The therapist guides the patient's work on focused awareness and shares his/her own phenomenological perspectives. The sharing of phenomenological perspectives is a workable definition of dialogue.

The paradoxical theory of change provides a means of doing therapy while not aiming. This attitude of awareness through dialogue and phenomenological focusing and experimentation replaces the aim of changing the person as the main therapeutic orientation and does away with theory-derived interpretation as a main technique. The dialogic therapist operates by receiving the other's experience respectfully, trying to experience the world as the other experiences it (as closely as possible while still knowing one's autonomous experience), accepting the other's experience as equally valid to one's own, and allowing a mutually influenced change in both points of view to emerge.

It is especially important for the therapist to understand and live out phenomenological and dialogic principles when the patient has a different experience of the therapist than the therapist has of self. A true acceptance of the validity of both phenomenological perspectives enables the experience of both parties to be deepened and widened through the phenomenological exploration.

The Gestalt therapy orientation is to be more fully in touch with the present, including personal awareness and good interpersonal contact. Rather than aiming to be different, to manipulate oneself to reach a content goal, one grows to be different by identifying first with present reality and then with emerging possibilities. This process orientation is quite consistent with principles of dialogue, phenomenology, and field theory.

Gestalt therapy supports jointly constructed process goals. For example, the therapy is oriented toward staying in contact with the here-and-now process of figure formation, that is, what is important to the patient at each continuing moment. This includes learning to use this process to explore any aspect of life—whether problematic, a matter of positive expansion, or just an object of curiosity. Our experience has been that this leads to deeper emotional connections, insight, and healing.

Meeting the patient where the patient is and helping the patient be in touch with self and other in a manner consistent with the paradoxical theory of change replaces any therapist constructed end goal. Gestalt therapists dialogue about the patient's feelings, desires, aspirations, values, and situation. The effective therapist contributes a knowledge of how to proceed in sequential steps that do not exceed the patient's external or self-support and that take into account the structure of the patient's personality as well as personal and cultural values. This means helping the patient identify both with what *is* and with what is *emerging*, so that the patient can grow without disclaiming or artificially pushing him-/herself.

It should be noted that dialogue is a guide for Gestalt therapists and it is not our goal to convince the patient to believe in or behave according to dialogic principles. To aim to move the patient to be dialogic would be a violation of phenomenological and dialogic principles. Therefore, we do not believe that the patient ought to practice dialogue—but it is a possibility. When the patient experiences the therapist's dialogic relating and builds support through the relationship and phenomenological experimentation, the patient may move toward being more dialogic. This is a happy outcome, but not one the therapist aims for as such.

## THE PHENOMENOLOGICAL METHOD

Phenomenology is a discipline guiding people to stand aside from their usual way of thinking so they can distinguish between what is actually being experienced (perceived and felt) in the current situation and what is residue from the past (Ihde, 1977; Spinelli, 1989). A Gestalt exploration seeks "naive" perception "undebauched by learning" (Wertheimer, 1945, p. 331). The discipline includes methods for discriminating between actual experience and experience clouded by preconceptions, assumptions, and filters of what reality is (Ihde, 1977). Data includes what is "subjectively" felt as well as what is "objectively" observed. Actual experience is a phenomenological reality and not a surface manifestation of some other, "real" meaning that can be found through the therapist's interpretation.

This phenomenological discipline of here-and-now exploration is a foundation of most existential thought; and sharing present experience is an indispensable component of an existential dialogue. In fact dialogue could be defined as shared phenomenology. A therapy that is truly experiential or dialogic must emphasize, clarify, and enhance present experience.

Phenomenological discipline helps the willing patient and therapist move from unrefined subjective experience to a more refined experience. Phenomenological processes are the mainstay of inclusion, empathy, and affect attunement, all of which are essential to experiential therapy. The experience-near reflections that are the most common intervention and means of contact in experiential therapies are based on phenomenological assumptions.

Gestalt therapy extends this shared phenomenological and dialogic approach by teaching the patient how to focus and experiment phenomenologically. This proactive attitude is one potent way for the therapist to be active in dealing with character pathology while maintaining a dialogic and phenomenological attitude. A further extension is the use in sessions of direct, active experiments that are phenomenological in their intent, design, and execution.

This awareness work focuses on the continuum of the patient's awareness, and on interruptions of this awareness. What is the patient in contact with? What is not allowed into focal awareness? The therapeutic work in the phenomenological frame moves from straightforward awareness to awareness of awareness, and from this to insight (Yontef, 1993). Great emphasis is put on how the patient constructs his/her sense of reality, especially his/her sense of self. This gives an alternative to either attacking defenses or supporting defenses, that is, being aware of defenses. Experiments help clarify and separate variables. In time, this attitude and skill set become integrated into the patient's everyday functioning, that is, phenomenological ascent (Spinelli, 1989; Yontef, 1993).

To summarize, learning to grow by accepting who one is happens in a dialogic relationship. The phenomenological attitude supports dialogue, and it is through the dialogic relationship that the clinical phenomenological treatment occurs. In dialogic treatment two persons share their phenomenological perspective and work cooperatively in focusing, understanding, and experimenting with new behaviors and discovering experientially.

## INTEGRATING RELATIONSHIP AND TECHNIQUE

Some humanistic psychologists see using active techniques, such as "Gestalt therapy techniques," as inauthentic and manipulative and therefore inconsistent with a dialogic relationship. I believe this dichotomy to be spurious, naive, and unnecessary. Gestalt therapy envisions a relationship that includes but is not limited to empathic reflection and a vision of active methodology that is a cooperative effort at growing through experiential understanding. In this view the therapist does not relate by being an expert who can explain the real meaning behind the surface or by being a change agent who directly modifies patient behavior.

An authentic relationship emphasis can be integrated with an active methodology if the methodology is a phenomenological one. It is the thesis of Gestalt therapy that therapy which is the most effective and safe integrates a certain kind of relating to patients, i.e., dialogic, and a varied and active phenomenological methodology. Many modern experiential psychotherapies, including the Rogerian and the intersubjective self systems, have similar pictures of the therapeutic relationship. Practitioners of dialogic Gestalt therapy agree with these views that the most central aspect of psychotherapy is the relationship, but Gestalt therapists also believe that active focusing can not only make the therapy more effective but can also enhance the quality of the therapeutic relationship. Moreover, the relationship provides a supportive environment making the active experimentation safe for the patient, and it also directs the application of our knowledge and techniques.

Obviously there are a variety of active methodologies, with differing philosophies of therapy and differing stances on relationship. Techniques can be shared among the various methodologies, but the meaning, benefits, and dangers of the techniques are so different in different contexts that they are not equivalent. Using "Gestalt therapy techniques" in another framework may be useful for work in that framework, but it is not Gestalt therapy. Using behavior therapy techniques, say, desensitization, can be useful in Gestalt therapy, but it is not and should not be confused with systematic behavior modification.

For instance, an active methodology for therapeutic exploration can use body awareness in the service of systematic behavior modification, while it can be used in a phenomenological therapy such as Gestalt therapy in the service of understanding and growth that emerges out of the experimentation and therapeutic interaction and is not directed according to preset outcome goals. The latter is consistent with the principles of a therapeutic relationship according to existential dialogic principles; the former is not.

Gestalt therapy methodology includes focus on the unguided subjectivity of the patient, the guided subjectivity of the patient, the phenomenologically refined awareness of the patient, actively guided phenomenological experiments, and direct dialogue between therapist and patient. The patient receives reports of the Gestalt therapist's awareness (observations, affect, association from the therapist's history, feelings toward the patient, and so forth) and suggestions about new behaviors, for experimentation in or out of sessions.

The experiment involves a mentality of "try something new and see what you experience." A patient who races from thought to thought, feeling to feeling, getting agitated and anxious might be asked to experiment with putting a period after each sentence and taking a breath. A sexually inhibited patient might receive a suggestion of experimenting with just looking. The patient who splits complex thoughts/feelings into either/or dichotomies might be asked to experiment with combining "I love Joanne" *and* "I am scared to death of being with her" into one sentence.

## Example 3: Margaret

Margaret was a 35-year-old woman. In her first session she spoke rapidly, changed topics often. Multiple crises, each with life and death urgency, suddenly became her focus. Her manner and voice registered her sense of panic and urgency. She was having a fight with her neighbor, was angry with her boyfriend, was fighting with a department store over disputed charges, and had multiple medical complaints (headaches, tired, stomach pains) for which the physician could not find a clear cause. She had heard that I was a wonderful therapist, unlike her previous therapist. In response to questions about her immediate experience, she reported intense affect—chiefly panic and rage. Empathic reflections were acknowledged but seemed to have little effect. She was clear that she wanted a "magic pill," an instant solution from a master therapist, as if this was the only way she could imagine change.

It was clear to me that her process in the session was a micro-example of how she coped with life at the macro level. In each story she brought up, her behavior had the quality of her wanting to be rescued, avoiding rather than confronting difficulty, acting in panic, often making the situation progressively worse. In the work of the session, she did the same. If she was going to be able to do the work of regulating her life, we needed to interrupt this style in therapy sessions long enough for her to be aware of it and through directed focusing build up a reservoir of skills for improved self-regulation and coping with life problems. It was clear that while she very much needed a relationship with an empathic and accepting therapist who felt warmth or affection for her, she also needed an active teaching methodology as well.

As her speech was building up speed in the latter part of the first session, I said, "Try an experiment: Close your eyes, take three deep, slow breaths, with long exhales." As Margaret started the experiment, she closed her eyes and breathed rapidly, blowing out the air in a hyperventilating manner that did not release tensions. When she was finally able to do the breathing in the manner I was suggesting, she did slow down, breathing in a normal manner, and talking with less panic.

When she started to rev up again during the session, without contact with me, I looked at her and interrupted her monologue. "Try another experiment. Look right at me and go back to trying the slow breathing pattern." After I could feel some connection between us for the first time, I asked her what she experienced. "Right now I feel calmer and am glad to be here." Here the use of active experimentation aided the development of a contactful relationship—and my suggesting the experiments in a soft manner avoided the danger of the interruptions being perceived as antagonistic or combative. The centering activity introduced in the session would later become a tool she could use in her daily life.

That was our beginning. This kind of proactive, guided experiment that built self-support and supported good contact between us continued to be a frequent focus for several months. Her regular behavior in life out of the session helped clarify what needed to be done in the session; that is, she needed to learn how to regulate herself. Sometimes we focused on the moment in the hour; sometimes we focused on the events of the week both because she needed to do so and in order to gain understanding of the parallel processes that were going on in micro in the session and in macro in her regular life.

At the end of the first session, and once a second session was scheduled, Margaret asked what she should do about these multiple problems—again wanting to be rescued. I neither offered a suggestion to fix or solve the problems nor at the time did I directly interpret or confront this behavior. Instead I reflected to her that I guessed that she felt like she could not handle these problems herself, which she confirmed. I suggested she might like to learn and that we could do this in therapy. She nodded, as if this were a new thought. I suggested that for the moment she practice the centering activities we had been working with during the session as support for her finding the best solutions she could. Obviously, she still wanted and felt she needed more than that, which I acknowledged, but she could accept this answer for the moment. In large part this was due to my interacting at this point with firmness and clarity, but without giving her a verbal or nonverbal judgmental message.

Understanding borderline process helped me to react to Margaret in a way that would establish good contact and focus the awareness work in a sequence she could grow with. My picture of her ongoing process was clarified by her continued hypomanic buildup in reaction to simple empathic reflections, but also by her rapidly improved functioning in response to the more proactive, actively engaged, experimental interventions. Further clarification came from her expectation that she be rescued at the end of the session. Subsequent work confirmed that her self-interruption, failure to center herself, picturing herself as helpless, and expecting to be rescued was a regular part of her functioning. This changed in small but definite stages until the structure of her functioning was more self-supportive.

Therapy beyond that point focused on rather severe childhood intrusion and abandonment experiences that could be dealt with in a healing way now that her self-support had been improved and our relationship deepened. In her family any autonomy, independence, or competence resulted in attack and/or abandonment; the price of any semblance of nurturance was being merged with her mother as a pitiful, incompetent child. Before some therapeutic consolidation of self-processes, focusing on her intense, primitive affect and the historical experience creating it would have been more regressive than her self-support. At the beginning she did not have the ability to experience the regressive processes in the context of growth, healing, and insight but likely would have regressed into helplessness, being overwhelmed by affect, demanding rescue, with increasing crises between sessions. There would also have been a strong chance of suicidal despair or rageful acting out.

To summarize, learning to grow by accepting who one is happens in a dialogic relationship. The phenomenological attitude supports dialogue, and it is through the dialogic relationship that the clinical phenomenological treatment occurs. In dialogic treatment two persons share their phenomenological perspective and work cooperatively in focusing, understanding, experimenting with new behaviors and discovering experientially.

## Example 4: Nancy

This example illustrates the integration of many of the fundamentals of Gestalt therapy that we have been discussing.

Nancy is an attractive 30-year-old woman working on an advanced degree in counseling. Her presenting problem is relationships with men and low self-esteem. She wants love and commitment but only expects abandonment due to her self-perception of being inadequate, boring, loathsome, and unlovable. Her dating history has been with men lacking kindness toward women and fearful of intimacy and commitment.

From the beginning, Nancy reacted very positively to warmth and empathy in the therapeutic relationship but also constantly scanned for signs of the rejection, abandonment, and betrayal she expected from men. Early in the therapy I was 5 minutes late for her session. Her immediate thought was "Gary does not want to see me." She brought her reaction into the session for exploration. I told her that I guessed that while she was alone in the waiting room she felt anxious, a feeling of a great void, worried thinking filling the gap—and that it triggered old thoughts of hers that she was undesirable and other people only tolerate her as a burden. She nodded confirmation. I told her that I was really sorry, regretted being late and triggering all that, and that I actually looked forward to seeing her. She nodded and said that she had sensed that I liked her and she knew that she was being helped by me.

Finally, when the connection with her was reestablished following my being open, warm, and empathically attuned to her, and also telling her my feelings toward her, I told her that I had characterological difficulty with being on time. That disclosure of mine was the final step needed for her to engage in a deeper exploration of her assumption of rejection and abandonment, leading to work on her current and childhood experience with feeling that significant others thought of her as a burden. She did not need me to be without flaw, did not need more information about my difficulty, she only needed me to be honest, emotionally present, responsive, understanding, and accepting. Supportive, empathic interactions with me were almost always followed by Nancy's recovery of self-functions and a cohesive sense of self, a sense of self-acceptance, and a deeper self-exploration.

Here is the picture I had of her at the time:

Nancy gets so anxious about both the abandonment she believes is inevitable and possible future incidents of shame and humiliation that she goes into desperate panic. She is ashamed of her anxiety and panic, and of course the shame elicits increased anxiety. She is obviously narcissistically wounded and quite shame oriented. She carries with her a self-image that does not include her positive qualities, such as being bright, sensual, playful, vibrant, loving.

Nancy sees men as powerful, intrusive, and rejecting and herself as lost, lonely, scared, desperate, and empty. She dichotomizes confluence and isolation. As a result, when there is no contact, let alone confluence, she pictures herself alone forever—of course, due to her inadequacy. She tells herself that if a particular relationship does not work out, the situation is catastrophic and confirms her belief that no man will be interested in her since she is "fat, ugly, and unattractive." If "he" does not love me, I am unlovable, "I am a bother." Actual experience that men do find her interesting and attractive does not alter this sense of self.

When she is in a primary relationship, she needs the man to give her inner cohesion, safety, and to heal her feeling of shame and humiliation. When with a man who will not let her feel at all special, such as her current boyfriend (Joe), she asks, "What's wrong with me?" When he does not meet minimal wishes of hers, she believes it is because she wants too much. She has trouble picturing being both nurtured and competent. Nancy can tolerate being alone, and when she is not in a primary relationship she meets her contact needs with her friends. It is the rejection and abandonment by a man that she finds devastating. Her expectation of betrayal by men goes back to crushing disappointment and betrayal by her older brother and father (discussed below).

In a later session Nancy became aware of her shame, humiliation, and rage that was often retroflected against herself. Her boyfriend, Joe, had treated her badly and verbally attacked her without apparent cause or warning. She felt rageful, wanting to kick and hit him, to hurt him as she had been hurt. She also had a sensation of hurt in her stomach. I suggested she stay with a focus on the sensation without interpreting it. What emerged was her felt sense that the stomach pain was telling her not to act on the wish to hurt him.

I suggested that she imagine Joe was sitting in the empty chair and express her feelings to him either verbally or nonverbally. As is common with patients with a history of narcissistic injury and tendency toward global shame, Nancy had a very negative reaction to enactment techniques such as this. In Nancy's case, the reluctance does not seem related to an avoidance of the affect or insight that can come from such techniques. She brought significant issues/feelings to explore, and she was very responsive to focusing suggestions. She would do mental experiments, did get to real affects, talked with mobilized emotions, explored the background of current experiences, was able to do mental experiments to separate variables, and so forth. So we proceeded by phenomenological focusing without the empty chair.

The following picture emerged:

Joe demonstrates his longstanding avoidance of committed, intimate relationships by moving in and out of relationship with her. He attributes all problems in the relationship to her, including his distancing and exiting. Sometimes at tender moments he cruelly attacks her. He frequently does not follow through with promises and dates, without ever giving her warning, explaining, or apologizing. When he approaches her lovingly, he does not discuss or acknowledge his poor treatment of her. Inevitably he follows the loving connection by either distancing within the relationship or breaking off the relationship again.

In reaction, she feels shame, humiliation, hurt, grief, and rage. Being confluent with his negative judgment, she desperately clings, needing him to change so that her negative self-image is mollified. The relationship reinforces her life script of "knowing" that any man will leave or betray her.

She missed her next session, an unusual event for Nancy. When I saw her the following session, she said we had gotten too close, we had moved into her internal space. When she had thought between sessions about the previous hour and her experiment with giving up her retroflecting defenses, she feared that if she did not go along with my suggestions she would lose me—she was afraid that I would emotionally kill off our relationship.

As she realized that her experience was more important to me than any technique or program I offered, she stayed with herself, directing the anger outward, undoing the retroflection, sounding quite strong. Her therapeutic focusing was self-directed, and she did not emotionally lose me. She left feeling safer with me and stronger in the world.

This was an example of the textured interplay between relationship and technique, and between immediacy, past, and future.

Nancy continued to feel desperately alone and in need of maternal support to have a positive and cohesive sense of self. As a homework experiment I suggested she meditate on the sentence "Mommy and I are one." She was receptive to this focused awareness experiment, reporting next session some definite relief from this experiment—although also being aware of mourning the abandonment of her independent self by her mother.

The following material emerged from this:

Nancy was sexually molested by an older brother when she was 3 years old. Her father discovered this when she was four. His stern reaction did not feel emotionally supportive. His exhortation not to repeat the situation felt like blaming her for the event rather than lovingly supporting her right to say no. Her father's subsequent behavior was never as soft and loving as she had previously experienced it. At four she had been in the throes of Oedipal idealization of her daddy, and it felt like she had lost that "good daddy." In reaction to the chastisement he received and the loss of the sexual relations with Nancy, her brother became distant and unaffectionate. The intimate relationship with neither man was ever truly healed.

Her mother taught Nancy that her father was fragile, not to be counted on, easily stressed. Nancy's feelings were considered too much for men. Later her father developed a heart condition and Nancy was told that her emotionality would kill him.

Her mother was empathic, but only as long as they were confluent. With differentiation, her mother gave her a message that she was bad or selfish. Nancy became compliant with mother, repressed and retroflected her anger, and felt guilty when she did well. Her normal need for autonomy was balanced by a felt need for confluence with mother.

Nancy is caught in a bind between shame and guilt (Yontef, 1993, 1996). If she is independent (e.g., leaving the maternal orb), assertive (especially with brother or father), or sexual, she is bad. On the other hand, if she is dependent, accommodating, or not sexual, she feels shame and inadequacy. She has found it was easier to see herself as unattractive and inadequate than face the guilt of being independent of mother, assertive, vibrant, sexual, and cherished by a man.

Crushing disappointment and a tendency toward inflation or deflation are central issues for Nancy. She has a strong, primitive need for recognition, affection, and acceptance. She has needed a positive reaction from me to feel whole and OK with herself. But she does not need to be taken care of, takes responsibility for herself, in therapy does not pull for care beyond the therapeutic frame. In fact, sometimes she takes too much responsibility, blaming herself in self-shaming fashion for things that were not her doing. In therapy she needs a positive reaction from me to feel whole and OK and has a positive reaction to empathic interventions that do not ask her to do any "show and tell" experiments.

At first she projected her picture of powerful, intrusive, rejecting men onto me, and in reaction felt shame and envy. She was afraid I would be bored with her, judge her negatively, think her fat and ugly. She was afraid that I would make her vulnerable, and then the power would be mine: I could intrude, hurt her, leave her—at my will. There were obvious issues of safety, trust, and fear of betrayal. If I found her unattractive, it would confirm her self-view. If I found her attractive, she was afraid I would use her sexually.

On the other hand, she was also afraid that her emotions would be too much for me. Her mother's message that her anger might kill her father colored her contact with me. Nancy reports that father would "slap me with words," but mom said that father was fragile and that Nancy had to apologize for upsetting him. Anytime Nancy spoke up, her mother told her to go to her room and apologize, leaving Nancy feeling that she had to apologize to an abuser and that no one supported her. In her relationship with me she was afraid that merely bringing this up would result in her losing me emotionally.

After exploring this issue, she was late for her next appointment—unusual for her. She talked of being angry, but without focusing it in the room. I asked if she was angry with me. She said she was angry with me for exposing her shame and said she wanted to hide. She was even afraid that I would literally slap her—which had never occurred in either of our lives. She did maintain a sense that this would not occur literally, but the symbolism of it captured her fear of stinging rejection. She realized that she was projecting onto me the way father treated her when he verbally slapped her. At this session it was enough that she could stay in contact with me while sharing these feelings and associations, assimilating the material from the previous few sessions.

As therapy progressed, she came to trust and partially assimilate that I did not find her a bother, I was neither going to be turned off by her nor be sexual with her, that I was not betraying her, that perhaps she could be lovable.

She developed a more accurate appraisal both of her strengths and her contributions to relationship difficulties without being filled with shame. She developed a more accurate sense of her childhood and adult relationships. She broke up permanently with Joe and increased her ability to see potential difficulties early in dating relationships. She built a sense of confidence in herself, resuming creative activities that she had stopped long ago, and became more assertive and risk taking professionally. Part of the support for all of this was an ability to center herself when intense feelings arose, which included tools learned and practiced in the therapeutic relationship.

Work with Nancy illustrates the advantage of a dialogic relationship in which focused awareness experiments are used with discrimination, and in combining a narrow focus on the immediate with a wider focus on history and other background factors. Nancy grew in the context of a dialogic therapeutic relationship that used an experiential, directed, focused awareness methodology but without enactment techniques such as the empty chair.

Her here-and-now pattern of contact in therapy and in life clarified each other and developed in parallel. Exploration of the larger patterns of her life clarified what was happening immediately in sessions. The reverse was also true—that exploration of the immediate clarified her history and current functioning in the world.

## THE NEW MODEL OF GESTALT THERAPY

It is my experience that patients and trainees who worked in Gestalt therapy, training, or supervision in the late 1960s or the 1970s and then worked in or observed that framework again in the late 1980s and the 1990s have seen dramatic changes. Both the relationship and the quality of awareness have been much deeper and broader, change has been more profound, there have been fewer side effects such as narcissistic injury, and there has been a more consistent repair as breaches occur in the relationship. There has also been a much more differentiated approach to patients according to their personality style and character structure. Therapists report improved work with their own patients.

As the therapist is clear about what is happening, and also warm and accepting, patients react less to the therapist as an intruder, a threat, or someone who abandons them at critical moments. This has made patients feel safer and enabled them to engage more fully not only with the therapist but with others in groups, intimate relations, and the community. Equally important, patients and trainees have reacted less to the therapist or trainer as a charismatic figure whose power they can only vicariously experience through identification with the idealized figure but never claim for themselves, and more as a good person they can relate to horizontally. The capacity of patients to claim their choice, acknowledge alternatives, and take risks in terms of new behavior are better supported with this new attitude.

Ideally the therapist relates with firm and clear boundaries; focuses on how the patient behaves and what the patient experiences; acknowledges context; and admits his or her own flaws, weaknesses, fallibility, and mistakes. Any particular experiment is suggested as only one of many ways of exploring whatever is the object of study, and the patient's help in directing the work is invited. Patients are carefully trained to treat therapist statements about them as hypotheses that they can and should correct or disconfirm to the extent that they perceive them as inaccurate.

When patients interrupt, resist, and pull back from staying in contact with their own feelings, the modern approach is gently, insistently, and respectfully to make clear the interruption, and that the interruption has an important function that needs explication. The attitude and demeanor of the therapist is crucial. If it turns out that the therapist has a role in triggering the interruption, this too needs to be clearly acknowledged. The inadvertent triggering of an interruption may happen through the therapist posing a question in a manner encouraging speculation rather than description of actual experience, coldness or harshness of tone which might trigger shame, or by the therapist's failure to understand accurately the patient's experience (Yontef, 1995, 1996, 1997a, 1997b).

One of the regular activities in Gestalt therapy is to suggest and encourage the patient to try new behaviors as an experiment. This encourages patients to get data on their own reactions to new behaviors, how they go about it, what is experienced in the new behavior, what resistances come up, what unfinished business from earlier periods of life emerge from the background as a result of the new activity, and so forth. For example, in working with Amy, the woman mentioned earlier who wanted a relationship with a man and averted her eyes in the therapy sessions, I suggested an experiment of just looking at men.

New behavior in the session included "staying with" (maintaining focus on an experience that emerges as long as it continues to operate), mental/fantasy/imagination experiments, empty-chair and two-chair experiments, physical experiments (breathing changes, movement, expressive experiments, sensory focus, and so forth). "Staying with" is a direction or suggestion by the therapist when observing an emotion emerging into awareness and the patient is encouraged not to interrupt or interpret the feeling, to keep sensory and mental focus on the feeling, to allow the feeling to change, transform, complete itself without conscious intervention or direction by the patient. These can often be used in coordination with "homework" assignments.

## SUMMARY DISCUSSION

Focusing on processes emerging at each moment together with focusing on historical and repetitive characterological patterns form an integrated whole. When the here-and-now work is informed by the larger gestalten, it is safer and more effective. The knowledge of Margaret's borderline personality organization supported an interaction in which boundary skills were built and the dangers of treatment with borderline individuals avoided. Knowing Nancy's history of betrayal and abuse sharpened my emotional response to her. At the same time, observing and exploring her reaction in the therapeutic relationship clarified the sense of self she brought into her romantic relationships.

Working with tools of phenomenological experimentation is in polar integration with relating dialogically. The dialogic relationship is in itself a phenomenological experiment, one that makes it safe to do other work with focused awareness, to experiment, and to learn how to explore one's life experientially. The tools of phenomenological experimentation help clarify exactly what is happening in the therapeutic relationship, thus strengthening it. When Nancy started thinking and feeling that I did not want to see her, clarification required (1) my empathic response and disclosure of something about my feelings of caring and regret, and my characterological difficulty with being on time, and (2) narrow lens focusing on her continuum of awareness led to awareness of factors in her history that she was projecting onto me. This enabled her to restore her sense of being valued by me. Effective experiential therapy works with here-and-now process and with larger gestalten of history and characterological structure; and it works with a relationship focus as well as active, directed focusing of awareness.

## REFERENCES

Beisser, A. (1970). The paradoxical theory of change. In J. Fagan & I. Shepherd (Eds.), *Gestalt therapy now.* Palo Alto: Science and Behavior Books.

Hycner, R. (1985). Dialogical Gestalt therapy: An initial proposal. *The Gestalt Journal, 8*(1), 23–49.

Hycner, R., & Jacobs, L. M. (1995). *The healing relationship in Gestalt therapy: A dialogic/self psychology approach.* Highland, NY: Gestalt Journal Press.

Ihde, D. (1977). *Experimental phenomenology: An introduction.* Albany: State University of New York Press.

Jacobs, L. (1989). Dialogue in Gestalt theory and therapy. *The Gestalt Journal, 12*(1), 25–67.

Lee, E., & Wheeler, G. (Eds.). (1996). *The voice of shame: Silence and connection in psychotherapy.* San Francisco: Jossey-Bass.

Lewin, K. (1936). *Principles of topological psychology.* New York: McGraw-Hill.

Lewin, K. (1951). *Field theory in social science: Selected theoretical papers* (D. Cartwright, Ed.). New York: Harper.

Perls, F. S. (1992). *Ego, hunger and aggression.* Highland, NY: Gestalt Journal Press. (Original work published 1942, Durban, South Africa: Knox.)

Perls, F. S., Hefferline, R., & Goodman, P. (1994). *Gestalt therapy.* Highland, NY: Gestalt Journal Press. (Original work published 1951, New York: Dell.)

Spinelli, E. (1989). *The interpreted world.* Newbury Park, CA: Sage.

Wertheimer, M. (1945). *Productive thinking.* New York: Harper.

Yontef, G. (1993). *Awareness dialogue and process: Essays on Gestalt therapy.* Highland, NY: Gestalt Journal Press.

Yontef, G. (1995). Gestalt therapy. In A. S. Gurman & S. B. Messer (Eds.), *Essential psychotherapies: Theory and practice.* New York: Guilford Press.

Yontef, G. (1996). Shame and guilt in Gestalt therapy: Theory and Practice. In R. Lee & G. Wheeler (Eds.), *The voice of shame: Silence and connection in psychotherapy.* San Francisco: Jossey-Bass.

Yontef, G. (1997a). Relationship and sense of self in Gestalt therapy training. *The Gestalt Journal, 20*(1), 17–48.

Yontef, G. (1997b). Supervision from a Gestalt therapy perspective. In C. E. Watkins (Ed.), *Handbook of psychotherapy supervision.* New York: Wiley.

Zinker, J. (1977). *Creative process in Gestalt therapy.* New York: Brunner/Mazel.

# 5

*****

# Existential Processes

## Kirk J. Schneider

## THE TRADITIONAL EXISTENTIAL POSITION

The aim of existential therapy is to "set clients free" (May, 1981, p. 19). Freedom is understood as the capacity for choice within the natural and self-imposed limits of living (Schneider & May, 1995).

The freedom to do or to act is probably the clearest freedom that we possess; the freedom to be or to adopt attitudes toward situations is another less clear but even more fundamental freedom (May, 1981). Freedom to do is generally associated with external, physical decisions, whereas freedom to be is associated with internal, cognitive, and emotional stances. Within these freedoms we have a great capacity to create meaning in our lives—to conceptualize, imagine, invent, communicate, and physically and psychologically *enlarge* our worlds (Yalom, 1980). We also have the capacity to separate from others, to transcend our past, and to become distinct, unique, and heroic (Becker, 1973). Conversely, we can choose to restrain ourselves, to become passive, and to conform to others (May, 1981; Rank, 1936). We can choose to be *a part* of others or *apart* from others—*a part* of our possibilities or *apart* from our possibilities (Bugental, 1981).

Notwithstanding the possibilities there are great limitations on all these freedoms. We can only do and be so much. We can only expand and contract so far. Whatever we choose, moreover, implies a relinquishment of something else (Bugental, 1981). If I devote myself to scholarship, I relinquish athleticism. If I indulge in business affairs, I minimize spiritual pursuits. Moreover, every freedom has its price: if I stand out in a crowd, I become a larger target for criticism; if I acquire responsibility, I court guilt; if I isolate myself, I lose community; if I merge and fuse with others, I lose individuality; and so on (Becker, 1973; May, 1981). Finally, every freedom has its counterpart in destiny. May (1981) defines four kinds of destiny (or "givens" beyond our control): cosmic, genetic, cultural, and circumstantial. Cosmic destiny embraces the limitations of nature (e.g., earthquakes, climatic shifts); genetic destiny entails physiological dispositions (e.g., life span, temperament); cultural destiny addresses preconceived social patterns (e.g., language, birthrights); and circumstantial destiny pertains to sudden situational developments (e.g., oil spills, job layoffs). In short, our vast potentialities are matched by crushing vulnerabilities. We are semiaware, semicapable, in a world of dazzling perplexity.

How then, shall we deal with these clashing realities according to existential theorists; and what happens when we do not? Let us consider the latter first. The failure to acknowledge our freedom, according to existential theorists, results in the dysfunctional identification with limits, or repressed living (May, 1981). This dysfunctional identification forfeits the capacity to enliven, embolden, and enlarge one's perspective. The reticent wallflower, the pedantic bureaucrat, the paranoid reactionary, and the robotic conformist are illustrations of this polarity. The failure to acknowledge our limits, on the other hand, results in the sacrifice of our ability to discipline, discern, and prioritize life's chances (May, 1981). The aimless dabbler, the impulsive con man, the unbowed hedonist, and the power-hungry elitist exemplify this polarity.

The great question, of course, is how to help clients become emancipated from their polarized conditions, how to help them *integrate* freedom and limits? This question strikes at the heart of another existential problem—that of identity. Whereas reprogramming clients' behaviors, or helping them to understand the genesis of their concerns, leads to partially rejuvenated identities for existential theorists, *experiential* encounters with these concerns are the great underappreciated complements to the aforementioned change processes (Schneider & May, 1995). The experiential modality for existential theorists embraces four basic dimensions—the immediate, the kinesthetic, the affective, and the profound or cosmic (Schneider & May, 1995). The road to a fuller, more vital identity, in other words, is to help clients *embody* their underlying fears and anxieties, to help them attune, at the deepest levels, to the nature of those issues, and in so doing, to help them respond to, as opposed to react against, those issues. The net result, according to existential theorists, is an enhanced capacity for intimacy, meaning, and spiritual connection in one's life (Bugental, 1978; May, 1981).

The classic case of Mercedes, reported by Rollo May (1995), illustrates this standpoint. Mercedes lived much of her life in subordination to others. Her stepfather was a pimp and her mother a prostitute. Mercedes herself was coerced into prostitution to enable the family to subsist. Yet Mercedes bristled at her subservient position. She harbored tremendous resentment toward her "clientele" and even more toward her "caretakers." She was frequently depressed, impaired in her love life, and unable to carry her pregnancies with her husband to full term. Dr. May utilized many approaches to help Mercedes confront and integrate her rage (which in his view portended her freedom). These efforts, however, invariably failed to spark her, until one day when he encountered her experientially. Instead of encouraging *her* to acknowledge her resentment, however, *he* acknowledged it for her. *He* vented his fury on her stepfather; *he* unleashed his indignation toward her mother; and *he* embodied the bitterness she had harbored. In turn, Mercedes was finally able to affirm and express these qualities—directly and bodily—in herself. The upshot, according to Dr. May, is that Mercedes integrated her freedom: She quit prostitution, revived her marriage, and carried her pregnancy to term.

The experiential mode is diversely interpreted by existential theorists. For example, Yalom (1980) appears to stress the immediate and affective elements of his therapeutic contacts, but he refers little to kinesthetic components. Bugental (1987) stresses kinesthetic elements of his encounters but places lesser emphasis on interpersonal implications of those elements. Tillich (1952) and Friedman (1995) accent the interpersonal dimension of therapeutic experiencing but convey little about the kinesthetic aspect, and so on.

There are also differences among existential theorists regarding verbal and nonverbal channels of communication. May, Yalom, Tillich, and Friedman, for example, rely relatively heavily on verbal interventions, whereas Bugental (1987), Gendlin (1978), and Laing (1967) draw upon comparatively nonverbal forms of mediation.

Finally, there are differences among existential theorists with regard to philosophical implications of therapeutic experiencing. Although most existential theorists agree that clients need to confront the underlying givens (or ultimate concerns) of human existence during the course of a typical therapy, the nature and specificity of these givens varies. Whereas Yalom (1980), for example, focuses on the need for clients to experientially confront death, freedom, isolation, or meaninglessness, Bugental provides a more elaborate schema: the need for clients to confront embodiment–change, finitude–contingency, action–responsibility, choice–relinquishment, separation–apartness, or relation–being a part of (Bugental & Kleiner, 1993). And whereas May (1981) unites these positions with his notion of freedom and destiny (or limitation), as previously suggested, there is only a vague explication of this synthesis in his work.

## AN EXISTENTIAL–INTEGRATIVE MODEL AND EXPERIENTIAL LIBERATION

Existential therapy, as I view it, is an integrative therapy. Indeed, each of the conventional therapies, for example, pharmacological, behavioral, cognitive, analytic, and interpersonal, can be seen as liberation strategies within an overarching ontological or experiential context. But although each of the above strategies "liberate" clients at corresponding levels of consciousness,

I view the ontological or experiential domain as the most liberating context (see Schneider & May, 1995, pp. 136–137). In this chapter, my primary focus is on the experiential domain of therapeutic interaction. The clients for whom this chapter is primarily written, in other words, have the desire and capacity for immediate, kinesthetic, affective, and profound therapeutic change. For those readers interested in the full explication of this model, and the coordination of a diversity of approaches within this integrative framework, I refer you to Chapter 5 in *The Psychology of Existence* (Schneider & May, 1995).

## THE CONSTRICTIVE–EXPANSIVE CONTINUUM OF CONSCIOUSNESS

Within this existential–integrative framework, there are three phenomenologically based characteristics that help guide my work.[1] They are constriction, expansion, and centering. These characteristics guide my understanding of clients' freedom as well as limitation at each of the previously discussed levels and regions of consciousness. Put another way, constriction, expansion, and centering help me to understand functional and dysfunctional physiology, behavior, cognition, psychosexuality, social interaction, and experiential contact. They also help me to understand functional and dysfunctional encounters with death, isolation, meaning, change, contingency, responsibility, relinquishment, and separation/attachment (Schneider, 1990/1998).

Constriction, expansion, and centering are basic configurations of consciousness. The Chinese Taoists, for example, characterized consciousness in similar terms of yin and yang; Søren Kierkegaard used an analogous metaphor of inhalation and exhalation; William James, in his classic *Principles of Psychology* (1890/1950), seized upon the more scientific analogue of inhibition and excitation; and Gestaltists, finally, utilized the comparable metaphors of focal and peripheral awareness. For the purposes of this framework, constriction is understood as the perceived "drawing back" and confinement of thoughts, feelings, and sensations, whereas expansion is signified by the perceived "bursting forth" and extension of thoughts, feelings, and sensations. Constriction is characterized by a sense of retreating, diminishing, isolating, falling, emptying, or slowing; expansion is associated with a sense of gaining, enlarging, dispersing, ascending, filling, or accelerating. Centering, finally, is the capacity to be aware of and direct one's constrictive and expansive potentialities.

Constrictive and expansive awareness lie along a potentially infinite continuum. The term "potentially" here is a key one. I believe, with William James (1904/1987), that consciousness is perpetually surrounded by a "more" that it can but vaguely apprehend (p. 1173). The capacity to constrict or expand, therefore, is delimited. One may achieve provisional integration of the polarities, but probably not absolute or ultimate integration (Schneider, 1987, 1989, 1996).

Elaborating, then, only degrees of the capacity to constrict or expand are accessible to consciousness. Constrictive or expansive dream fantasies, for example, where victimization or, on the other hand, perpetration play a role may be *sub*conscious. At the furthermost horizons, constriction and expansion appear to be associated with the groundlessness of the infinitesimal and the infinite (see Grotstein, 1990). The further one constricts, in other words, the more one feels wiped away, obliterated. The further one expands, the more one perceives explosiveness, chaotic derangement (Laing, 1969). These polar eventualities, obliteration and chaos, smallness and greatness, contextualize a vast range of behaviors, symbols, and experiences (Schneider, 1990/1998, 1993; Schneider & May, 1995). When therapy clients are traumatized, for example, I often find obliterating smallness or chaotic greatness at the trauma's core. Rigid, demeaning family structures, for example, or repressive bosses, spouses, peer groups, and cultural contexts conjure up dissolution fears for many clients, whereas unpredictable and disorganized family structures or reckless, indulgent associates foster anarchy fears for other clients. There are also, of course, many genetic, economic, and ecological correlates of the above obliterating and chaotic scenarios.

My point here is that because of trauma (see Schneider, 1990/1998, and Schneider & May, 1995, for a discussion of its acute, chronic, and implicit forms), constriction and expansion, smallness and greatness, become associated with their furthermost expressions of dread—obliteration and chaos. In turn, these dreads set entire psychological dysfunctions into swing. The dread of constriction (obliteration), for example, appears to foster an equally extreme counterreaction to that dread, that of relentless expansion. The dread of expansion (chaos) tends to promote the equally extreme counterreaction of constriction. One will do everything one can, including becoming extreme oneself, to avoid the polarity that one dreads.

These "hyper" reactions, moreover, figure into the variety of defensive configurations commonly labeled psychopathologies. Depression, for example, is often a defense against the expansive risk taking or responsibility that proved unmanageable to one at some critical juncture; antisocial personality and narcissism are often defenses against some form of terrifying smallness or invalidation (Schneider & May, 1995, p. 143).

Stated in terms of the classic psychodynamic formulation, *drive–anxiety–defense*, this experiential model posits: *awareness of potential for obliteration or chaos–anxiety–defense* (compare with Yalom's schema, 1980, pp. 9–10).

The second tenet of this model is that the confrontation with or integration of one's constrictive (obliterating) or expansive (chaotic) dreads fosters vital, invigorating functioning. This functioning can also be described as maximally centered, fluid, and discerning. One who achieves such integration experiences a deeper sense of presence within oneself and toward others. There is at this juncture an enhanced ability to "occupy" the side of oneself that one formerly split off. There is an enhanced capacity to pause over this formerly estranged side of oneself and, as a result, to creatively respond to, as opposed to reflexively react against, constrictive or expansive possibilities. There is also a beneficial physiological component to such integration. This component has been variously termed "physiological resilience" and "hardiness" (Antonovsky, 1979; Kobasa, 1979).

As straightforward as this theoretical formulation may be, it is not until we examine the real-life circumstances under which it operates that we fully appreciate its relevance. Accordingly, let us consider the following case formulation to illustrate the above experiential model. To protect confidentiality, this case—which is a typical clinic or private practice case—is a composite drawn from my practice. Any similarity between this example and actual clientele is purely coincidental.

## EMMA: HYPERCONSTRICTION AND COMPLEXITY

Typically, there is a tenuous link between a client's initial presenting behavior and core (constrictive or expansive) dread. Generally, it takes months, even years, to unpack the layers of fears and defenses overlaying a client's core terror and basic defensive stance. This core condition, however, may suggest itself the moment that therapy begins. Such was the case with Emma, a dynamic and multifaceted woman.

Emma entered my office on a bright and cloudless day. She was of medium build, approximately 40 years old, and Caucasian.

Emma was charming. She was vibrant and articulate—and it was clear that she had "been around." She dressed with style, spoke in clear, firm tones, and got right to the point (as she understood it at the time). "There is something terribly wrong with my life," she declared. "I am at the end of my rope."

As I "sat" with this last statement and with Emma herself, I saw a person of solid conventional resources. She knew the societal "game" and how to play it. There was a hardness to her look and her makeup was formed by sharp and careful lines. It was clear that Emma—if she so desired it—had weight in the world.

There were, however, signs of strain beneath Emma's tough veneer. There was a fearfulness in her eyes and a melancholy about her face. Her otherwise resonant voice was interrupted by moments of urgency and breathlessness. It became increasingly evident to me that somewhere, deep in the recesses of her world, Emma was in turmoil.

When I invited Emma to elaborate on what was "wrong" in her life, this is what I discovered:

She derived from a family of four—her mother, father, and slightly younger brother. When Emma was 3 years old, her father deserted the family, never to be seen again. It was at this point that her paternal uncle, roughly the same age as her father, gradually began to replace his brother as "head of the household." Although Emma's mother was devastated by the desertion of her husband, in her weakened state she accepted and even encouraged the uncle's developing new role. The mother and uncle exchanged some romantic feelings, according to Emma, but this was short lived. Basically theirs was an arrangement of convenience, which everyone in the family grew to recognize.

Although Emma's memories of those early years were vague, by age four she knew something was askew. She felt like she experienced something with her uncle that no one else in the family had experienced and that to the degree they did experience it, they suppressed it. According to Emma, the uncle possessed a terrifying demeanor. He was very tall—well over 6 feet—of stocky build, and bullish. Her main memory of him at this early age was that of his booming voice and rancid breath.

Emma's memory clarified significantly as she recalled her late childhood (e.g., age nine) and early adolescence. In no uncertain terms, Emma conveyed that she had been brutalized by her uncle at these ages. She literally recalled him throwing his weight around with her—bellowing at her, pushing her, shoving her on her bed. She had a clear memory of him forcing a kiss on her and of being enraged when she rebuffed him. Although she did not recall being overtly sexually molested by her uncle, her dreams teemed with this motif and with many other sinister associations.

As I and others have found typical, Emma's reaction to these brutal scenarios was complex. The terms "helpless" or "hopeless" are too facile to describe this reaction. Indeed, virtually all words—from the ample lexicon of modern psychology—fail to address her layers of response. The closest she could come to describing her earliest feelings was a sense of paralysis. Beyond being an oppressor, her uncle acquired a kind of metaphysical status before Emma, and she, in turn, felt virtually microbial before him.

Yet Emma was no "shrinking violet." By adolescence, she became "wild," as she put it, displaying a completely new character. She became heavily involved in drugs, smoking, and seducing young men. She would leave home for days, periodically skip school, and associate with a variety of "bad boys." Speed (methamphetamine) and cocaine became her drugs of choice because they made her feel "wicked"—noticed, special, above the crowd. She didn't "take any shit," as she put it, and she occasionally exploded at people (usually males) if they got in her way. She even began raging at her uncle for brief periods, despite his continued dominance of her.

Emma's hyperexpansions, however, were short lived. They were blind, semiconscious, and reactive. Beneath them all, her world was collapsing—narrowing, spiraling back on itself. The clearest evidence of this was the essential vacuity of Emma's life. She concealed herself behind makeup and laughter. She felt ashamed around peers and classmates. While she was popular for a period, her substantive relationships were a shambles. The men she involved herself with would beat her. She, in turn, would lash back at them, but with woefully limited results.

Emma was condemned by her past. As desperately as she endeavored to escape that past, she chronically reentered it. She repeatedly sought out boys and men like her uncle, repeatedly hoped that something—perhaps she or some magic—could "save" (or redeem) them from being violent men like her uncle, and repeatedly felt let down by such men and fantasies.

In sum, Emma was traumatized by hyperexpansion. The godlike power of her uncle made Emma feel wormlike. He came to symbolize her world— perpetually alarmed, perpetually confined, perpetually depreciated. Emma found ways, albeit transient and semiconscious, to counter this wormlike position, but her basic and unresolved stance remained wormlike, permeated by dread.

Emma's chief polarization, therefore, clustered around hyperconstriction. Her secondary polarization clustered around hyperexpansion and many gradations in between. In keeping with my theoretical stance, I attempted to help Emma confront her polarized states as they emerged, gradually proceeding to their core. Before describing my approach with Emma further, however, let us turn now to the applied portion of my model: the healing conditions of experiential liberation. We will then return to the results of my encounter with Emma.

## THE HEALING CONDITIONS
## OF EXPERIENTIAL LIBERATION

One of the best illustrations of experiential liberation is Dante Alighieri's "Inferno," from *The Divine Comedy* (see May, 1991; Schneider & May, 1995). In this classic parable, Dante finds himself lost in a dark wood. He is alone and middle aged. Soon he encounters Virgil, who will accompany him into his "hell." It is no accident that I use the term "accompany" in connection with Virgil. Virgil does not advise Dante about going into his hell, nor does he attempt to explain that hell to Dante. Furthermore, he does not talk *about* the hell to Dante. Nor does he rationally restructure, reprogram, tranquilize, or cheer Dante up about his hell. By contrast, Virgil joins, stays present to, and makes himself available for Dante as he proceeds on his labyrinthine journey.

For me, Virgil epitomizes the experiential therapist. This is because through Virgil's presence Dante is able to discover the resources within himself to deal with and work through his hell. Put another way, Virgil neither directs Dante nor abandons him, but steadfastly contains, evokes, and reflects Dante back to himself. Virgil holds up a series of mirrors to Dante that help him to see what he struggles with, what blocks him from that struggle, and what resources he can muster to overcome that blockage. Through Virgil, Dante is able to face himself, to face the chaotic and obliterating levels of his suffering, and to "occupy" new ranges of himself (as exemplified by the third and final installment of *The Divine Comedy*, "Paradise").

Let us turn now to the more formal explication of this model. The aim of experiential liberation, it will be recalled, is to optimize constrictive/expansive choice. Choice at this level is characterized by immediate, kinesthetic, affective, and profound (or spiritual) dimensions of oneself. It is further characterized by vigor, creativity, and purpose.

There are four therapeutic subconditions or stances that promote experiential liberation. They are presence, invoking the actual, vivifying and confronting resistance, and meaning creation. Depending on clients' readiness and capacity for change, these stances may be sequential (as ordered above) or they may be in varying order. Generally they follow the aforementioned pattern.

## Presence

Presence is the sine qua non of experiential liberation. It is the beginning and the "end" of the approach, and it is implicated in every one of its aspects. Presence serves three basic therapeutic functions: it "holds" or contains the therapeutic interaction; it illuminates or apprehends the salient features of that interaction; and it inspires presence in those who receive or are touched by it. Let us consider this definition in greater depth.

Presence is palpable. It is a potent sign that one is "here" for another. "I will be with you," Virgil says, in effect, to Dante, "as long as I can be of help to you" (Schneider & May, 1995, p. 25). Being with another, "clearing a space" for another, and fully permitting another to be with and clear a space for him- or herself are all earmarks of presence (see Hycner & Jacobs, 1995). Another way to define presence is by its absence. When a therapist is distracted, when she or he is "occupied" by matters other than the person sitting before her/him, there is a distinct weakening of the relational field. From the standpoint of the client, the field feels porous, uninviting, precarious, cold, and remote. However, when a therapist is fully present, the relational field alters radically. Suddenly, there is life in the setting. The therapist acquires a vibrant, embracing quality. The therapeutic field becomes a sanctuary, to use Erik Craig's (1986) fine term, and the client has a sense of being met, held, heard, and seen. These qualities, in turn, invite the client to feel met, held, heard, and seen within himself. It is in this sense that even before a word is exchanged, the therapist becomes a mirror for the client and helps that client to "disarm."

Presence also illuminates a client's (and therapist's) world. This illumination is closely connected to empathy, but not to diagnostic assessment (Greenberg, Rice, & Elliott, 1993; Bohart, 1991). The therapist becomes a barometer not just for what is happening in the client but for what is happening in the field between her/him and the client (Friedman, 1995). Put another way, presence illuminates the entire atmosphere of therapist–client interaction. It is reflected in the following (silent) questions: What is really going on here? What is palpable? Where is the charge in this relationship? It is through this prism of inquiry that a deep and holistic gestalt begins to emerge about a given relationship. The therapist begins to sense not merely what the client is saying but *how* the client is being *while* he or she is saying it.

Presence reveals much more about clients than can be accessed by standardized assessments. It allows for surprise, self-correction, and moment-to-moment unfolding. But it also, significantly, allows for a rich and panoramic understanding of the therapeutic encounter.

The moment I meet with someone, for example, Emma, I immediately attune to how we are together. What is the "taste," feel, and texture of our contact? How do we sit with one another, position ourselves, and make eye contact? How does this person before me sit, move, and gesture? Is she "in my face," or is she soft, pliable? Is she effusive, or is she subdued? Does she quiver, or is she composed? How does she dress? What vocal fluctuations does she display? What is her energy level and where do I feel pulled in this relationship? All of these questions are clues for me, microcosms of a dynamic, evolving picture, and portents of challenges to come.

Finally, the presence of the therapist to her/his own fears and anxieties serves as a model to clients. To the degree that therapists can tolerate and accept a wide variety of experiences within themselves, clients too are inspired to acquire such abilities. As a result, therefore, clients are able to deepen as therapy proceeds, to become more accessible, expressive, and intentional (Bugental, 1987; May, 1969), which is very different, typically, from that which clients derive by pharmacological means, behavioral or cognitive reprogramming, or intellectual explanation.

In sum, presence holds and illuminates that which is palpably (immediately, kinesthetically, affectively, and profoundly) relevant within the client and between the client and therapist. Presence is both the ground and eventual goal of experiential work.

### Invoking the Actual

The next stance of experiential liberation is *invoking the actual*. Invoking the actual invites and encourages clients *into* that which is palpably (immediately, kinesthetically, affectively, and profoundly) relevant. If presence holds a silent mirror to clients' depths, invoking the actual holds a more active and vocal mirror to those depths. Borrowed from Wilson Van Dusen (1965), invoking the actual calls attention to clients' *ways* of speaking, gesturing, feeling, and sensing. It is an attempt to alert clients to what is "alive" and charged in the relationship. The following is a leading question of invoking the actual: What is really going on here (within the client and between myself and the client) and how can I assist the client into what is really going on?

As previously suggested, that which is frequently going on cuts beneath the client's (or therapist's) words and discursive content. The therapist's job is to be attuned to these processes and, as appropriate, call clients' attention to them. This calling of attention helps clients to experience the expansive rage, for example, beneath their constrictive sadness, or the contractive melancholy beneath their expansive bravado. Or it helps clients experience their polarizations in relation to the therapist and the therapist's responses to them. Turn by turn, this unlayering supports clients on their Dantean journey.

Some of the verbal invitations to invoke the actual include *topical focus*, *topical expansion*, and noting *content/process discrepancies*. Topical focus is usually initiated toward the start of given sessions and includes such comments as these: "Take a moment to see what's present for you." "What really matters right now?" "Can you give me an example?"

The focus on *personal* experience, moreover, is also a salient entrée into the actual. Encouraging clients to make "I" statements and to speak in the present tense illustrate this focus.

Topical expansion helps clients to elaborate on and deepen their experiences. Prompts like "Tell me more," "Stay with that (feeling) a few moments," or "You look like you have more to say," all can facilitate further immersion in one's concern (Bugental, 1987).

Content/process discrepancies are notable differences between what a client says and how she or he says it. Here are some examples: "You say you are fine, but your face is downcast"; or "Your body hunches over as you talk about your girlfriend—I wonder what that's about"; or "When you talk about that job, your eyes seem to moisten."

Inviting clients to "be with" their most intimate expressions requires great sensitivity. The therapist must be attuned not only to process issues but to clients' abilities to encounter those issues. I always make an effort to "check in" with clients who seem to be struggling with these intimate awarenesses. I might inquire, for example, how this style of approach is going for them, or suggest that they can signal me if our encounters become too intense. There is always room for flexibility with invoking the actual, and for clients to take charge of the format. Of course, there are times where I will reflect back to clients their need to shift out of our intensive process, but I genuinely try to gauge the usefulness of such feedback and to be as empathic as possible when I provide it.

One of the great values of invoking the actual is the wealth of information that it provides, even when clients decline to engage it. Raising clients' consciousness about their feelings, bodies, styles of existing, at the very minimum "plants seeds" for clients, helps them to see where they may want to continue the invocation at some future date, and may well even jar clients into presently reengaging their intensive contact. When I invited my client Emma to vent her animus toward her uncle in a role play, she was not initially able to do so. However, she learned a great deal about herself from that invitation and in a subsequent role play exploded at her uncle.

Invoking the actual can be understood in terms of a spectrum of intensity. I view the invocations I described above as orienting invocations. They spur clients to be present to their sufferings, but they frequently require supplemental offerings to deepen and consolidate that which has been achieved. In this regard, I have found silence, gentle prompts to "hang in" with the pain, guided or embodied meditation, and interpersonal encounter to be vital. Before delving into these areas, however, there is one key area of invoking the actual that has yet to be addressed—trust.

One recent evening, a jittery supervisee stepped into my office. He was deeply intrigued by the experiential concepts we had been exploring but had one overarching question: "What do you do after the client is immersed?" The panic exhibited by this student is not uncommon among beginning trainees (not to mention seasoned veterans at times!). To sit with clients in pain, to have no idea where that pain will lead, or whether it will dissipate, is unsettling indeed. The cultivation of trust, however, is one of the primary experiential tasks. Without therapeutic trust, no therapist could have the steadiness, patience, supportiveness, and stark belief in the healing powers of the client that experiential work demands. Among trusting experiential therapists, there is a refusal to equate clients with their dysfunctions. Further, such therapists are continually open to the *more* of consciousness, the *more* of living. From this standpoint a client is more than a "depressive," but a dynamic, unfolding person. My advice to the supervisee?—Do not withdraw from the situation too hastily. Gently suggest to the client to stay present, that more may emerge, and that come what may, you are "here" for her. In my experience, too many trainees (and professionals) do not heed this advice and rob the client of three illuminating scenarios: the experience of deepening, the experience of an inability to deepen, and the experience of resistance to deepening.

*Guided (or "embodied") meditation* is one of the most transformative forms of invoking the actual of which I am aware (see Schneider & May, 1995, for a full explication of this modality). Guided meditation entails concerted invitations to clients to enter embodied, meditative states. I try to be flexible about how I structure guided meditation. Sometimes I suggest a sequence of simple breathing exercises, attunement to and identification of a somatic tension area, and invitations to physically self-contact the identified tension area. I follow up this sequence with an invitation to clients to associate to the feelings, fantasies, and images aroused by the tension area. At other times, I directly invite clients to attune to bodily tension areas and to free associate to these areas. At still other times, I invite clients to solely make physical (e.g., hand) contact with their anxiety and experience what emerges. In short, I cannot overestimate the impact of this style of experiential immersion for certain clients—it cuts through to the core.

The field that occurs *between* client and therapist is another salient opening for invoking the actual. The interpersonal *encounter*, as I (and other existential theorists) call it, possesses three basic dimensions: (1) the real or present relationship between therapist and client; (2) the future and what can happen in the relationship (vs. strictly the past and what has happened in relationships); and (3) the "acting out," or experiencing to the degree appropriate, of relational material (Schneider & May, 1995, p. 165). While I cannot possibly do justice to the rich and nuanced texture of encounter on these pages, I will provide a few observations. The encounter enables clients to open up their deepest fears and fantasies directly in the living relationship. The encounter enables clients to work through those fears and fantasies in an intensive but safe relationship. Finally, the experiential dimension of the encounter can be enhanced and deepened through timely invitations to stay present to the feelings, sensations, and images brought up by the encounter (see Schneider & May, 1995, and Hycner & Jacobs, 1995, for an elaboration on each of these points.)

While there are many other ways to invite and encourage clients into the palpably relevant (see Schneider & May, 1995, for a fuller discussion), the challenge is to cultivate them, tailor them to the situation, and creatively refine them.

## Vivifying and Confronting Resistance

When the invitation to explore, immerse, and encounter are abruptly or repeatedly declined by clients, then the delicate problem of resistance must be considered. Resistances are *blockages* to that which is palpably relevant.

There are several caveats to bear in mind about experiential work with resistances. For one, therapists can be mistaken about resistances. What I label resistance, for example, may simply be the refusal on the part of the client to follow my agenda. It may also be a safety issue for the client or an issue of cultural or psychological misunderstanding. It is of utmost importance, therefore, to bracket our attributions of resistance and to clarify their pertinent roots. Second, it is crucial to respect resistances. Resistances are lifelines to clients and as miserable as clients' patterns may be, they are the scaffoldings of their existence, both known and familiar.

Resistances, moreover, demarcate the monumental battle that clients experience. This battle consists of two rivaling factions: the side of the client that struggles to emerge and the side of the client that struggles to suppress that emergence, that remains entrenched. It is crucial, in my view, to name this battle with clients; it is the most important battle with which they contend.

Resistance work is mirroring work. Whereas invoking the actual mirrors clients' struggles to emerge, resistance work, as previously indicated, mirrors clients' barriers to that emergence. Resistance work must be artfully engaged. The more that therapists invest in changing clients, the less they enable clients to struggle with change. By contrast, the more that therapists help clients to clarify how they are willing to live, the more they fuel the impetus (and often frustration!) required for lasting change.

*Vivifying* resistance is the amplification of clients' awareness of how they block themselves. Specifically, vivification serves three therapeutic functions: (1) it alerts clients to their defensive worlds; (2) it apprises them of the consequences of those worlds; and (3) it reflects back the counterforces aimed at overcoming those worlds. There are two basic approaches associated with vivifying resistance—*noting* and *tagging*. Noting acquaints clients with initial experiences of resistance. Here are some examples of noting: "Your voice gets soft when you speak about sex." "You were sad, and suddenly you switched topics." "It is difficult for you to look at me when you express anger." Tagging alerts clients to the repetition of their resistances. Here are some examples of tagging: "Whenever we discuss this topic you draw a blank." "Everytime you explore your career goals you look resigned." "You repeatedly appear to want to blame others for your misery." In addition to noting and tagging, there are also a variety of other verbal and nonverbal vivifications of resistance (see Schneider & May, 1995, pp. 168–170). It is even sometimes helpful to simply support clients' resistance, particularly when such clients are immovable. This support alleviates the pressure on clients to self-disclose and can, paradoxically, accelerate renewed self-disclosures (see Schneider, 1990/1998, pp. 194–198).

In exceptional circumstances clients need more than a mere acknowledgment of their defensive patterns; they need a *confrontation* with those patterns. Whereas vivifying resistance *alerts* clients to their polarized stances, confrontation *alarms* them about those stances. While confrontation has its benefits, usually toward the latter stages of therapy, it is imperative that therapists be selective about it. If confrontation is too intense, the therapist may rob the client of responsibility for facing a life decision; or, correspondingly, he may lose the client altogether. Perceived correctly, confrontation is an amplified form of vivification. It still mirrors clients' self-sabotage, but it does so dramatically, with life or death significance. Although there are no clear-cut criteria for confronting, two elements are generally present: chronic client entrenchment (or polarization) and a strong therapeutic alliance.

Here are some examples of confronting: "You say you can't stop drinking, but you mean you won't!" "How many times are you going to keep debasing yourself with men?" "You'd rather argue with me than get on with your life!"

There are, of course, times to acknowledge the fatigue, torment, and basic helplessness that clients feel before their resistances. This is especially true as clients approach liberation, which can be the most resistant period of all. Such acknowledgments provide perspective and the room for clients to regroup.

## Meaning Creation

As clients face and overcome the blocks to that which is palpably relevant, they begin to discern the meaning of their odysseys. This meaning is not abstract or intellectual, but *embodied*—the result of a hard-won self-encounter. The meaning created by experiential liberation, furthermore, yields new shapes, textures, and priorities to clients' lives. Whereas formerly a given client may have hidden herself in the world, now she is capable of standing forth in the world and pursuing her aspirations. Other clients find meaning in scholastic or athletic pursuits, religiosity, or romance. The key here is not the discovery of particular meanings but what clients bring to those meanings—their passions, creativities, and imaginations. Whereas before clients were precluded from those avenues of motivation, now they are able to occupy them, fully range within them, and implement them in their lives. It is not that all symptoms or problems are eradicated through such a process, it is simply that the major barriers to choice in a given area are removed. The result for such clients is that they experience more centeredness, less panic, and a greater capacity to respond to rather than react against their fears.

What is the therapist's role in this experiential creation of meaning? Beyond what she or he has already provided with her/his presence and invitations to aliveness, the therapist's role is a relatively small one. However, that small role can be integral. The therapist, for example, can provide a timely "sounding board" to echo and refine clients' discoveries. In turn, these discoveries can be implemented in the outside world, and refined once again, if need be, in therapy.


## EPILOGUE

Let us return now to our client Emma. I will then offer a few closing observations. Emma's experiential liberation unfolded over four arduous years. We experienced the gamut of emotions during our intensive contact, from searing personal vulnerability, to panic, to rage, to bottomless grieving, to disappointment with, fury at, and terror of me. I worked with her to personally and intensively stay present to these feelings and to use role play, rehearsal, journal writing, exploration of our relationship, embodied meditation, dream analysis, and even a 6-month stint of emergency medication, to facilitate this engagement. I also struggled with Emma over her tenacious resistances. First I assisted her to explore these resistances, then to mobilize her frustration with them, and finally to overthrow and transcend them.

The core of Emma's dysfunction was the dread of standing out. The closer we came to this core, the more Emma fought to deny it. This was understandable: not only did Emma fear standing out before her uncle, she feared the fuller implication of that fear—standing out before life. While the former fear was explainable and discussible, the latter fear exceeded explanations and words; it had to be experienced. By tussling with and remaining steadfastly present to this fuller fear, Emma was able to enter a new part of herself. She was able to "hold" that which was formerly unmanageable. As a result, she became more resourceful, trusting, and bold. She was also able to declare herself—not merely before me and her abusers—but before life itself. Today, Emma is in a nourishing and committed relationship, is active in her community, and asserts firm boundaries with her uncle. She still suffers, but she does not equate herself with that suffering. She equates herself with possibility

In sum, experiential liberation provides the seedbed for major client transformation. Through its four subconditions—presence, invoking the actual, vivifying and confronting resistance, and meaning creation—experiential liberation optimizes clients' capacities to respond to (rather than merely react against) their fears. In turn, clients acquire a markedly greater capacity to constrict or expand, as appropriate, within the natural and self-imposed limits of living.

Experiential liberation is gaining support from unexpected quarters. There is an increasing recognition among traditional researchers that therapeutic outcome depends "far more on the client's resources, . . . therapist's style, attitude, and interpersonal relationship with the client" (Duncan & Moynihan, 1994, p. 300) than it does on preconceived techniques. It may be, therefore, that along with the trends toward standardizing and manualizing our field, an experiential countertrend is emerging (Mahrer & Fairweather, 1993; Schneider, 1998). That trend would be welcome not merely to experiential therapists but to growing numbers of clients (*Consumer Reports*, 1995; Seligman, 1995).

## NOTE

1. My use of the term "guide" in this sentence is noteworthy. I view my framework as a touchstone or guideline, and not as a "cookbook" or manualized formula. My implicit position is *not* whether a given person fits my framework but whether my framework accords with a given person.

## REFERENCES

Antonovsky, A. (1979). *Health, stress, and coping.* San Francisco: Jossey-Bass.

Becker, E. (1973). *The denial of death.* New York: Free Press.

Bohart, A. (1991). Empathy in client-centered therapy: A contrast with psychoanalysis and self-psychology. *Journal of Humanistic Psychology, 31*(1), 34–48.

Bugental, J. (1978). *Psychotherapy and process: The fundamentals of an existential–humanistic approach.* Reading, MA: Addison-Wesley.

Bugental, J. (1981). *The search for authenticity: An existential–analytic approach to psychotherapy* (enlarged ed.). New York: Irvington.

Bugental, J. (1987). *The art of the psychotherapist.* New York: Norton.

Bugental, J., & Kleiner, R. (1993). Existential psychotherapies. In G. Stricker & G. Gold (Eds.), *Comprehensive handbook of psychotherapy integration.* New York: Plenum.

*Consumer Reports.* (1995, November). Mental health: Does therapy help? pp. 734–739.

Craig, E. (1986). Sanctuary and presence: An existential view of the therapist's contribution. *The Humanistic Psychologist, 14*(1), 22–28.

Duncan, B., & Moynihan, D. (1994). Applying outcome research: Intentional utilization of the client's frame of reference. *Psychotherapy, 31*(2), 294–301.

Friedman, M. (1995). Dialogical (Buberian) therapy: The case of Dawn. In K. J. Schneider & R. May (Eds.), *The psychology of existence: An integrative, clinical perspective.* New York: McGraw-Hill.

Gendlin, E. T. (1978). *Focusing.* New York: Bantam.

Greenberg, L. S., Rice, L. N., & Elliott, R. (1993). *Facilitating emotional change: The moment-by-moment process.* New York: Guilford Press.

Grotstein, J. (1990). Nothingness, meaninglessness, chaos, and the "black hole." I. *Contemporary Psychoanalysis, 26*(2), 257–290.

Hycner, R., & Jacobs, L. (1995). *The healing relationship in Gestalt therapy: A dialogic/self psychology approach.* Highland, NY: Gestalt Journal Press.

James, W. (1950). *Principles of psychology* (2 vols. bound as one). New York: Dover. (Original work published 1890, New York: Holt).

James, W. (1987). *William James: Writings.* New York: Literary Classics/Viking. (Original work published 1904).

Kobasa, S. (1979). Successful life events, personality, and health: An inquiry into hardiness. *Journal of Personality and Social Psychology, 37*, 1–11.

Laing, R. D. (1967). *The politics of experience.* New York: Ballantine.

Laing, R. D. (1969). *The divided self: An existential study in sanity and madness.* Harmondsworth, Middlesex, UK: Penguin.

Mahrer, A. R., & Fairweather, D. (1993). What is "experiencing"? A critical review of meanings and applications in psychotherapy. *The Humanistic Psychologist, 21*(1), 2–25.

May, R. (1969). *Love and will.* New York: Norton.

May, R. (1981). *Freedom and destiny.* New York: Norton.

May, R. (1991). *The cry for myth.* New York: Norton.

May, R. (1995). Black and impotent: The case of Mercedes. In K. J. Schneider & R. May (Eds.), *The psychology of existence: An integrative, clinical perspective.* New York: McGraw-Hill.

Rank, O. (1936). *Will therapy.* New York: Knopf.

Schneider, K. J. (1987). The deified self: A "centaur": response to Wilber and the transpersonal movement. *Journal of Humanistic Psychology, 27*(2), 196–216.

Schneider, K. J. (1989). Infallibility is so damn appealing: A reply to Ken Wilber. *Journal of Humanistic Psychology, 29*(4), 495–506.

Schneider, K. J. (1993). *Horror and the holy: Wisdom-teachings of the monster tale.* Chicago: Open Court.

Schneider, K. J. (1996). Transpersonal views of existentialism: A rejoinder. *The Humanistic Psychologist, 24*(1), 145–148.

Schneider, K. J. (1998). *The paradoxical self: Toward an understanding of our contradictory nature* (2nd ed.). Buffalo, NY: Prometheus Books. (Original work published 1990, New York: Plenum/Insight.)

Schneider, K. J. (1998). Toward a science of the heart: Romanticism and the revival of psychology. *American Psychologist, 53*(3), 277–289.

Schneider, K. J., & May, R. (1995). *The psychology of existence: An integrative, clinical perspective.* New York: McGraw-Hill.

Seligman, M. (1995). The effectiveness of psychotherapy: The *Consumer Reports* study. *American Psychologist, 50*(12), 965–974.

Tillich, P. (1952). *The courage to be.* New Haven, CT: Yale University Press.

Van Dusen, W. (1965). Invoking the actual in psychotherapy. *Journal of Individual Psychology, 21,* 66–76.

Yalom, I. D. (1980). *Existential psychotherapy.* New York: Basic Books.

# 6

\*\*\*\*\*

# Focusing Microprocesses

## Mia Leijssen

## THE ESSENCE OF FOCUSING

Focusing is a special way of paying attention to one's felt experience in the body. By carefully dwelling on one's bodily experience, which often is quite vague at first, one can get in touch with the whole felt sense of an issue, problem, or situation. Through interaction with symbols, the felt experience can become more precise, it can move and change, it can achieve a felt shift: the experience of real change or bodily resolution of the issue.

Focusing is a client process, discovered and developed by Gendlin (1964, 1968, 1981, 1984, 1990, 1996) partly out of his theory of personality change and partly out of his research on the process of psychotherapy. Comparing successful with unsuccessful therapies made it clear that successful clients were using a specific form of self-exploration (Gendlin, Beebe, Cassens, Klein, & Oberlander, 1968; Hendrick, 1986; Klein, Mathieu-Coughlan, & Kiesler, 1986; Mathieu-Coughlan & Klein, 1986). This process was subsequently studied in depth by Gendlin in the hope of discovering principles that could be used in teaching these crucial skills to less successful clients.

Focusing is characterized by, and can be distinguished from other activities by, two aspects: (1) the specific object of attention being the *felt sense* and (2) the attitude adopted by client and therapist being the *focusing attitude* (Iberg, 1981). Before describing these essential aspects any further, we will give an example from psychotherapy practice:

A 32-year-old woman has been depressed since the birth of her child 3 years ago. She has read a great deal about postnatal depression, but the explanations don't touch her. She thinks, "That is probably what I have," but doesn't feel that it fits. The therapist invites her to stop looking for explanations, to direct her attention toward the center of her body and remain with the question "What is really the matter with me?" Tears well up in her eyes. She wants to give an explanation for it but the therapist encourages her to wait and remain silently attentive to her body. She spontaneously crosses her arms over the region of her abdomen and heart. The therapist lets her fully feel this gesture. Suddenly an image appears of her little daughter being carried away immediately after birth. "I don't want them to take away my daughter!" she shouts. This verbal expression is obviously right; her body recognizes that this is it, and it obviously relieves her to repeat the expression several times. But that is not all yet; further tension remains in her body. The therapist asks her to keep her attention on her body and to see what else there is. Then she sees herself standing behind glass with, in the distance, her baby in the incubator. She despairs deeply of ever being able to reach the helpless little being in the distance; she cries but with pain and anger at the gynecologist (while in reality she had behaved "reasonably"). She now discovers that she was forced to accept the situation of leaving the child behind in the maternity ward. When, 2 weeks later, she was allowed to take the baby home, it "wasn't hers anymore." Although these were painful experiences, she now feels very relieved when bringing them into the open. For 3 years her body has carried this along without finding a proper expression for it. The woman herself had "forgotten" the events, but her body kept carrying them in the form of a depression. Now that this bodily knowledge has been opened up, the woman feels liberated. Her energy returns and, for the first time, she feels love for her daughter.

## Object of Attention: The Felt Sense

Rogers (1961) sometimes refers to this specific object of attention, for example, in the following statements: "Therapy seems to mean a getting back to basic sensory and visceral experience" (p. 103); "The client is hit by a feeling—not something named or labelled—but an experience of an unknown something which has to be cautiously explored before it can be named at all" (p. 129); "The referent of these vague cognitions lies within him, in an organismic event against which he can check his symbolization and his cognitive formulations" (p. 140).

This internal point of reference is further described by Gendlin at first as "experiencing": "The process of concrete, bodily feeling, which constitutes the basic matter of psychological and personality phenomena" (Gendlin, 1964, p. 111); later as the "felt sense": "The edge of awareness; a sense of more than one says and knows, an unclear, fuzzy, murky sense of a whole situation, that comes in the middle of the body: [t]hroat, chest, stomach, abdomen" (Gendlin, 1984, p. 79); and more recently: "The body referred to here is not the physiological machine of the usual reductive thinking. Here it is the body as sensed from inside" (Gendlin, 1996, p. 2).

Thus, therapy is restoring contact with the meaning–feeling body in which existence manifests itself, a process in which the arrested experience is touched upon again so that it can once more start moving and reveal and further unfold itself to complete its meaning. The implicit organismic experiencing, which the client feels but cannot yet express, must at one time or another become the object of attention in therapy. It is this inner knowing which will open itself in the therapeutic interaction and from which new meanings will emerge.

## The Focusing Attitude

The vague, the unformed, the unspeakable can only let itself be known when it is approached in a specific way. Dealing with this inner object of attention requires an attitude of waiting, of quietly and friendly remaining present with the not yet speakable, being receptive to the not yet formed. To achieve this, it will be necessary to suspend temporarily everything that the person already knows about it and to be cognitively inactive. This kind of attention can also be found in Zen meditation and Taoism, but in therapy it is directed toward a specific object, the felt sense. However, many clients offer resistance because they experience this inner process as threatening. The focusing attitude presupposes tolerance for uncertainty, an ability to give up control and to be vulnerable, since neither the therapist nor the client can anticipate what will emerge from the implicit. Not knowing exactly what is going to emerge is very frightening to people who have been used to keeping emotions down and under strict control. It is obvious that a person will only dare to adopt such an attitude if there is already a good deal of interpersonal security. The focusing attitude emerges spontaneously in some people in a safe milieu. In others, this way of giving attention inwardly is not spontaneously used but something which they can nevertheless discover in contact with the therapist. (For the development of the focusing attitude, see Leijssen, in press.) The therapist interacts with the client in an attitude of acceptance and empathy; gradually, in this corrective therapeutic milieu the client learns to adopt a focusing attitude by interacting with the bodily felt experience (the client's inside) in the same friendly and listening way.

Before differentiating types of focusing processes, I would like to emphasize that focusing can only happen if the interpersonal conditions are right: "One can focus alone, but if one does it with another person present, it is deeper and better, *if* that relationship makes for a deeper and better bodily ongoing process. If not, then focusing is limited by the context of that relationship" (Gendlin, 1996, p. 297; his emphasis). Wiltschko (1995) points out that "The relational space between client and therapist is the living space in which the client's developmental process can occur. In fact, internal and interpersonal processes are not separate, rather they are two aspects of one process" (p. 5). Moreover, if the relational conditions are not good, focusing is almost useless because the inner process is very much a function of the ongoing interactional process" (p. 1). "Focusing is not an intrapsychic process to be contrasted with interpersonal relating. Such distinction misses the fact that we are alive in our situations and relationships with others, and that we live bodily our relations" (Gendlin, 1996, p. 297). The essentially *interactive* nature of the formation of a bodily felt sense in the client is what Rogers (1961) stressed when he said that the client must to some degree perceive the empathy, genuineness, and positive regard from the therapist. The inner process is always a function of the interpersonal process.

## Microprocesses

Focusing is a process of finding felt senses and then interacting with them in a friendly way so as to feel movement (Friedman, 1995, p. 8). Successful clients know how to make contact with a vague but bodily felt sense. In order to teach focusing, Gendlin (1981, 1984, 1996) described a model which involves six process steps, with many details grouped under each: (1) clearing a space; (2) getting a felt sense; (3) finding a handle; (4) resonating the handle and felt sense; (5) asking; and (6) receiving. Focusing training pays due attention to each step separately in order to show people how to proceed through the focusing process.

I will cover the different steps not for the purpose of teaching focusing but in order to describe them as microprocesses or task-relevant processes offered at certain moments in psychotherapy. "They help to establish the working conditions that are optimal for facilitating particular kinds of self-explorations" (Rice, 1984, p. 182). It is important for a therapist to learn when and how specific microprocesses can be used at various moments in therapy. This requires a process diagnosis in which the therapist recognizes the signals heralding the emergence of a microprocess in need of facilitation. My description of the microprocesses is inspired by Gendlin's manuals (1981, 1996) and *The Focusing Guide Manual* of Weiser Cornell (1993). Also the writings of Armstrong (1993), K. McGuire (1993), and Müller (1995) were helpful in developing a differentiated view on several microprocesses.

I have grouped the various microprocesses into three comprehensive processes that require several skills on the part of the client: (1) finding the right distance to a felt sense; (2) developing a felt sense in all its components (body sensations, emotions, symbols, life situations); and (3) fully receiving the felt sense. Clients can sometimes stall at different stages and are unable to let fruitful self-exploration take place. The difficulties that clients may encounter at each stage can be described as follows: (1) the client is unable to find a proper relationship with the felt sense—the client is either too close to what is felt (overwhelmed) or too far from it (out of touch); (2) the client remains stuck in one of the components of the felt sense instead of allowing the full felt sense with its four components to emerge; and (3) the client is led astray by interfering ways of reacting (the inner critic, superego) that prevent her or him from receiving the felt sense. The therapist will have to intervene differently as a function of the specific *difficulties* in the client process. I will thoroughly examine each phase in succession and indicate how the therapist can proceed to keep the client on the right track or, where difficulties arise, can introduce the necessary skills in a more directive manner. I will illustrate how each principle may be applied in experiential therapy practice.

The three phases sometimes appear in *hierarchical* order: the client first finds the proper way of relating to the problem before a felt sense in all its components unfolds and is fully received. However, they may appear in a *different order*: thus, work with an interfering way of reacting may be necessary if the client is initially unable to make any contact at all with certain feelings; or the search for a right distance may appear at the end when assigning a more appropriate place to an interfering behavioral pattern. Or each process may *by itself* take up a complete session, or a specific process may be used as *part* of other therapeutic approaches. We are thus dealing with different skills that may be used only every now and then and may come to the fore with varying emphasis.

## FINDING THE RIGHT DISTANCE

*Right distance* means making contact with the experience without coinciding with it. In a first phase we don't work with the content of a problem but with *relating to it*: the client learns to create space between her-/himself and the problem so as to relate to it as an observing self instead of coinciding with it. Often the client's difficulties have to do with a *wrong way of relating*, a wrong distance between her-/himself and the experience. Either the distance is too large and the client remains *too far* from the experience, thus "feeling nothing," or else the distance is too small and the client is *too close* and flooded by the problems so that no "self" remains to relate to what is felt. "We can describe a continuum of client process from Close Process (overwhelmed) to Distant Process (out of touch), with Middle Process, the Ideal Focusing distance, in between" (Weiser Cornell, 1996b, p. 6). The therapist will intervene differently according to whether the client is too far or too close in relation to the problems.

Finding and keeping a proper way of relating is an important therapeutic process that may be applied in different contexts, for example, at the start of a therapy session, during the therapeutic process, in crisis situations, or as a moment of contemplation.

### The Client Is Too Far

The client is in this process when he or she does not know what to talk about, feeling but little or always doubting the feelings, needing a long time to contact a feeling, losing that contact easily, concentrating on intellectual processes and speaking from there, explaining a lot of things to the therapist, rationalizing the problem, predominantly quoting external authorities, or engaging in dead-end discussions. In such cases, the therapist should actively help the client to discover new ways of relating to him-/herself. A question such as "How does that feel?" is mostly not enough for such clients because they don't know how to feel in their bodies for meaning. They look for meaning "outside" of themselves: at other authorities, in theories, or in books. Introducing an approach addressed to the body is often a necessary step in bringing such clients in contact with a new source of knowledge: their own inner authority.

For example, Oskar, 48, tends to talk about events from the past week in a very rational way. He often consults books, looking for an explanation of what happens to him. He starts the 22nd session with a long talk about a friend and tells in much detail how he "thinks" he should feel furious:

THERAPIST: You think you should feel furious . . . but you don't feel any contact with it . . . Now, could you set aside for a moment everything you thought and we will start with your body and see what comes from there . . . I will direct your attention through your body . . . Take your time to close your eyes and take a few deep breaths . . . (*The therapist lets the client fully feel his body, from the feet up, and invites him every time: "What are you aware of in that part of your body?," letting him simply be the observer of what emerges.*) . . . Just notice what you experience . . . (*When the whole body has been covered, the therapist asks the client to bring his attention into the center of his body.*) . . . What strikes you most after you have covered your whole body?

CLIENT: That feeling in the region of my stomach . . . that tension there . . . that is the most powerful.

A valuable way of assisting the client in achieving an inner relationship may be to direct *attention* first *into* the body. Gendlin (1996, p. 71) describes several "preliminary instructions" in order to learn to sense the body from inside. Usually it is sufficient to invite the person to do so at the beginning of the session, using a few simple instructions such as the following: "Take your time to feel how you are inside your body . . ."; "Follow your breathing for a moment, simply breathing in and out, without wanting to change anything about it . . ."; "What strikes you when your attention scans your body?" The therapist can also ask the client, at the beginning of the session, to close his or her eyes for a moment and see how the different areas in the body feel. Breathing and sensations in the throat, chest, stomach, and abdomen receive full attention. Should the therapist choose to let the client start with some form of relaxation, the former should see to it that the relaxation does not become too deep; indeed, focusing demands full concentration and keen receptivity. When working with a group, I sometimes start with music and movement, something which carries the participants immediately to a more bodily level of awareness.

A client who does not know what to talk about is sometimes invited to check out whether he or she would be able to say: "I feel totally well." Such a provocative request usually elicits a protest in which mention is made of the issue that prevents the client from feeling totally well. A similar *contrast experience* may also be elicited by asking the client to state: "All my problems are solved," whereupon problem areas still outstanding often come to the fore and can be used as topics of exploration. It may also be helpful to review with the client what is currently happening in his or her life and ask what each topic evokes in the body. Among those, the topic provoking the strongest sensation is chosen. The therapist looks here for minute bodily reactions in the client. Indeed, eye movements, facial expressions, breathing, small gestures, or changes of posture may all be signs of an underlying emotional charge that the client may fail to notice unless the therapist draws attention to them.

The client may not only be too far removed from feelings at the beginning of the session but may also lose this contact *during the session*. The therapist may handle this by the following suggestions and/or quotations: "Take your time to feel how this lives in your body . . . What do you sense there?"; "Can you say whether the problem is totally solved?"; "How is your breathing while you talk about that?"; "You say 'it doesn't touch me,' but at the same time you make a stamping movement with your leg . . . What quality of bodily feeling do you find in there?"; etc. It is by means of such questions that the therapist redirects the client's attention inward and more specifically to those sensations that are likely to emerge from the body. I sometimes ask clients to put their hand on the spot where they can feel it in the body. In this way, I ask them literally to "*hold on to*" the experience. And I add an invitation to direct the *breathing* toward that spot.

By the process directives described above, attention is shifted from "outside" to "inside" and an inner relationship is initiated whereby the client learns to move into the position of an observing, nonjudgmental self capable of sensing certain events inside itself. Gradually the transition is then made from observing simple phenomena such as breathing to complex ones such as conflicts.

## The Client Is Too Close

The opposite position can be seen when a client shows, verbally or nonverbally, that too much is coming his or her way or that the experience is too intense. It is not even unusual to see a client switch round from "too far" to "too close." The client is then likely to show aversion for what emerges, or feel anxiety or tension, or feel flooded by something in which she/he is drowning or losing her-/himself, or else the client may totally identify with the experience—all *markers* that the therapist's help is needed in creating more distance. Indeed, some distance between oneself and one's problem is needed to make an inner relationship possible.

When dealing with "too close a way of relating," the therapist calls upon the natural human capacity to "*split*" and on the enormous power which may be contained in one's *imagination*. The therapist encourages the client to distinguish "*parts*" in her-/himself over which a certain amount of control can be developed or to which special care can be given. The use of *metaphors* to make these processes more concretely present is paramount here. (Talking about "creating distance" or being "too far" or "too close" is already using metaphors to describe these processes.) According to the nature of the problem with which the client coincides or which floods her/him, the therapist's way of facilitating disidentification or creating distance will vary. The metaphors used should suit the client's world. There are several ways of helping a client find the right distance.

We first give an example of a complete (albeit abbreviated) therapy session in which the client, who is "too close," is helped to achieve a better way of relating.

Sonia, 39, arrives extremely tense for her 24th session; she is bumping into everything and is unable to think. She does not understand why she should be so tense. Indeed, it is the first day of her holidays:

THERAPIST: Let's look at that together, quietly . . . Take your time and follow your breathing for a moment—you may close your eyes if you wish—and simply follow the rhythm of you breathing the air in and out . . . (*silence*) . . . You said you were very tense . . . Ask your body what it is that makes you so tense. . . .

CLIENT: Well, it is indeed vacation, but I have to do an awful lot of things in the next little while. If I don't watch it, the month will be over and I will have gotten nowhere.

THERAPIST: OK, we will have a look at what it is that demands your attention . . . Here you have a notepad . . . Each problem that makes you tense will receive a name which you will write down on a sheet of notepaper, and next, you will assign the sheet—and thus the problem—a place in this room here, at a comfortable distance from yourself. So, what is it that comes to you first?

CLIENT: There is load of work in the house, and various things need repairs . . . The carpenter should come; there is a problem with the heating system; the electrical system needs checking; I have to buy lamps; the curtains need washing . . .

THERAPIST: Yes, this is a lot all at once. Take a little sheet for each of these worries, one for the carpenter, one for the heating, one for the electricity, one for the lamps, one for the curtains . . . and write on each that key word . . . (*silence; client writes on notepaper*). . . . Now assign each of these a place on the floor or somewhere else in this room, but while doing so try to feel how it is to really put aside each one of these worries for a while. You don't forget them but you let them rest, you give them a place . . . (*Client deposits the notes on the floor, within reach, and sighs deeply.*) OK, there they are. Now have a look at what else makes you tense. (*silence*)

CLIENT: I have to make an appointment with the dentist; a tooth is hurting me quite a bit and I always postpone it.

THERAPIST: So, you have to contact the dentist to have your tooth repaired . . . Write that down on a sheet of paper . . . (*Client writes.*) and give that a place as well . . . (*Client deposits the note next to her on the table.*) . . . What else? (*silence*)

CLIENT: I urgently have to talk to my cleaning lady. (*Client gives a lengthy explanation of the problem with the cleaning lady during which the therapist helps her clarify what exactly needs to be made clear to the cleaning lady.*) . . . I want to tell her clearly that she has to stick to what I ask her . . .

THERAPIST: Make another note of your conversation with the cleaning lady . . . and put that down too. (*Client deposits the note on the floor on the other side; there follows a deep sigh.*) Is there anything else? (*Several practical problems follow, all of which are similarly given a place.*)

CLIENT: Now I feel my loneliness weighing heavily on me . . . I miss hugs . . .

THERAPIST: Tell your body that you hear that it misses hugs . . . and try to breath in a friendly way around the spot where you feel the lack . . . Give it a soft, friendly breathing space in there . . . (*silence*)

CLIENT: That feels good . . . I seldom acknowledge that and harden myself . . . This feels better . . . (*silence*)

THERAPIST: Anything else?

CLIENT: I get frightened because I suddenly come face to face with my father! He is old and needy. I am supposed to take care of him but I cannot after all he has done to me (*There was incest with the father.*) . . . I don't even feel like visiting him . . . Now that I am on vacation, I don't have an excuse any more to postpone it . . . It's like a mountain which I dread . . . It is not by accident that I come out with this after everything else . . . I always avoid this by keeping very busy.

THERAPIST: You don't have to start "climbing" that mountain right away . . . We don't have the time now to deal with it . . . If you wish, we could take more time for the problem with your father in the next session . . . Have a look now and see if you can step back a bit and let this mountain lie in front of you for a while without having to start your vacation with this heavy climb . . .

CLIENT: It's good though that I briefly touched upon it, but I feel indeed that I have to give myself the time to catch my breath first . . . I notice that it relaxes me to step back and leave this mountain where it is, for the moment . . .

THERAPIST: Our time is almost up . . . You deposited these various notes here . . . Have a look and see what you want to do with them, what you would feel good rounding off with?

CLIENT: I'll take them home and put them on my notice board in the order in which I want to tackle them. (*Client carefully picks up the notes, one after the other, loudly voicing what she wants to do with them and puts them away in her handbag.*)

THERAPIST: Why don't you take briefly the time now to feel how you are and whether it needs something else. (*silence*)

CLIENT: I feel I lost 20 kilos! I have this wonderful feeling that I also have room to enjoy myself. . . I'll first go and sit on a terrace and have a drink to celebrate my vacation . . .

The most usual way of creating distance when the client's way of relating is too close is to ask the client to assign the problem *a place outside* of her- or himself. Sometimes the simple request to let "it" go a little further away may be enough. In most cases, however, the therapist may have to help the process along more firmly by giving, for example, instructions such as "Could you give that problem a place somewhere in this room? . . . Have a look around where you would like to put it."

It may be very helpful as well to carry this out *concretely*, for instance, by having the client write down on a piece of paper the name of the problem or by drawing it and then depositing the paper somewhere in the room. Even with sophisticated clients this may have a very liberating effect and is often more effective than just indicating at fantasy level where something should go. In this way, several of the client's problems may be assigned a place in the therapy room. This process of creating distance may be helped along even further at fantasy level by using various metaphors. When a client happens to feel an overload, especially on the shoulders and back, one may work with the following image: "Imagine yourself carrying a heavy rucksack full of problems and having a look at its contents; and imagine that you take the problems out, one at a time, and deposit them here . . . Notice how you feel each time you unload a specific problem and put it down." Or another metaphor when a client feels the center of the body to be stuffed up or feels that something grabs him/her completely: "Try to imagine that you have a space inside of you, a sort of room which is filled that you can no longer move around in it . . . Let us make some room in there . . . Have a look what is in there that takes up too much room . . . Imagine that you put it out of that room for a moment and give it a place elsewhere where you can still see it but where it does not sit on top of you any more . . . How does it feel inside when this space is vacant?" Should the problem be very *threatening* or frightening, it may not be enough to put it at some distance but one may have to put up a fence between it and the client. Thus a client who is overwhelmed by anxiety when trying to speak about her aggressive father may imagine not only that her father is put away in the most remote corner of the therapy room but also that a "cage" has been built around him, as is sometimes done in court with dangerous criminals. Or another client may draw something which he finds very threatening and stick the drawing on the outside of the therapy room window. However when the client is overwhelmed by something "childlike" in quality or something which is very *dear*, then other metaphors may have to be called upon to create the proper distance. Thus it would hardly be compassionate toward the client who coincides with wounds received in childhood to just put these away somewhere in the therapy room. Indeed, the place assigned should be "outside" while it should also be taking care of that part of the client. Thus one might ask, "Could you take that wounded child on your knee," thus introducing distance while still respecting the sensitivity of the issue.

In brief, the request to put away at some distance what is too close can never be stereotyped. It will always imply a search—in interaction with the client's reaction—for a form adapted to the client's needs, while firmly and inventively promoting distance between the client and the problem.

Another way of making distance is by *having the client*, in actual fact or in imagination, "*step back*." For example, the therapist might say, "Leave everything where it is for the moment and take a step back so that you get some distance." Or, when a client speaks predominantly about being flooded, the following metaphor might help: "Can you imagine stepping out of the water for a moment and sitting on the beach looking at the waves instead of drowning in them?" To illustrate this, here is a brief fragment from a therapy session in which the suggestion to "put the problem at some distance" does not work but where having the client "step back" does.

Isabelle is 40 and is working on her fear of dying in her third therapy session. Halfway through the session she gets a stabbing pain around the heart:

CLIENT: There is a terrible pressure here (*indicating her breastbone*); I cannot take it any more . . . It is such a strong counterforce preventing me from living . . . I can hardly go on breathing!

THERAPIST: Could you try to push this counterforce a bit further away?

CLIENT: I wouldn't know how to do that.

THERAPIST: Could you give me an idea of how you experience it? Apart from preventing you from living, how are you getting along underneath it or what sort of feeling does it give you?

CLIENT: It is an enormous, heavy block of concrete on top of me; I don't get any air under there!

THERAPIST: OK. Now I understand that you cannot push away something like that! We'll leave the heavy block where it is, and you may try to imagine that you yourself step back . . . Try to imagine making a step which gets you from under this block. (*Client nods while therapist suggests it; such small bodily signs are an indication that we are on the right track.*)

CLIENT: Yes, that feels good (*deep sigh*) . . . I can breath again (*silence*) . . . and all of a sudden I also see that the block of concrete is my mother who has always prevented me from living!

In case of strong (painful) body sensation, a third way of creating distance may be indicated, namely inviting the client "*to breath around the spot in question.*" Creating a breathing space in the body often provokes a tangible shift in the way the problem is experienced. With a client suffering from serious stomach pain that prevents him from concentrating on anything else, the therapist could suggest, "Let your stomach know that you will take care of it . . . Go around this painful spot with your breath, as if you were putting a soft bandage around it . . . Now try to find out whether this pain needs anything else before you let it rest for a while."

The same way of creating space may also be more firmly indicated than simply "putting it away" in case of something precious or tender facing the client. The client tries to find a good spot in the body for the problem while not coinciding with it any longer. For example, the client who feels an enormous lack in her abdomen after the death of her baby shortly after birth is asked by the therapist, "Could you breathe toward that painful spot in a friendly way . . . Could you make a space with your breath where this lack has a place? . . ." Sometimes this "space" created by breathing may even be imagined concretely by means of a metaphor such as a "cradle" in which "it" can be put down.

A fourth possibility of helping along the process of creating distance from an overwhelming problem consists of the therapist asking the client to make contact with a "*good spot.*" This good spot can be retrieved in fantasy from the client's past and be connected with an experience in which the client can remember feeling very happy—for example, "In my grandparents' garden there was a big tree in which I felt safe." It could also be something which the client simply imagines, such as lying on a beach or being occupied with one's favorite activity like riding a motorcycle (M. McGuire, 1982/83, 1984; McDonald, 1987). From this favorite spot or activity, in which the client finds enough relaxation, the client is then asked to observe the previously overwhelming problems. Similarly, a good spot may be searched for in the body itself, as with a rheumatoid arthritis patient who is totally overwhelmed by pain and is asked to find a spot in her body that does not hurt. She discovers that her face feels good. While keeping her attention on her face, she is able to continue working on her problems without being overwhelmed by pain. This method of concentrating on a good spot and keeping the positive sensations connected to it in the foreground is very helpful in cases of real physical pain. It is even said that experiencing the good spot does not only have a pain-killing effect but also a healing one, for example, with some cancer patients (Kanter, 1982/83; Grindler, 1985).

Whichever way one chooses to create distance, in no event is creating distance the same as "putting the problem away," "forgetting it," or "repressing it." It is rather a friendly search for a good spot for it in consultation with the client's feelings and images. It is an attempt at establishing a better relationship, whereby the client gets space to look at problems instead of coinciding with them and whereby the energy and healing power of the observing self becomes free to face the problems and get a hold of the situation. By extricating oneself from the problem, one gets a better view of the exact nature of the problem (one sees more when not too close by) and becomes capable of taking good care of it when needed. Thus, no longer coinciding with the "hurt child" creates the opportunity for the "adult part" in oneself to care for the "child part." "Those familiar with inner child work will see the similarity. The difference is that there is no need to personify the felt sense as a child. If it feels like a child to the client, that is welcome, but if not, it can still be given gentleness, acceptance and listening" (Weiser Cornell, 1996a, p. 100). "In fact, real progress seems to involve maintaining a part of oneself that is apart from the intensity, and supporting that part as one explores the intense emotion" (Iberg, 1996, p. 24). Only when a state of "having-contact-without-coinciding" is achieved will it become possible to work on the content of the problem.

The therapist helps the client to be *with* the feelings, not *in* them. Focusing works best when the client can "sit next to" his or her feelings instead of plunging into them. Weiser Cornell (1996a, p. 17) gives various tips to facilitate this *being with* instead of letting the client feel engulfed, proposing the use of Inner Relationship techniques instead of Finding Distance techniques (1996b). "Disidentification is often the first step toward establishing the Inner Relationship. The essence of disidentification is to help the client move from 'I am this feeling' to 'I have this feeling.' In most cases, disidentification can be facilitated simply with empathic listening or reflection, in which the therapist adds phrases like 'a part of you' or 'a place in you' or 'something in you'" (Weiser Cornell, 1996b, p. 4). When, for example, the client says, "I am sad," the therapist can slighty change the verbal expression to "You're aware of something in you that feels sad." By this special way of formulating the expression, the client is invited to turn to the content, to get in touch with this content, to establish a relationship between "I" and the content. The content has an explicit part, the part that is already known, already communicable ("sad"), and an implicit part, an aspect that is as yet indefinite, not yet unfolded, which is noted by the therapist by use of the word "something." By saying "in you," the therapist indicates that besides the content, there is an "I" that has a content, that it is not the content, that this "I" is bigger than the content (see also Wiltschko, 1996, pp. 61–

62). Another kind of listening response to help the client stay separate from and in relationship with his or her experience, instead of identifying with the experience, includes in the reflection what the client is doing or experiencing right now, by adding a verb—something like "sensing," "realizing," "noticing," "are aware of," "feeling"—to describe his or her current experience. When, for example, the client states, "It's heavy," the therapist gives the client a place to be with it by reflecting, "You're noticing it's heavy." This *disidentification* is a step toward gentleness: it brings in the possibility of empathy and compassion, and it helps the client to develop a relationship to an inner part.

## Clearing a Space

Even when the client is neither "too close to" nor "too far from" the problems, it may make sense to start with the process of "clearing a space" in order to grant the body openly the time to reveal what it brings along. The client's attention is first given to being seated comfortably and is then turned to the body by following his/her breathing. Then the client asks inwardly, *"How am I right now?* What am I bringing along with me at this moment? What comes to my attention?" Every perception, topic, or feeling coming to the fore is acknowledged. Each is briefly touched upon and given a place without its content being dealt with as yet. This may be done, for example, by naming it out loud, or by writing some aspect of it down as one would on a shopping list, without doing the actual shopping yet. The client may thus put into words those issues that preoccupy him/her, and the therapist reflects them briefly. Here, too, a more forcible effect may be had by writing each topic down and giving the paper an actual place in the therapy room. One can go on with this until one feels sure all worries have been acknowledged and temporarily put down. After all problems have thus been given a suitable place, clients may experience a deep feeling of peace, rest, life energy, and being centered, which may come near to a spiritual/religious/transcendental experience. "Transcendent means moving beyond one's former frame of reference in a direction of higher or broader scope. The transcendent dimension, found in all human beings, involves moving beyond one's own unhealthy egocentricity, duality, and exclusively towards more healthy egocentricity, inclusively, unity and capacity to love" (Hinterkopf, 1996, p. 10). Hence one experiences the satisfaction obtained from practicing this step separately, even if not a single problem is subsequently looked at.

The focusing step of clearing a space is comparable to certain techniques of *meditation*. Attention is shifted from outside to inside, from speaking to silence, from thinking to experiencing, and the body is given the opportunity to bring to the surface what it (often unwittingly) carries along. Everything which comes up is briefly given attention but nothing is dealt with. Then everything is put down, the person extricates him-/herself from the problems, thus creating room for an influx of positive energy and lightness.

This process is in itself a healing one; it creates the experience of a "new me," untouched by difficulties but capable of finding a better way of relating to the person's problems from the position of the observing self.

As a therapist, I find it very useful to go briefly (10 minutes) through this focusing step myself before receiving my clients. This brings me in touch with the various experiences that live in me at the beginning of my work. Any chances of mixing up my own topics with those of the client are thus decreased. It also helps me to put my worries aside so as not to be preoccupied by them when I should be giving my full attention to my clients. I do the same thing at the end of my workday. It helps me to put my client's problems down instead of carrying them home as a big burden. The step of clearing a space may thus be a form of "mental hygiene" for the therapist as well.

The space-clearing phase being completed, one may *choose one problem from the list* to work with, should one wish to do so. This introduces the next process in the focusing movement.

## UNFOLDING THE FELT SENSE

The usual way of gaining access to the felt sense is through a vague bodily sensation, such as a feeling of tension, heaviness, shakiness, pressure in a specific area of the body—throat, chest, stomach, abdomen—or a vague feeling of discomfort tgat is difficult to locate but does not go away.

In the earlier example of Oskar, the client who was initially "too far" from his experience, the client, after letting his attention go through all parts of his body, gets in touch with a feeling of tension in the region of his stomach. We will show here how the therapist assists him in getting in touch with the felt sense in it:

CLIENT: That feeling in the region of my stomach . . . that tension there . . . that is the most powerful.

THERAPIST: There you experience something powerful . . . Why don't you remain there and look what else will come out of it . . .

CLIENT: It wants to jump out of it, as a devil out of a box . . .

THERAPIST: Something wants to jump out . . . *(silence)*

CLIENT: Hate . . . but that would be very unusual for me.

THERAPIST: You hesitate to use the word "hate," but that is what jumps out at you?

CLIENT: Yes, hate . . . that feels powerful . . . that is it.

THERAPIST: Hate . . . that word suits your feeling best . . .

CLIENT: It also gives me power!

THERAPIST: You notice that your hate is accompanied by a feeling of power.

CLIENT: I always withdrew from my friend because he has hurt me so often. (*Client tells about an incident in which he felt deeply humiliated.*)

THERAPIST: You don't want this to happen again . . . Something in you wants to keep facing him with power?

CLIENT: Yes, that feels good . . . that is it . . . (*sighs, sits more relaxed; silence*) . . . This was the last time that I'll give him so much power over me . . . I see him tomorrow and will make it very clear that I won't let myself be pushed aside any more . . . (*Client sits up straight and considers further what he wants to tell his friend.*)

In the above example, the client starts with tension in the region of his stomach and uses the word "powerful" for it. The therapist values this bodily *sensation* by reflecting it and letting the client stay with it, introducing in this way the focusing attitude. Then, more comes up; the meaning unfolds through *symbols/images*, such as "jump out of it," "as a devil out of a box." Again the therapist takes these images over as they are and then leaves room for silence in order to give the internally felt experience time and space to unfold further. Then "hate" comes to the fore, an *emotion* contained in this experience. The therapist leaves the client the time to sense whether the words he uses really correspond to the feeling. The therapist repeats these "handles" literally. This is important since the slightest change in wording may introduce a nuance which no longer corresponds to what the client experiences. When the client sees his expressions mirrored, he can resonate them against his experience in order to see if they reflect it exactly. He can either agree with the expression or correct or complete it. Next, the client establishes the connection with the *situation* which evokes the feelings. He acknowledges that his friend has often hurt and humiliated him. The therapist leaves the client some room to talk about that situation and brings together some elements mentioned earlier by the client. From this the growth step, the "new," emerges, whereupon the client clearly experiences (sigh, relaxation of the body) that something in him is changing. This *felt shift* is a sign that the meaning has been fully expressed and that symbolization of the implicitly felt experience has resulted in an essential step of bodily felt change.

A *full* felt sense usually unfolds through different *components*: (a) bodily sensations; (b) emotions; (c) external situation; and (d) symbols/images. Their order of emergence is not that important. Clients have their own preference for starting with a specific component and for stressing certain elements. A *felt sense comes to completion* by letting the connection between bodily sensations, emotions, external situations, and symbols take place. This process of unfolding results in a feeling of relief, a bodily felt experience of something having been freed, whereby a new surge of energy is felt. Real therapeutic change always carries with it the characteristics of this process.

When the various elements do not unfold spontaneously, the therapist has to *evoke the missing components* in order for the felt sense to become fully present. Often the conversation comes to a halt because the client and therapist remain stuck in the same component(s) long after it (they) has (have) ceased to be productive. A therapist who is alert to (a) missing component(s) is able to lead the stagnating process toward renewed movement.

When the *bodily sensation* is missing, the client can, for example, be helped along by a suggestion such as "Could you try to sense how all that feels in your body?" or "How does your body react to that?" or "Is there a sense in there about . . ."

A client who does have bodily sensations but nothing else may be asked, "Which emotional qualities are present in this sensation? Does it feel like something threatening, or pressing, or pleasant, or which emotional tone does it have?"

The link with the situation in the client's life should always be established if one does not want to get stuck in a series of vague sensations which lead nowhere. The *situation* can be elicited by questions such as "What in your life feels like that?" or "Do you have a feel for what this is about in your life?"

*Symbols* often emerge by themselves. When a client does not find any expressions, the therapist may ask whether certain words, images, colors, shapes, or movements come to the surface (working with drawings, clay, bodily expression, and the like may at this stage be an inviting alternative to a strictly verbal approach, especially with clients who have difficulty finding symbols or who fall back readily into rationalizations; see Leijssen, 1990, 1992, 1996, in press).

The therapist gives the client the opportunity to test whether the expressions of the client or the therapist put "it" accurately:

> Many people are not so clear about the authority their feelings should have over the words that are spoken about them. Some people have an attitude that "if you say so, it must be right." This is especially true for some people who as children were consistently told how they felt. . . . You may detect this problem by watching carefully to see the client's reactions to your 'less than your best' responses. . . . Take the initiative to say something to the effect of "I don't think I got that quite right. It doesn't seem to fit. Did my wording seem incorrect somehow?" In this way you can invite the client to seek more precision of expression, and you model an attitude of respect for the authority of their own experiencing (Iberg, 1996, p. 25)

In the focusing process checking with the body, over and over, all through the session is an important way to look for confirmation of the words from the felt sense of the client. In this *resonating* step we ask the body, "Does this word fit? Is it like this?," or we simply reflect the expression of the client with the implicit invitation to offer it back to the felt experience. During expression, the feeling may change and new expressions may emerge that help the felt sense unfold further. The criterion of accuracy always lies in the client's bodily reactions. The power of the symbol does not only lie in the fact that through it the implicitly felt sense is externalized. Symbols are also *handles*: they contain the whole feeling, which can then be evoked again by means of that expression. Clients often remember the image that accompanied an important shift in their experience and recall it later in order to contact that feeling again.

When the right symbols that fit the experience are found, the client feels a satisfying sense of rightness. This is a *"felt shift"*: a physical sensation of something moving in the way the problem is experienced. There are many kinds of shifts (see Friedman, 1996, pp. 24–25; Weiser Cornell, 1996a, pp. 30–32, 90). On the continuum of *intensities* at the low end there are "small shifts" which may be very minimal, very subtle; one could easily skip over them if one didn't know about them. At the high end the shift is intense, dramatic, obvious; it's a "big shift"—no one would miss it. There are also different *kinds* of shifts: sometimes the client feels a release or a relief in the body (e.g., a sigh, tears); sometimes it is a sharpening of some vague experience or the sense becomes stronger (e.g., a general feeling of confusion becomes a clear feeling of anger); sometimes the client feels something moving from one location in the body to another (e.g., a choking sensation in the throat becomes a warm feeling around the heart); sometimes it is an experience of more energy, excitement, enthusiasm, personal power, or new life awakening and stirring in some parts of the body or the whole body; at other times it's a feeling more of peace, clarity, groundedness, a warm spacious sense of well-being. The client might also have a new insight about an issue, but we consider this only as a felt shift or a new step if the insight doesn't happen only in the mind but is also in some way a bodily felt resolution. As long as a feeling of tension, tightness, confusion, etc. remains (visible in the facial expression, breathing, and posture), elements are still lacking or the proper expression has not yet been found. In that case, a friendly wait for what is still unclear or wants to move forward is indicated.

The therapist may facilitate further exploration by *asking other questions*. The choice of whether or not to use questioning is made on the basis of a feeling that "more news" or a deeper release may be coming from what is implicitly felt. The questions aim at furthering or fully reaching the bodily felt relief which may already partly be present. These are open questions, directed at the felt sense and followed by a waiting time to see what else may emerge from there. Often, as yet unexpected meanings may still come to the fore. One has the choice between various kinds of questions:

1. General questions such as "What is it in all this that makes me feel this way?"; "If 'it' could speak, what would it say?"; "Is there anything else in that feeling that demands attention?"; "Does it want to say more?"; or "What prevents me from fully feeling it?"

2. Specific questions such as "What is the worst in it?"; "What is the most difficult part in it for me?"; "What is the best for me in it?"; "What is the core of that problem?"; or "What is dearest to me in there?"

3. Movement questions such as "What does it need?"; "What might bring relief?"; "What else am I missing in there?"; "How would it look if it were resolved?"; "If I were not stuck with this issue, what could it then become?"; "What actions need to be taken?"; or "If I contact my 'wise place,' what kind of advice would it give me?"

All these questions should be asked in a friendly manner and be introduced with something like "Could you ask that feeling . . ." or "You could try and see whether it wants to answer this. . . ." Asking such questions can be a natural next step if the client seems not to know what to do. The purpose of the questions is to maintain an attitude of friendly interest and respectful curiosity, and to direct attention to what more is there. Asking them implies that the client is the one who can best feel what the next step should be. The "response" from the felt sense takes some time; it can take a minute before it opens up and reveals a new step. "Old information" will be there immediately, but what the felt sense can create is infinitely better, more creative, and far richer than anything the conscious mind of the client (or the therapist) can think up. The questions create a welcome for new ways of being, a new meaning, new action steps. The bodily felt sense does not "have" to give an answer; the questions only provide the opportunity for the inner knowledge to fully open up. Clients may not need such questions. It may then be enough to suggest, "You may remain with it in a friendly way and see if anything else comes up."

The following four *illustrations*, in which each client starts from a different component, will make clear how the full felt sense may unfold in verbal psychotherapy.

## Starting from the Body Sensation

This example comes from the 18th session with Erna, 44:

CLIENT: I feel my heart pounding terribly!

THERAPIST: Something makes your heart pound . . . (*silence*) . . . How is it to feel your heart like that?

CLIENT: (*sigh*) It feels like anxiety, but it isn't anxiety.

THERAPIST: Anxiety isn't the right word . . . Try to remain with the sense of it . . .

CLIENT: It is rather some sort of nervousness . . .

THERAPIST: Something that makes you nervous . . . (*silence*) . . . Have a look and see if that is the word that suits it best . . . whether other words may still emerge?

CLIENT: Tense expectation . . . that is it! My heart pounds like drums announcing something!

THERAPIST: You feel a tense expectation . . . any idea what is being announced? (*silence*)

CLIENT: I know what it is . . . the party I have to go to tomorrow . . .

THERAPIST: That party evokes tension . . .

CLIENT: Now I feel my heart pounding even harder . . . I, ugh . . . I hardly dare admit it, but I'm going there expecting to meet the ideal man . . .

THERAPIST: That makes it exciting! But it isn't a pleasant excitement?

CLIENT: No . . . (*silence*) . . . the excitement is also fear that it will again go wrong . . .

THERAPIST: It wouldn't be the first time that your expectations don't come out . . .

CLIENT: That makes it even more painful . . .

THERAPIST: Could you perhaps ask your body what it would need here in order to relax?

CLIENT: (*silence*; *sigh*) That I simply go to the party and enjoy the company without wondering whether there is a marriageable man around . . .

THERAPIST: Have a look inside and see whether it agrees: simply going to the party without expecting to meet the man of your life . . .

CLIENT: (*laughs*) Then it even looks like it could be fun . . . I know a few people who will be there and that may just do . . . (*sits visibly more relaxed*).

## Starting from Emotions

This example comes from the sixth session with Ivo, 32:

CLIENT: I always feel guilty, ashamed and restless.

THERAPIST: How are you aware of these feelings in your body?

CLIENT: It presses in my chest . . .

THERAPIST: A feeling of pressure . . . as a pressure looking for a way out?

CLIENT: Yes . . . (*silence, blushing shyly*) . . . I even have an image with it of a huge mother's breast with lots of milk . . .

THERAPIST: As if you needed plenty in order to give . . .

CLIENT: Yes, that's it! It suits me so well . . . (*sigh, silence*) . . . when I don't share with others I feel uneasy about what I have.

THERAPIST: It needs to share with others . . . Is there more inside that asks to be noticed? (*silence*)

CLIENT: Yes . . . there is more . . . I notice I am getting sad but don't know what it is.

THERAPIST: Just give it some time to clarify itself . . .

CLIENT: I suddenly think I'll never have children. (*Client is gay.*) I never realized before how much this affects me. That is it! (*deep sigh*)

## Starting from the Situation

Maria, 56, suffers from habitual low self-esteem. In the 23rd session she tells about a situation during a trip where another woman in the group seeks her company. She had advanced several hypotheses as to why this woman should have been interested in her:

THERAPIST: What about taking the time to put aside everything you have thought around that and so to speak develop a fresh feeling on how it is for you, what you sense in your body when you recall the event with this woman on your trip . . .

CLIENT: (*silence*) It is some sort of warmth (*laughing*).

THERAPIST: It gets warm inside of you . . .

CLIENT: Yes, and also . . . a kind of cosy tenderness but . . . very quiet and slow . . .

THERAPIST: Something warm, cosy, tender, quiet . . .

CLIENT: Yes . . . even touching . . . (*silence*) . . . yes, a kind of slowness, as if sitting down on the ground . . . on a clump of clay . . .

THERAPIST: It is touching to encounter yourself as being rooted, which has something slow about it . . .

CLIENT: Yes, and it touches me also that this is allowed . . . here (*sigh*) . . . It was like that too with this woman on my trip! . . . We had similar roots, which isn't what I usually encounter in my environment. (*silence*)

THERAPIST: Perhaps there is more around that which wants to come out . . . Could you ask your feeling whether it would like more or how it wants to proceed? (*silence*)

CLIENT: If I dared, I would let this woman know how great it was with her . . . but I am not sure it wouldn't be too much of an imposition . . .

THERAPIST: Could you first leave some room for that idea . . . How does it feel when you imagine yourself telling her that you found it great? . . . (*silence*)

CLIENT: Exciting . . . in fact, wonderful . . . It also feels wonderful to do that to her.

THERAPIST: It seems like an exciting, wonderful idea . . .

CLIENT: The longer I stop at the thought . . . the nicer it feels . . . oh . . . you don't find me stupid, do you?

THERAPIST: Did you really think so?

CLIENT: Not really . . . It is just that I haven't felt so young in ages . . .

### Starting with Symbols

Rudy, 28, often uses metaphors when speaking. The therapist usually has a hard time at helping him reach a full bodily felt experience. This is the 29th session:

CLIENT: I live with a shadow which I cannot amputate.

THERAPIST: Could you tell a little more about what you experience around that?

CLIENT: Simply that it is always there.

THERAPIST: Something of an unpleasant feeling which you cannot get rid of?

CLIENT: Always something dark that accompanies me.

THERAPIST: What is it in your life that you feel is always with you as something dark? (*silence*)

CLIENT: I don't know if it is that . . . but the first thing that comes to mind . . . is my father's suicide.

THERAPIST: Your father's suicide . . . that feels like a shadow hovering over your life . . . Could you take the time and check whether your body agrees with that? . . . (*silence*)

CLIENT: Yes . . . that has influenced me so much, marked me so badly; I can never undo it . . .

THERAPIST: How do you feel this influence, this mark in your body?

CLIENT: I just feel the lack . . . as if I had no backbone . . . no direction in my life.

THERAPIST: In your body you become aware that your father is missing— no backbone, no direction, you call it . . .

CLIENT: Yes, and his suicide remains present as something dark, like something that is hanging over my head . . . as if I, too, may end up committing suicide . . .

THERAPIST: It hangs over you—you say—and it seems like it is whispering in your ear that suicide is also your final destination. We may have to go further into this soon. But I would first like to ask you: How does it feel there, inside you? (*silence*)

CLIENT: That is a big empty space.

THERAPIST: A big empty space ... where does this feeling mostly sit?

CLIENT: Hmm (*silence*) ... Here in my abdomen mostly (*shows the spot with his hand*).

THERAPIST: Yes, why don't you put your hand on the spot where you mostly feel it ... (*silence*) ... Do other characteristics of this space strike you? (*silence*)

CLIENT: Cold ...

THERAPIST: May I suggest something? Can you try to go into that space with your breath, as if to warm it up with your breath? ... Would you try?

CLIENT: Hmm ... (*silence, deep sigh*) ... that feels good ... as if I were making a little fire in this room ... yes (*smiles*) in this way it could even be a place to come home to ...

The above fragment puts the therapist in a dilemma as to whether to follow the client in the image of what is hanging over his head or to delve further into the inner bodily felt sensations. In this example, the therapist gives priority to "rooting" the client in his own body and promoting there the development of a good spot.

Words coming from the "deeper inner voice" are easily identified: not only do they come from the center of the body, but they also arrive much more slowly, a few at a time, often sounding surprisingly new and sometimes irrational, and most of all producing a feeling of relief and new energy. The difference with "voices coming from outside" is further elaborated in the following section.

## RECEIVING AND DEALING
## WITH INTERFERING WAYS OF REACTING

This process consists of receiving everything that emerges in the experiencing process. In order to give a new experienced element a decent chance, the client has to maintain a friendly, welcoming attitude. Remaining present in an interested and friendly manner does not mean approving or liking everything. The client may, for example, dislike something painful but nevertheless remain friendly toward the part of him-/herself that suffers the pain; or the client may not approve of a solution involving aggressivity toward someone else yet continue to listen with interest. Therapist and client remain attentively present (maintain a focusing attitude) with what is about to be expressed. If a client has a tendency to gloss over something or does not take it in, then the therapist may invite more receptivity by means of suggestions such as "Give yourself some more time to remain with that and to see how it feels, without judging it immediately or fitting it into what you already know."

However, emerging changes and new developments may encounter tough resistances in the client. In focusing terminology, the obstacles most often encountered are called the *inner critic* or *interfering characters*. Gendlin (1996, pp. 247–258) identifies the part that attacks from within and interrupts a person's every hopeful move as "the superego": "The superego absorbs the aggression and violence that the conscious person rejects. . . . Many lovely, sensitive people are inwardly brutalised and oppressed by their superegos. They would never treat others as their superego treats them" (p. 249). He adds, "When thought of as a manner of experiencing, the superego is inherently 'not me.' What we call 'me' pulls back, defends itself, hides, and becomes constricted under the attack" (p. 250).

These "disturbing" ways of reacting demand special attention and guidance as they put the client on a sidetrack and, when they become dominant, lead to an unproductive process. They are ways of reacting that have once helped the client but have now become "structure bound," which means that they show up anytime, whether appropriately or not, regardless of the situation; they perpetuate old patterns of behavior that are no longer adapted to the current situation. Should the therapist not deal with them right away, then the client may keep getting stuck, always in the same way. Recognizing, exploring, and making ineffective such nonhelpful ways of reacting is a complex and often recurring process in which different steps must be taken with the utmost care. The therapist has to intervene actively in order to assist the client in (1) identifying interfering ways of reacting; (2) disidentifying from them; (3) visualizing them or giving them a concrete form or putting a "face" to them; (4) exploring what function they had or still have; (5) assigning a new place to them; and (6) returning to that part of the person that was/is in the grips of the interfering character.

## Identifying Interfering Characters

Interfering ways of reacting can appear as self-criticism, self-doubt, distrust, rationalizations, denying, ridiculing, and so on. They are characterized—and can thus be distinguished from a felt sense—by their predictability and stereotyped expression. For example, they are like a recurring voice saying "Don't be silly," "Be reasonable," "It will fail anyway," "This isn't allowed," "You must be independent," "You're no good at anything," "Be peppy," "That is stupid," "That is not a solution," etc.; or recurring negative thoughts and feelings such as "I am worth nothing," "I was born under an unlucky star," or "Nobody likes me." As Gendlin (1996) put it, "The pattern is characterized by guilt, shame, humiliation, blame, fear, the inability to act freely, the avoidance of competition, the wish to give up one's power, the conviction that one can never get what one needs, the habit of stopping oneself from acting to get what one wants, and many other variants. These avoidances of life and living are related to superego attacks" (p. 256). Also, "The superego . . . has attitudes. It is usually negative, angry, hostile, attacking, mean, petty; it enjoys oppressing a person" (p. 255). Interfering reactions are character-ized by their unfriendly, demanding, humiliating, depressing, nagging, sharp, fast, loud tone of voice, thus smothering or suppressing the softer, more ten-der voice of inner knowledge. They make sure that the client will feel worse; they keep one below one's potential, inhibit one, prevent one from fully liv-ing, or else they let one feel good only after having satisfied their demands. They do not take care of the child's best interest or of its vulnerable or vital aspects, as inner knowledge often does. The difference in manner of speak-ing between the two becomes obvious when a client hesitates, for example, to perform a task and hears the interfering voice say, "You are lazy, you are no good at anything!," whereas the voice of inner knowledge might react in a much friendlier way: "You seem to have a difficult time at this task." The therapist should first and foremost be capable of recognizing the interfering character when it emerges. This being done, the therapist can then choose to leave the interference aside for the time being and direct attention to the more central experience of the still developing felt sense, by trying to get back to what the client was feeling just before the attack. "It comes down to simply bypassing the superego's attack. . . . The main procedure is to move the superego out of the way of the process" (Gendlin, 1996, pp. 257–258). But often this simple strategy doesn't work and more long-range ways to process the inner critic are necessary. The therapist can follow the client in focusing attention on the interfering character while helping the client develop an alternative coping strategy, as will be described in the following steps.

## Disidentifying or Distancing Oneself

A client who is confronted with the voice of an interfering character has to be helped by means of a message or instruction that should enable self-detachment from that voice or should these negative thoughts and feelings to be seen as only a part of the self, not the whole. Simple rephrasing by the therapist may already change the emphasis and invite the client not to coin-cide any longer with the interfering reaction. The client who says, "I hate to be so weak," may hear the therapist reflect, "There is a part of you that does not tolerate the idea of you having weaknesses . . . Could you have a look and see what is in there that wants your attention?"

Apart from naming it "a part" of the person, the therapist may make the disidentification more concrete by asking the client to imagine putting "it" in front of him/herself. In this way, most clients reach an insight fairly quickly. They gradually see something meaningful emerge. Discovering meaning is strongly encouraged by the following step, which usually follows very closely after disidentifying or distancing oneself.

## Putting a "Face" to It, or Giving It a Concrete Form

The client is invited to describe what she/he sees when the critical voice or negative thoughts are put at some distance—whether there is a particular figure, face, person, or shape that fits the image. The client may be asked to draw it or mold it in clay or to get up and portray the character, using her/his whole body. Or, in group therapy, one group member may instruct another to take the role or to keep the character safely away. Usually clients are remarkably responsive in giving a concrete description of the figure that emerges. Such figures may be their real-life parents. Often they are figures that symbolize the severe, hard, and demanding, but also the solid, protecting, and safe, such as schoolteachers, policemen, soldiers, or old aunts. Sometimes the client sees an animal such as a parrot, a snake, or a watchdog, or a more abstract shape such as a block of granite, a high wall, or a waterfall.

## Exploring the Past and Present Function of the Interfering Character

Interfering characters are powerful parts of a person who either were taken over from a parent or important authority figure (introjected parts) or else were created for protection or survival in difficult or painful circumstances (self-protection parts). Many times the interfering characters are unhealed parts of the client that have been cut off from love and acceptance. They often served the important function of helping and protecting the "vulnerable child" or keeping unbearable feelings from emerging but have continued doing so even when no longer required. They do not differentiate nor do they see things in perspective, but they act in an all-or-nothing way. With the therapist's help, the client discovers how the interfering character came into being and how it has served its function. When exploring the interfering character, one first lets it know that one has heard what it has to say. This often allows the client to take a more relaxed attitude toward the "disturbing part." The "good intentions" of the voice or the thoughts are looked for. These will provide additional knowledge about how to tackle the next step.

## Assigning a New Place to It

In the case of introjection of what has been seen at home, clients usually feel relieved quickly when they see through it and they may have few problems letting go of it or putting it aside. A simple instruction from the therapist to put "it" further away or a request to leave "that" out is generally responded to positively. However, when it refers to a part that was created to protect the vulnerable child, the therapist will have to exercise more caution. It would bespeak little respect to simply put aside a part that has been the client's ally. In such cases, acknowledgment of how the interfering character has helped the client is needed first and it makes sense to express gratitude for it. Subsequently, the client will have to decide to what extent that character is still needed; he/she should learn to differentiate between circumstances where the character's protection or help is still required and those in which that same way of reacting may become troublesome. This process mostly consists of a shift of power, the client acquiring the final say over the character rather than remaining in its grip. The client decides again in which circumstances the reaction of a specific character is appropriate.

## Returning to That Part of the Person That Was/Is in the Grip of the Interfering Character

Here the transition is made to the part of the client that was dominated by the interfering character and to how it feels to be in the grip of such a severe, demanding, critical part. Here the question is also asked what the dominated part really needs. Often a great deal of anger or sadness comes to the surface, and the discovery is made that one would like a comprehensive, loving, supportive part instead. It may help some clients to find a metaphor for this substitute, such as a warm comforting mother, a supporting father, a friendly elephant preparing the way, protective wings around oneself, etc.

In clinical practice it may not be possible to separate these various aspects of working with interfering characters as neatly as we have done here. It may not even be necessary to go through all these steps. It is important that the therapist offers alternative ways of reacting to the interfering character instead of letting the client react in his or her structure-bound way. Certain aspects may receive more attention than others, according to the nature and origin of the interfering character. On the one hand, the therapist may have to steer a bit and make sure that the client develops a new kind of interaction; on the other, the therapist should always follow the emerging new meanings and put the authority of what "feels right" with the client.

A few examples of how interfering characters appear during therapy sessions and how the therapist may respond by emphasizing various aspects may illustrate how the above looks in clinical practice. The fragments are reduced to the essential steps of working with a particular disturbance and thus give a simplified picture of what is sometimes a difficult attempt at putting an interfering character at some distance and getting to know it better while keeping it separate from the deeper-lying felt sense which the client carries in him or her.

Brigit, 28, was sexually abused by her father between the ages of 6 and 16. In one therapy session she gets in touch with "a deep feeling of hurt inside." While talking about it, a sharp mocking voice comes up in her, saying: "Don't exaggerate! Are you sure it's true, everything you are telling here?" (step 1). She knows this voice very well because that is the reaction with which she usually erases her feelings. The therapist asks her to put the voice in front of her for a moment (step 2) and see whether she can put a face to it (step 3). Almost immediately the client sees the picture of her mother, who reacted like that every time the young girl tried to inform her of what father did. The therapist now asks the client to put the image of her mother saying such things still further away (step 5) and provides an alternative message: "You felt deeply hurt inside; try to give that more space; let's listen to that some more . . ." (step 6). The client succeeds subsequently in expressing her anger and pain.

Hans, 38, tells how annoyed he is with his partner. He senses anger coming to the surface but immediately cuts the feeling off with "That's not fair toward her, it's not right to be angry with her" (step 1). When the therapist asks him to put in front of him that part of himself that is not allowed to be unreasonable (step 2), he answers, "But that's all of me! I cannot put it in front of me because that is precisely what I am, that reasonable man!"

THERAPIST: You feel you are totally coinciding with that reasonable part . . . As if the unreasonable part were totally pushed away underneath it. Is that how it feels?

CLIENT: Yes, that's right.

THERAPIST: How does that unreasonable little boy feel underneath it? (*step 6*)

CLIENT: In fact, he is very angry but is not allowed to show it. (*Client starts crying.*)

THERAPIST: Go ahead and let the little boy express his anger.

CLIENT: Goddamn, at home nobody was ever angry; only sadness was allowed . . . (*cries again*) . . . I feel so alone.

THERAPIST: When you felt something like anger, you got yourself in an isolated position at home?

CLIENT: No one in the family ever showed anger; mother cried a lot, especially after father's death (*Client was eight at the time.*) . . . and I was seen as the smart, reasonable boy . . . especially after father passed away, I behaved very reasonably . . . Everybody found it great that I, as the eldest, could also support my mother. (*step 4*)

THERAPIST: But, in fact, this boy was also angry at father, at mother? (*step 6*)

CLIENT: I knew I was not supposed to feel it that way because father couldn't help it that he was dead, but nevertheless, yes, I was very angry indeed that he left us to fend for ourselves, and angry at mother because she cried so much; she remained totally stuck in it and kept repeating what a good man he was ... (*deep sigh, silence*) ... I am fed up with being nothing but the reasonable and smart one! This has lasted long enough! (*step 5*) Damn, after all I was only a little boy myself and wanted an ordinary father, not a dead ideal!

Gus, 42, speaks enthusiastically about a new plan that he just came up with. Suddenly his mood changes and he says, "O well, it wouldn't work out anyway." (step 1)

THERAPIST: Where does that suddenly come from?

CLIENT: I always get this. I'm so used to it. I think, "Don't get your hopes up, it won't turn out well anyway!"

THERAPIST: Could you also visualize what comes up then? (*steps 2 and 3*)

CLIENT: In the past, I totally sank away in it, but recently I started noticing because you asked me to, and now it always feels like a parrot sitting on my shoulder pecking at my ear.

THERAPIST: Thus you don't coincide with it any longer, but it keeps bothering you.

CLIENT: Yes, and I can't get it to shut up.

THERAPIST: Could you ask it why it always wants to be with you? (*step 4*)

CLIENT: It pecks exactly at my weak spots ...

THERAPIST: It feeds itself with whatever is vulnerable in you?

CLIENT: It prevents me from being hurt, being disappointed ... It always anticipates that.

THERAPIST: Aha ... it protects you against disappointments ... Could you let it know that you heard exactly that it tries to protect you from being hurt or disappointed?

CLIENT: (*relaxes, silence*) Yes ... but it also prevents me from being enthusiastic; it drags everything down.

THERAPIST: It has ended up with a lot of power.

CLIENT: I just don't have the power to silence it.

THERAPIST: How would you feel about portraying it in clay or in a drawing? (*step 3*)

CLIENT: I could draw it because I see it clearly in front of me.

Therapist gives client a big sheet of paper and colored crayons, and clients starts drawing a parrot. It gives him obvious pleasure to draw it.

CLIENT: Already by drawing it, I start to find it grotesque, not as powerful as I had expected . . . I'll surround it by a cage too . . . And in the margin I'll write—as in a comic strip—all the rubbish it is saying. I find it funny to see it like that, as a comic strip figure . . . (*step 5*)

THERAPIST: Now it feels like you have more power over it?

CLIENT: Yes, I find it ridiculous now.

THERAPIST: Do you still want to keep it, or what would you want to do with it?

CLIENT: In the cage, it's all right. I can put it away when it exaggerates . . . I don't want to get totally rid of it yet because I sometimes find it funny. It has a sense of humor which makes me popular with my colleagues.

In fact, the whole gamut of therapeutic skills is required when one is working with interfering ways of reacting. The client has to feel exceedingly safe in the relationship with the therapist before dismantling an interfering character. Indeed, it is an important defense against interpersonal threat. The therapist should communicate strongly the Rogerian basic attitudes whenever an interfering character comes to the fore; here empathy and respect for both the interfering character and the underlying part of the client are necessary. Interfering characters have often served the function of keeping overwhelming emotions under control; thus, these will come up again once we open up what is hidden under the interfering character. The principle of finding the right distance from the interfering character is an essential element in letting the client work with it without coinciding with it, while nevertheless having enough contact with it to make exploration possible. The different elements with which a felt sense can be completed also apply to exploring an interfering character: an image evoking emotions and bodily sensations comes up and is usually followed by the memory of the situation in which the interfering character originated. The return to the underlying part of the client is also marked by the situation in which that part got suppressed; in the process, certain emotions and bodily sensations come to the fore and often a new image or symbol is called upon which suits the underlying part better. During the whole working process with an interfering character, the therapist's authentic presence is very important: the therapist's solidarity is needed to hold both the powerful interfering character and the deeply hurt "little child"; also the therapist often has to give an authentic and lively counterargument that provides room for the client's healing process.

Remarkably, the sessions devoted to working with an interfering character are always experienced by the client as an *important turning point*. Immediately afterward, mention is made of noticeable changes in the client's life and at the end of therapy, that process is often vividly remembered as a key event of the therapeutic process.

# CONCLUDING REMARKS

In concluding a therapy session, the focusing attitude of taking care of what is present can be emphasized once more. The therapist could, for example, suggest, "Would you let the feeling know that we will end soon and see whether it needs something else before we can end?" When the process is not yet fully completed and session time is up, the session's final experience can be specially highlighted, or an expression which appeared to be very meaningful during the session may be drawn into the foreground—for example, "The expression: 'face him with power' seemed to touch you particularly . . . If you wish, you could hold on to it and try to find out how it goes on from there, or we could return to this next time." Often an image used during the session seems to stick and can be worked with during several sessions.

Sometimes the client is asked to conclude by seeing what wants to be remembered from the session or what in particular wants to be taken home. In this validation process, the road covered during the session is sometimes briefly gone over to help the client internalize the therapeutic events and use the therapeutic tools for him-/herself. Attention should also be given to helping the client preserve a friendly attitude toward the process once the session is over. For that purpose, a metaphor can sometimes be used. Thus, when something vulnerable remains present with the client at the end of the session, the therapist may suggest that the client carry it along with him/her as "a child in a carrier," or something precious may be taken along in a "jewel box." New material emerging at termination is no longer dealt with, but the client may be assisted in providing a good place for it where it can wait until later. Finally, it may make sense to say a word of appreciation for the process which just took place, even though only a small step has as yet been made.

By now the reader will have become well aware of the fact that focusing consists of a multitude of complex processes. In practice, the therapist should not try to review all the steps with the client because this generally would result in overlooking what the client really needs. It is, however, important for the therapist to be in full command of the microprocesses in order to refer to them should the client's process require it to do so. The spirit of working in focusing-oriented therapy can thus be described:

> We do not abandon the client-centered axiom that the client is the final authority about what is "really" going on. . . . I hope to guide the client to more effective introspection. Ideally the interaction should be nondirective: the client makes improvements, rather than being directed to do so by the therapist. The specific method I use to minimize directiveness is a two step approach. The first step is a simple empathic reflection of the event. . . . The second step may not be needed, since when a process event is well reflected, the problem may resolve itself. . . . If the client does

not find an improvement in the process, I then make guiding suggestions. . . . The kind of process improvement in question here is evaluated by the client. . . . I recommend reaching a confirmed understanding of a process event to give the improvement every chance to come spontaneously from within the client, but if it does not, I make a suggestion, rather than letting the client proceed oblivious to a small change which might bring improvement. (Iberg, 1996, pp. 22–23)

Adding focusing suggestions may be totally consistent with the way many therapists are already working, or it may represent somewhat of a shift in attitude and language:

The combination of any therapeutic method with Focusing is not as easy as it seems at first glance, because the point with Focusing is not the technique but rather specific Focusing attitudes, and they cannot be achieved so easily. . . . A Focusing therapist is in contact with his/her body, with his/her bodily resonance, the felt sense, about the whole person of the client, the client's ongoing experiencing and self-expressing. This is because all therapeutic "techniques" emerge from this implicit resonance. The therapist's felt sense is the source of Focusing Therapy techniques (provided that the therapist is exactly perceiving the client's verbal and non-verbal expression). These "techniques" are not only listening and guiding methods but also *authentic responses* towards the client's person. (Wiltschko 1995, pp. 2, 6, emphasis in original)

Moreover, "Focusing-oriented therapy is not therapy that includes brief bits of focusing instruction. Rather, it means letting that which arises from the focusing depths within a person define the therapist's activity, the relationship, and the process in the client" (Gendlin, 1996, p. 304). In a focusing process the therapist models and repeatedly encourages the client to listen with friendly attention to him-/herself and to take care of what emerges from his/her felt sense. In this way, the client gradually learns to take over the therapist's task and to acquire the attitudes by which he/she can become his/her very own therapist.

## REFERENCES

Armstrong, M. C. (1993). Sexual abuse, dissociation and multiple personality disorder. *The Folio: A Journal for Focusing and Experiential Psychotherapy, 12*(2), 35–43.

Friedman, N. (1995). *On focusing: How to access your own and other people's direct experience.* (Available from the author, Arlington, MA).

Gendlin, E. T. (1964). A theory of personality change. In P. Worchel & D. Byrne (Eds.), *Personality change* (pp. 100–148). New York: Wiley.

Gendlin, E. T. (1968). The experiential response. In E. Hammer (Ed.), *Use of interpretation in therapy* (pp. 208–227). New York: Grune & Stratton.

Gendlin, E. T. (1981). *Focusing* (rev. ed.). New York: Bantam.

Gendlin, E. T. (1984). The client's client: The edge of awareness. In F. R. Levant & J. M. Shlien (Eds.), *Client-centered therapy and the person-centered approach: New directions in theory, research and practice* (pp. 76–107). New York: Praeger.

Gendlin, E. T. (1990). The small steps of the therapy process: How they come and how to help them come. In G. Lietaer, J. Rombauts, & R. Van Balen (Eds.), *Client-centered and experiential psychotherapy in the nineties* (pp. 205–224). Leuven, Belgium: Leuven University Press.

Gendlin, E. T. (1996). *Focusing-oriented psychotherapy: A manual of the experiental method*. New York: Guilford Press.

Gendlin, E. T., Beebe, J., Cassens, J., Klein, M., & Oberlander, R. (1968). Focusing ability in psychotherapy, personality and creativity. In J. M. Shlien (Ed.), *Research in psychotherapy* (Vol. 3, pp. 217–241). Washington, DC: American Psychological Association.

Grindler, D. (1985). Research perspectives on "clearing a space" with someone who had cancer. *The Focusing Folio*, 4(3), 98–124.

Hendrics, M. N. (1986). Experiencing level as a therapeutic variable. *Person-centered Review*, 1, 141–162.

Hinterkopf, E. (1996). A process definition of spirituality: Implications for focusing therapy. *The Folio: A Journal for Focusing and Experiential Therapy*, 15(1), 9–12.

Iberg, J. R. (1981). Focusing. In R. J. Corsini (Ed.), *Handbook of innovative psychotherapies* (pp. 344–361). New York: Wiley.

Iberg, J. R. (1996). Finding the body's next step: Ingredients and hindrances. *The Folio: A Journal for Focusing and Experiential Therapy*, 15(1), 13–42.

Kanter, M. (1982/83). Clearing a space with four cancer patients. *The Focusing Folio*, 2(4), 23–27.

Klein, M. H., Mathieu-Coughlan, P., & Kiesler, D. J. (1986). The experiencing scales. In L. S. Greenberg & W. M. Pinsof (Eds.), *The psychotherapeutic process: A research handbook* (pp. 21–71). New York: Guilford Press.

Leijssen, M. (1990). On focusing and the necessary conditions of therapeutic change. In G. Lietaer, J. Rombauts, & R. Van Balen (Eds.), *Client-centered and experiential psychotherapy in the nineties* (pp. 225–250). Leuven, Belgium: Leuven University Press.

Leijssen, M. (1992). Experiential focusing through drawing. *The Focusing Folio*, 11(2), 35–40.

Leijssen, M. (1996). Characteristics of a healing inner relationship. In R. Hutterer, G. Pawlowsky, P. F. Schmid, & R. Stipsits (Eds.), *Client-centered and experiential psychotherapy: A paradigm in motion* (pp. 427–438). Vienna: Lang.

Leijssen, M. (in press). Focusing: Interpersonal and intrapersonal conditions of growth. In B. Thorne & E. Lambers (Eds.), *Person-centred therapy: A European perspective*. London: Sage.

Mathieu-Coughlan, P., & Klein, M. H. (1984). Experiential psychotherapy: Key events in client-centered interactions. In L. N. Rice & L. S. Greenberg (Eds.), *Patterns of change: Intensive analysis of psychotherapy process* (pp. 213–248). New York: Guilford Press.

McDonald, M. (1987). Teaching focusing to disturbed, inner city adolescents. *The Focusing Folio*, 6, 29–37.

McGuire, K. (1993). Focusing inner child work with abused clients. *The Folio: A Journal for Focusing and Experiential Psychotherapy, 12*(2), 17–33.

McGuire, M. (1982/83). "Clearing a space" with two suicidal clients. *The Focusing Folio, 2*(1), 1–4.

McGuire, M. (1984). Part II of an excerpt from: "Experiential focusing with severely depressed suicidal clients." *The Focusing Folio, 3*(3), 104–119.

Müller, D. (1995). Dealing with self-criticism: The critic within us and the criticized one. *The Folio: A Journal for Focusing and Experiential Psychotherapy, 14*(1), 1–9.

Rice, L. N. (1984). Client tasks in client-centered therapy. In R. F. Levant & J. M. Shlien (Eds.), *Client-centered therapy and the person-centered approach: New directions in theory, research and practice* (pp. 82–202). New York: Praeger.

Rogers, C. R. (1961). *On becoming a person.* Boston: Houghton Mifflin.

Weiser Cornell, A. (1993). *The focusing guide's manual.* Berkeley, CA: Focusing Resources.

Weiser Cornell, A. (1996a). *The power of focusing.* Oakland, CA: New Harbinger.

Weiser Cornell, A. (1996b). Relationship = distance + connection: A comparison of inner relationship techniques to finding distance techniques. *The Folio: A Journal for Focusing and Experiential Therapy, 15*(1), 1–8.

Wiltschko, J. (1995). Focusing therapy: Some basic statements. *The Folio: A Journal for Focusing and Experiential Therapy, 14*(3), 1–12.

Wiltschko, J. (1996). Focusing therapy. II: Some fragments in which the whole can become visible. *The Folio: A Journal for Focusing and Experiential Therapy, 15*(1), 55–78.

# 7

*****

# Interpersonal Processes

## Wim van Kessel
## Germain Lietaer

### RELATIONAL CHANGE PROCESSES

Opinions about how and to what extent the therapist–client relationship influences the client's process of change vary among basic therapeutic paradigms as well as among subdivisions within paradigms (Clarkson, 1995). This also applies to the "experiential family" where the views of, say, Carl R. Rogers, Frederick S. Perls, and Alvin R. Mahrer are in certain respects quite different. What we intend to discuss in this chapter will thus inevitably be colored by our own therapeutic background. We both see ourselves as therapists of client-centered denomination, be it with slightly different "added affinities": for the first author a predominantly psychodynamic one; for the second an experiential–existential one. In this chapter, we intend to focus on the ways in which the here-and-now client–therapist interaction is explicitly explored and worked through on a metacommunicative level. However, by way of introduction, we will first mention certain other forms of interpersonal impact and describe how the interactional point of view has gradually staked a claim within the evolution of client-centered therapy.

#### The Relationship as Context and as "Tacit" Interpersonal Healing Process

When the central role of the relationship in client-centered therapy is pointed out, reference is usually made, first and foremost, to the Rogerian basic attitudes, which are meant to provide a safe *context* for in-depth self-exploration. Indeed, these "therapist conditions" form the first part of Rogers's process equation: "The more the client perceives the therapist as real or genuine, as empathic, as having an unconditional regard for him, the more the client will move away from a static, unfeeling, fixed, impersonal type of functioning and the more he will move toward a way of functioning which is marked by a fluid, changing, acceptant experiencing of differentiated personal feelings" (1961, p. 42). We see this contextual influence as comprising three layers. First, as crucial ingredients of the relational bond, the Rogerian basic attitudes exercise an appreciable influence on what the client can let seep through in his pre-explicit experiencing. Secondly, they offer the client the support and safety needed to communicate and explore openly what is present at a felt-sense level. Thirdly, the therapist conditions and the responses that spring from them guarantee a constructive run of the client's exploration process. It is perhaps this three-way influence that causes the working alliance to be the most powerful predictor of therapeutic success in all orientations (Horvath & Greenberg, 1994; Gelso & Carter, 1994; Orlinsky, Grawe, & Parks, 1994).

Apart from that, the therapeutic relationship not only functions as a context or a condition for other task-oriented therapeutic processes but also serves as *medium* for corrective interpersonal processes: the client lives in the here-and-now relationship with the therapist, something that breaks through previously established interpersonal patterns (see, e.g., Yalom, 1980). Contrary to past experience, clients may, for instance, feel that the therapist really believes in their capacities, that their experience is taken quite seriously, that they are not rejected when expressing aggressive feelings, that their therapists remain stable when they express feelings of despair, that their limits are respected and so on. Rogers repeatedly refers to this process in his therapy comments; thus he describes as a crucial therapeutic moment the time when Jim Brown is able to allow the therapist's warm concern:

> In this relationship there was a moment of real, and I believe irreversible, change. Jim Brown, who sees himself as stubborn, bitter, mistreated, worthless, useless, hopeless, unloved, unlovable, *experiences* my caring. In that moment his defensive shell cracks wide open, and can never again be quite the same. When someone *cares* for him, and when he feels and experiences this caring, he becomes a softer person whose years of stored up hurt come pouring out in anguished sobs. He is not the shell of hardness and bitterness, the stranger to tenderness. He is a person hurt beyond words, and aching for the love and caring which alone can make him human. (1967, p. 411; emphases in original)

Together with this kind of corrective interpersonal experience, a process of internalization of the therapist attitudes takes place. Rogers describes the consequences of an empathic climate as follows. "Thus, the persons have become, in their attitudes toward themselves, more caring and acceptant, more empathic and understanding, more real and congruent. But these three elements are the very ones that both experience and research indicate are the attitudes of an effective therapist" (1975, p. 9). We find the same thought in the concluding remarks of Mia Leijssen's Chapter 6 (on focusing microprocesses, in this volume): "In a focusing process the therapist models and repeatedly encourages the client to listen with friendly attention to him-/ herself and to take care of what emerges from his/her felt sense. In this way, the client gradually learns to take over the therapist's task and to acquire the attitudes by which he/she can become his/her very own therapist." We believe this to be a very essential form of personality change, albeit mostly a "silent" one, that is, one which is not explicitly talked about in the verbal interaction.

## The Relationship as an Arena for Explicit Interactional Work

Besides functioning as the context and as the silent medium for corrective interpersonal experiences, the client–therapist relationship can also function as an open arena in which to explore explicitly the client's interactional style. This process occupies a central position primarily within the interpersonal wing of psychodynamic psychotherapy; but it has gradually come to be seen as an important process by other orientations as well, certainly those with integrationistic tendencies (e.g., Anchin & Kiesler, 1982; Andrews, 1991; Safran, 1993; Safran & Segal, 1990; Teyber, 1992; Yalom, 1995). Although the concrete treatment procedures by which this interactional perspective is given shape may differ from one orientation to the next, the nuclear identity of this approach may nevertheless be described in a few general terms:

- The aim of this sort of treatment is to have clients recognize that their complaints are related to their own typical way of relating to others.
- The psychotherapeutic process consists of clients acquiring a larger margin of freedom to vary their way of relating by acquiring more insight into, and more recognition of, their own specific way of relating and of the appeal to others persons that results from it.
- Because the client is mostly not conscious of these ways of interacting, the words "insight" and "recognition" should be read here as ways of becoming conscious. This is achieved by means of metacommunication.
- The medium through which to achieve this consciousness is the therapeutic relationship. In it, the client not only reports about his/her way of interacting with others but also demonstrates his/her specific preferred style in the relationship with the therapist, thus making it visible to both client and therapist.

The option to "preferentially" treat the client's problems within the here-and-now relationship with the therapist has only reluctantly been granted a place in the evolution of client-centered therapy. This initial reticence had, we believe, two reasons. First, the process smelled all too much of the psychoanalytic process of working through the transference. Rogers always refused to view this process as the "pure gold" of therapy. He was opposed to any attitude resembling a "blank screen" but rather emphasized the importance of the real relationship as a healing factor and believed that the client's transference reactions did not require special treatment: "The client-centered therapist's reaction to transference is the same as to any other attitude of the client: he endeavours to understand and accept" (Rogers, 1951, p. 203). John M. Shlien even goes a step further by claiming that "transference is a fiction invented and maintained by therapists to protect themselves from the consequences of their own behavior" (1987, p. 15). This extreme position, which we also find in Szasz (1972), is not shared by many. Or, as Gendlin says,

> If the client is a troubled person, he cannot possibly fail to rouse difficulties in another person who relates closely with him. He cannot possibly have his troubles all by himself while interacting closely with the therapist. Necessarily, the therapist will experience his own version of the difficulties, twists, and hang-ups which the interaction must have. And only if these do occur can the interaction move beyond them and be therapeutic for the client. (1968, p. 222)

So, even in client-centered therapy, the client repeats his past in the present relationhip with the therapist. The question remains, however, whether or not to give priority in principle to working through a problem in the here-and-now relationship with the therapist. And here opinions differ. Rice, for example, believes the vividness of the experience of a certain type of problem to be the criterion for deeper self-exploration, and not the position of the experience in the triangle "here–elsewhere–in the past":

> In a real sense, any member of a [problem] class is as worthwhile exploring as any other. Neither the past nor the present has priority, but rather the vividness with which an experience can be recounted by the client. After all, the more vividly an experience is recounted, the more likely it is to be an experience that is emotionally important to the client. More adequate processing of any one experience should lead to more adaptive responses in a whole range of specific situations. (1974, p. 303)

In Rice's view, working through the transference reaction in the here and now is not a *must* but a possibility, a subprocess among others. Other authors, on the contrary, show a marked preference for this process: thus Carkhuff added "immediacy" to the Rogerian therapeutic conditions (1969, Vol. 1, p. 38, and Vol. 2, p. 94ff.); van Kessel (1975), van der Linden and van Kessel (1991), and Kiesler (1982, 1988) all made a clear choice for the interactional approach. This is not to say that they disagree with Rice—quite the contrary. They believe, however, that the immediacy of the therapeutic relationship guarantees a maximum of vividness if anxiety does not interfere too much.

Another source of initial reticence had to do with the therapist's more directive position in interactional therapy, a position in which the therapist is not only following but also steering. There is, first of all, a selective attention to the interactional aspect of the messages conveyed in the client–therapist interplay. This was felt to clash to a degree with the principle that the client him-/herself should determine the session content. Besides, the metacommunication about the here-and-now interaction implies a number of interventions originating largely from the therapist's own frame of reference: feedback, confrontation, interpretation, and self-disclosure. These interventions clashed with the basic principle of client-centered therapy, which is to stay within the client's frame of reference on a *continuous* basis. Between 1955 and 1962, however, an important shift occurred: client-centered therapy evolved from a "nondirective" to an "experiential" approach (Lietaer, 1997). What was not allowed on account of the nondirectivity principle—the so-called *don't* rules—now disappeared into the background and emphasis was put on what really mattered: "maximizing the client's experiential process, using our own to do so" (Gendlin, 1970, p. 549). Now the therapist was "allowed" to bring in something from his/her own frame of reference as long as he/she steadfastly kept returning to the client's experiential track. This made client-centered therapy more interactional: the therapist was no longer just an alter ego but became a separate pole of interaction who, at certain moments, could present his/her own here-and-now experience to the client (Finke, 1994; Lietaer, 1993; Lietaer, Rombauts, & Van Balen, 1991; Van Balen, 1990; Pfeiffer, 1995; Tscheulin, 1990).

In the following section (and its subsections) we will describe, from a theoretical point of view, the core ingredients of this interactional process as it can be assimilated into the experiential paradigm. Later, a third major section ("Clinical Guidelines") will be devoted to the differences between the experiential and psychodynamic orientation concerning the working-through process of "transference reactions" and to how the therapist's interactional work can be embedded in the Rogerian attitudes.

## THE INTERACTIONAL PROCESS: CORE INGREDIENTS

The fundamental axiom of the interactional process may be described as follows: there is a mutual link between a person's psychological problems and complaints, on the one hand, and his/her specific approach to others around him/her, on the other. A client's problematic style of interaction differs from that of other people by being one-sided and incongruent in its communication and by the fact that this pattern is kept going by selective attention to, and influencing of, the other. Hence we have the question of how a client's conversation with the therapist differs from his/her everyday conversation with others. In other words, how does the therapist steer clear of following the client's preferred style of interaction in a complementary way? Indeed, should the therapist do this, nothing new would happen in therapy and the therapeutic dialogue would serve no other purpose than to reinforce the client's preferred interactional style and, insofar as this style is instrumental in perpetuating the client's typical complaints, would contribute to perpetuate these as well.

There are four *specific* characteristics of the therapeutic dialogue that may prevent this from happening, characteristics that set apart the therapeutic dialogue from the everyday one and that constitute the very moments within the therapeutic process which are likely to generate change in the client. We will now discuss these characteristics one by one and point out how Rogers's basic therapeutic conditions can be understood in the light of each of them.

## First Moment: Reversing the Priority between Levels of Communication

In human communication, the content aspect—exchange of information—may be distinguished from a level at which suggestions are given about the relational position of each of the conversation partners. The first level, exchange of information, clearly takes precedence in everyday conversation while the interactional aspect generally remains in the background and undiscussed, mainly because signals about the desired type of relationship are given in nonverbal ways (Bateson, 1972; Watzlawick, Beavin, & Jackson, 1967). The therapist will, however, try to reverse the importance of these two levels and not primarily pay attention to the communication content but rather to the signals defining the relationship between the client and him-/herself.

When a client, for instance, opens a conversation by saying in an accusing tone of voice, "I find you don't help me much with my problems," the therapist will not respond to the content and defend him-/herself or explain that, at the moment, he/she is not able to help any more than he/she does. He/she may rather pick out the client's accusing tone of voice and suggest that she/he may feel small and powerless in contrast with the powerful therapist who refuses to meet her/him halfway. By clarifying and explicating the client's feelings and by making explicit their relative positions as perceived by the client, the therapist gives priority to the interactional over the content aspect of the communication.

This example may create the impression that the content aspect of the client's conversation is of no importance in therapy. This would, however, be an overstatement. The therapist does pay attention to the client's tales such as those concerning her/his relationships with others, her/his role in these relationships, or her/his feelings about others and the outcome of the interaction. Special attention will be paid, however, to eventual parallels between the described relationships and what the therapist sees and feels in the present therapeutic situation.

Giving priority to relationship aspects means that the therapist will listen to the content of the stories in a special way, namely, with special attention to the interpersonal connotations in the content. Thus, when a client reveals secret aspects of her/his sexual fantasies, the therapist will not only pay attention to the content of these fantasies but also to the fact that the client is now able to tell him/her about them. He/she may understand them as a sign of increasing trust or as a seductive maneuver using erotic material. Something similar applies to a client relating dreams: not only is information about the dream content revealed but also, for example, the fact that the client is now capable of relinquishing some control within the relationship; indeed, she/he may sense that, by telling the dream, she/he is revealing more than she/he is aware of.

There is yet another way in which the content may reveal something about the relationship. We refer here to the power of reference in the client's content: thus, when a client expresses, say, dissatisfaction with her/his family physician, the therapist should be aware of the fact that this *may* imply an indirect underlying reference to the present therapeutic relationship.

Another description of the same basic therapeutic attitude is given by Sullivan's description (1953) of his own role as participant observer in a dialogue: the therapist is not only supposed to participate as a conversation partner but should be attentive to his/her own feelings and observations in relation to the conversation and the client. This means that he/she will not only lend an ear to the content expressed by the client but will simultaneously observe his/her own reactions as a listener: whether he/she feels invited to agree, provoked into opposition, moved by pity, or incited to give advice, say. To put it differently, the observing attitude is directed at the interpersonal aspects of the dialogue, which thus become the focus of attention.

## Second Moment: The Therapist Avoids Reinforcing the Client's Habitual Style of Interaction

The client's typical style of communication calls for a response from the other which will allow this typical form of communication to continue: the "complementary opposition." By adopting a noncommittal stance in the therapeutic dialogue, the therapist creates room for him-/herself to steer clear of the role that the client is trying to force on him/her by means of her/his own interactional slant in which the client almost "trains" her/his conversation partners. Instead of responding to the client's appeal and playing along, the therapist tries to find out what sort of appeal is being made here and how the client is trying to get the other, that is, him-/herself, hooked. The therapist does this by trying to feel what role he/she has been pushed into and not responding to the appeal made. He/she may instead opt for a certain amount of metacommunicative explication about this role appeal. Such a noncomplementary intervention produces a certain degree of anxiety and confusion in the client because it upsets the stereotyped style of interaction that she/he desperately wants to hold onto. Beier (1966, p. 55ff) has called this therapeutic attitude "asocial reaction." He speaks in this respect of *bene-*

*ficial uncertainty*, which indicates, on the one hand, the presence of enough tension and uncertainty in the conversation to stimulate the client to reflect and, on the other, the absence of incapacitating anxiety by which the client would no longer be capable of reflection.

When the therapist upsets the client's habitual style of interaction, the client may be expected to oppose this and show "resistance." We doubt that this resistance can be avoided in therapy. Even the so-called facilitating therapeutic conditions do not always seem to have an anxiety-lowering effect; in fact, they may even have an anxiety-enhancing effect. Thus, a very controlled norm-setting young woman admits feeling ill at ease with the therapist's permissive and accepting attitude: "Because you accept without reservation all these strange thoughts and feelings of mine, I feel I'll end up having no norms of good and bad myself and will allow myself just anything." The dependent client states that she feels well understood but protests against the lack of instructions from the therapist and against being held responsible for what she thinks and feels by the therapist. Just because the therapist fails to honor the rigid setup, the client may hold onto it even more firmly. The therapy situation often magnifies the client's specific patterns; thus an intervention that may at first look counterproductive may in fact be quite effective because it "artificially" magnifies the client's specific behavior and thus makes it more available for discussion.

Similarly, the therapist should guard against responding with a "counterattack" to a client who is picking a fight but will instead try to discuss the provocative character of such action. He/she will do well not to respond to a client's dependent silence by taking the initiative him-/herself and will not go along with the *social talk* in which another client will engage in order to play down or avoid the seriousness of her/his problems (Sachse, 1997). Instead of giving the socially expected response, the therapist will endeavor to answer in a surprising and unexpected way that will make it difficult for the client to continue her/his habitual communication pattern. These examples are intended to show that the asocial aspect of a therapeutic reaction is not only made up of what is explicitly said; even in his/her preverbal attitude the therapist frustrates the client in her/his rigid way of setting up the situation.

It is especially this "asocial" element in the approach to the client that has given interactional thought the dubious fame of being a set of manipulative strategies that lack all respect and acceptance of the client (and her/his suffering) and cause her/his resistance against change to increase. It is no doubt true that such an attitude on the part of the therapist will frustrate the client, but it may, we believe, also speak of trust in the client's capacity to transcend her/his limited style of interaction and to communicate with others in a more all-round and consistent way. By transmitting this trust to the client, the therapist will strengthen the cooperative relationship based on mutual respect, and the resistance that her/his asocial reactions are likely to elicit may become nameable and workable. However, establishing and maintaining such a cooperation contract is, we believe, essential in any form of uncovering psychotherapy and is not specific to the interactional approach. Therefore we only mention it in passing in response to an often-heard criticism on this working method.

## Third Moment: Elucidating the Interactional Pattern

The client creates her/his own interactional scenarios with the therapist, and (as said earlier) these will be characterized by communicative one-sidedness and contradiction. These scenarios constitute the point of departure for elucidation in an interactional perspective. To the client, they have their own logic and obviousness. But as we have already mentioned in discussing Beier (1966), the therapist's attitude is likely to create an uncertainty that leads the client to self-questioning about this logic and obviousness and makes her/him receptive to any new meaning which she/he or the therapist may give to it. Traditionally, client-centered thinking has limited the therapist's role to providing the right conditions for the client to give new meaning to the experiences her-/himself. We believe however that renewal that originates in the client is always limited. The stronger the reliance on a stereotyped style of interaction and the more fixed one's experience of oneself or the other, the more a therapist will be needed in order to arrive at new meaning.

Because the therapist does *not* allow to happen what repeats itself over and over in everyday interaction, room for interpretation is created within the therapeutic dialogue. When a therapist helps a client see what she/he evokes or elicits in others, the client may come to recognize that this attitude is not only limited to her/his specific interaction with the therapist but how it has become a familiar repetitive pattern with others as well. The therapist here uses his/her own feelings as a compass; by always consulting his/her own experience about the interaction, he/she is able to assess the communicative value of the client's interactional behavior, its one-sidedness, and its contradictions.

This is also the moment at which the "interactional analysis of the complaint" may acquire a meaning for the client and at which she/he may recognize that her/his problems and symptoms are not mere accidents with irreducible meanings but are directly related to, and play their role in, a one-sided and contradictory way of interacting with others. The therapist may further illustrate this by examples of similar incidents taken from the client's story or by earlier incidents within therapy. In doing this, he/she will repeatedly make the link between what "happens" now in therapy and what "happens" outside of therapy in relationship with others, and will show the client how she/he plays an essential role in such "happenings."

Although authors like Watzlawick et al. (1967) emphasize that the factual course of interactions can be sufficiently understood from the present behavior of the person in question—as a move in a chess game may be understood from the actual configurations of the pieces—it will almost always be necessary to also bring the client's past into the interpretation, and more particularly her/his relationship with key figures from the past. When we look at how a social system actually functions, it is easy to understand how the interaction between the various players keeps them imprisoned in their roles. Nevertheless, the game as such does not explain why each player with her/his own preferential role has entered it. The more firmly she/he holds onto her/his role, the more the question arises of how she/he has made that social role her/his own. Here we touch upon the question of the past, of the social antecedents that have formed her/him. By elucidation of these historical roots the experience of what seems to repeat itself over and over in the here and now acquires more substance and a greater obviousness. It not only shows the client her/his own specific contribution to the stereotyped course of her/his communication with others but may also get her/him to track down the reason why she/he got into it and what she/he avoids by it. By interpreting her/his present interaction pattern as a repetition of something which she/he acquired through past interactions, the client may start considering the possibility that her/his typical style of interacting may no longer be necessary—that it could be different. This gives her/him room to experience the therapist and others in a new way and thus approach them differently.

When an adult woman is able to recognize that her depressive mother never paid proper attention to her story and that she had to replace her absent father as the recipient of her mother's worries and complaints, it may be readily understood that, on the basis of her experience, she will still hesitate to appeal to others and ask or expect something from them. Her difficulties with her partner who has "a thousand hobbies" but pays no attention to her, and the fact that at work she feels she should always be ready for others, by whom she then feels abused—all this comes to appear in a new light when the link with the past is made. And the same goes for her persistent feeling of boring the therapist and the belief that "of course he wouldn't know what to do about her attacks of migraine either." By making it clear to her (i.e., interpreting) that up to the present she experiences people in the same way as she experienced her mother, but that other people are not her mother, a possibility is created to arrive at new meanings.

The avoidance aspect that may play an important role in any stereotyped interaction may often be poignantly revealed by the exploration of past interactions. What a child has repeatedly experienced as impossible and unreachable in relationships with key figures may have come to be seen, little by little, as unknown and hence unsafe, something that may have caused the longing to be no longer felt and thus be "excommunicated." The stereotypical interaction has then acquired a protective function and makes it possible to avoid and escape from the unknown and hence unsafe range of interactions. Because the therapist confronts the present situations—in and out of the therapy room—with the past ones, the client may become more sensitive to this avoidance aspect and may get to see how her/his behavior may prevent others from reacting in a certain way. She/he may come to see how avoidance has caused these reactions to become threatening and may come to feel that, in this way, she/he is also missing out on something which she/he "deep down" needs and wants. Of course, such an "unknown longing" also manifests itself as built into the incongruence of the present communications but will often be demonstrated more clearly by a confrontation with the past.

In summary, it may be said that the interactional scenario proposed by the client and in which she/he tries to involve the therapist will be stripped of its obviousness along four different lines of approach and may thus acquire a new meaning for the client. First, the therapist chooses his/her own feeling as a compass to decode the appeal contained in the client's behavior. Secondly, he/she sensitizes the client to the fact that her/his complaints serve a function in the one-sidedness and contradiction that characterize the communicative aspect of the scenario. Thirdly, the client shows that the scenario which she/he tries to establish with the therapist presents similarities with her/his attitude toward others about whom she/he talks. And, finally, the therapist makes clear that the scenario contains anachronistic elements, which means that the present, while allowing the creation of such a scenario, is— contrary to the past—no longer requiring it as the only possible, logical, or obvious choice.

### Fourth Moment: The Therapeutic Relationship as a Medium for Generating Change

From the interactional point of view, psychotherapy is seen as a process of social influencing in which the client–therapist relationship is used as a medium for diagnostic elucidation and therapeutic change. Both these aspects are, we believe, intimately linked, as should be clear from the description above. Because the client starts to realize that she/he chooses a certain attitude in her/his relationship with the therapist and other people around her/him that largely predetermines and limits the possible responses by others, a feeling will ipso facto arise that a different attitude toward others might well be a possibility. This widening of possibilities is underlined by the fact that the client's pattern of interaction acquires the meaning of holding on to a way of behaving that was originally motivated by interactions with key figures from the past. The client's courage to start operating outside the stereotypical style of interaction will probably grow in proportion to her/his recognition of the fact that this typical attitude toward others perpetuates the problems from which she/he suffers and limits unnecessarily her/his possible experiences.

So, the desired therapeutic changes are already prepared during the diagnostic process, in the sense that the client may acquire the motivation to work on changing. The therapist validates the effectiveness of his/her interventions in this area by being sensitive to signs of increasing willingness to open up to different attitudes toward others. Thus a dependent client who has been annoyed at the therapist for not giving specific instructions, starts to get the idea that she/he can make choices in life, thereby validating the interpretations that the therapist has made about her/his dependency.

Hence, the therapist's asocial reaction should not only be seen as frustrating, as said earlier—because it blocks the client's current style of interaction—but also as having an appeal value that invites a renewal and widening of communication. Here a parallel with behavior therapy certainly comes to mind, with its in vivo practice of new behavior that was hitherto anxiety provoking and hence avoided.

The therapist's interventions and interpretations aim at elucidating the client's scenario and giving it new meaning. A change in experiencing the scenario may, we believe, be seen as an indication that the intervention or interpretation has contributed to that elucidation. This may, for example, be shown in the therapist suddenly feeling more involved with the client, looking at her/him with more understanding and recognition, and observing a change in the feeling that the client elicits in him/her because he/she hears more nuances in the client's story. All this contributes to the client becoming more convincing, more genuine, and more consistent. An example may illustrate this. A man tells how his only way of interacting with others is by bickering with them, and he is also constantly looking for an argument with the therapist. But he now gets to hear from the therapist that, with this self-revelation, he is also confiding something and indirectly asking for trust. To this the client reacts by telling how, at a very early age, he suddenly lost his father to whom he was very attached and that, for fear of another loss, he has not dared share anything with anyone again. The therapist is struck by the fact that the client's "bickering" tone of voice has just given way to a softer one, and suddenly he understands why his client has hidden behind this argumentative manner. The novelty of the scenario validates the therapist's intervention.

Another instance that validates the therapist's interactional interventions is the occurrence of a shift in the pattern of complaints. A woman whose predominant form of interacting is a mannered friendliness thanks the therapist at the end of every session and thus manages to irritate him by this exaggerated friendliness. He suggests that, with this excessive friendliness, she may be keeping her feelings of anger at bay, at which point she tells how afraid she is of being rejected by the therapist: "After all, there are ten others on your waiting list, ahead of me," she says. The therapist suggests that this is her personal view that casts him as a severe, readily sanctioning man and wonders whether this reminds her of anyone in her life. She then tells how her father answered every expression of dissatisfaction on her part by threatening to send her to boarding school ("the convent"). The therapist now suggests that she obviously expects something similar from him. Once she really starts recognizing this, the therapist is given the opportunity to concretely explore her anger—at people in her present life and at her father who has always oppressed her. In this phase of therapy, her basic depressive affect and her sleeplessness decrease and, for the first time, she meets a man by whom she does not feel abused.

In summary, the four ingredients discussed above should be understood as moments in a constantly recurring cycle that, as such, constitutes the gearbox of therapy as an interactional learning process. The client's complaint, the recent and remote events in her/his life, her/his tone of voice and even what appear to be passing remarks about the weather or about the therapy room decor, her/his obvious silence—all can provide the interactional therapist with an opportunity to start another cycle as described above.

## CLINICAL GUIDELINES

How does an experiential therapist proceed when focusing on the here-and-now interaction? First, we will describe two working procedures by which, we believe, the experiential approach acquires a coloring that is rather distinct from the psychodynamic one. And next we will discuss the integration of interactional work in the Rogerian basic attitudes.

### Two Experiential Accents

Although the concept of "working through of transference reactions" may appear to be a borrowing from the psychodynamic tradition, it is nevertheless rather what Lazarus and Messer (1991) would call a "partial assimilation." By this they mean that a therapeutic process or procedure is internally transformed to some extent once it is integrated in a new context (here experiential psychotherapy). A first important difference between the experiential and the psychoanalytic orientation has to do with the position and the importance of the here-and-now interactional process. For experiential therapists this is never the only process nor even the main one, as is also shown by research findings (Lietaer, Dierick, & Neirinck, 1985; Lietaer, 1992). It is an important part process, which is sometimes but certainly not always kept in the foreground. As Gendlin writes: "Simply because an aspect of therapy is essential for some clients, this does not mean that it should be imposed on all clients all the time. As with the other avenues, it is an error to try to turn every hour of therapy into a discussion of relational events. We need only respond overtly to issues of the interaction when they arise" (1996, p. 283). This process, then, is not deliberately elicited. The therapeutic relationship is not structured in such a way as to maximize regression and transference. In fact, this is considered as an unnecessary detour process within the experiential orientation. We opt for a model in which the client's growth is stimulated right from the start. We believe that certain transference reactions, which may indeed be seen as a client's security measures, will gradually melt away without explicit working through under the beneficial influence of a good working relationship. The interactional work is then "limited" to those "relational issues" that keep appearing as process blocks in the course of therapy.

How often this interactional process by explicit metacommunication will come into focus will depend on both the therapist and client. As mentioned earlier, there are large differences among therapists as to their "interactional attention"; while some will only tackle interactional problems that appear "spontaneously" and overtly in the here-and-now relationship, others tend to search selectively and actively for an interactional translation of the client's problem. But the client's problem is a major determining factor as well. From the literature and our own experience, we may distill the following in this respect: In crisis intervention and when dealing with psychotic problems, an interactional focus is generally not indicated (Teyber, 1992, p. 20). With lighter problems for which short-term therapy is generally sufficient, interactional blockages don't often appear and the interactional process is limited to a "safe context in the background." In more serious impasses and stagnations in the process, on the contrary, and with action-oriented clients with a low level of self-exploration (Tscheulin, 1990), the interactional approach may be very beneficial. The literature tends to show unanimously that interactional work is especially indicated in long-term therapy with clients with severe past interpersonal damage (Leijssen, 1996), notably narcissistic and borderline personality disturbances (Finke, 1994, p. 95; Sachse, 1997). The color and content of the interactional work will also depend on the stage that has been reached in therapy. So, in the initial stage, for example, an incipient break in the working alliance will often give rise to interactional metacommunication (Safran, 1993); in the final stage, interactional work may be centered around unresolved issues of parting and loss.

A second interactional working principle that we believe tends to receive more emphasis within the experiential than within the classical psychoanalytic paradigm may be stated as follows: The emphasis is not on working to achieve insight, which consists of recognizing and genetically understanding how the client distorts the therapist and relates to him/her in a structure-bound way, but on the corrective emotional experience:

> It isn't enough that the patient *repeats* with the therapist his maladjusted feelings and ways of setting up interpersonal situations. After all, the patient is said to repeat these with everyone in his life, and not only with the therapist. Thus, the sheer repeating, even when it is a concrete reliving, doesn't yet resolve anything. Somehow, with the therapist, the patient doesn't *only* repeat; he gets *beyond* the repeating. He doesn't only *relive*; he lives *further*, if he resolves problems experientially. (Gendlin, 1968, p. 222; emphases in original).

This "living further" sometimes requires more than neutral benevolence (Wachtel, 1987). It requires the therapist to present himself not as a blank screen but—apart from and in addition to his empathic interventions—to deal in a transparent way, at the right moment, with what lives in the interaction between the two of them, and to express *his* version of the interaction. We also find this view in the interpersonal branch of psychoanalytic therapy, where "countertransference" and "impact disclosure" are no longer seen as a "crack in the mirror" but as an aid in the analytic work (Maroda, 1991; Kiesler & Van Denburg, 1993).

We now illustrate this further living and greater visibility by an abbreviated transcript of an interactional event from a therapy by a colleague, together with her comments (Leijssen, 1995, pp. 96–97). This clinical vignette shows how she makes interventions that fit the client's frame of reference as well as interventions which originate in her own frame of reference: besides reflection of feelings (T2*b*, T3*b*, T5, T7), the therapist brings in her own experience (T2*a*, T3*a*), makes an interpretative link with what the client has experienced with her mother in the past, (T3*c*) and also uses humor (T9).

Griet, 36 and single, has come to therapy after a suicide attempt during a depressive episode. Her life is badly marked by a cold, demanding mother who would have preferred to have a son. The following happens in the 28th session:

C1: Yesterday I visited my girlfriend who just had a baby . . . And I thought that, perhaps, I would never have children. (Client starts to cry quietly. Suddenly she shouts.) I have the feeling that you're laughing at me!

T1: (*very surprised*) Where did you get that idea?

C2: I saw you laughing and sneering.

T2: I don't really recognize this in myself, and that is also not what I feel toward you (*a*), but there is something which gives you the feeling of being ridiculous with your sadness (*b*).

C3: Yes, I know it is ridiculous to cry for such a trifle.

T3: I don't find your sadness about not having children a trifle at all (*a*), but you feel a sneering look directed at you, under which your pain is reduced to a ridiculous trifle (*b*). (*silence*) . . . I could imagine your mother giving you such a feeling when you cried (*c*). Does that ring a bell?

C4: Mother wouldn't have it that I cry: "There goes our stupid girl again," she would say.

T4: That is ridicule.

C5: Oh, yes, she could make me appear so ridiculous. . . In front of everybody she would say, "Our little Griet is the most stupid girl on earth" . . . I would have liked to vanish from the earth for shame.

T5: No wonder you never forget this look again . . .

C6: No . . . I never cry again when people are around . . . I always run away quickly when tears are coming . . .

T6: And now you were not able to run away . . .

C7: But I didn't want to run away . . . but then I looked at you . . . and suddenly I saw again . . . (*shivers*).

T7: It must have been terrible to be pushed out in the cold by your own mother . . . (*Client starts to cry and sob again. Meanwhile she tells further fragments of painful memories. Therapist reflects and supports with warm, sympathetic interventions.*)

C8: The last time I cried in the presence of somebody else was on my twelfth birthday. On that day my mother said, "And soon we will have this nuisance with woman's ailments and you will see that our Griet will make an issue of it!" . . . Now I believe that this is the reason why I didn't get my first period until I was 18.

T8: Blood and tears . . . were not supposed to flow.

C9: Yes (*relieved, big sigh*) . . . it feels good that now I was able to allow it . . . You wouldn't laugh at me now, would you?

T9: I wouldn't dare.

When a client accuses me of reactions which—truly—I don't recognize in myself, I generally say in a few words what my real reaction is, but I certainly won't start defending myself with it. I return immediately to the client who feels something and I try to explore it. With my empathic ability I try to put myself in the client's shoes and to understand her/his reaction from this vantage point. I feed this understanding back to the client. Once contact with the source of the transference is restored, strongly loaded memories generally come to the fore and only now can the emotions related to them become fully lived through. Once a thoroughly felt insight has taken place, the client may look back at her/his reaction with a certain humor, but it generally is still a bit fragile. In the following sessions comparable feelings sometimes still pop up, but then she/he is able to recognize more quickly the original source of her/his reactions.

## Interactional Work and Client-Centered Attitudes

In this subsection, we will look more carefully at the *way in which* the therapist can insert his/her interactionally oriented interventions in the most constructive way. The suggestions given here all show how important it is that the interactional metacommunication—with feedback, confrontation, interpretation, and self-disclosure as main interventions—be supported by the basic attitudes.

The close bond with *congruence* is obvious: The feeling for what happens in the relationship, the interactional barometer, should function properly! This presupposes a close contact with one's own flow of experiencing and the meanings that it may contain; sufficient awareness of what may be one's personal contribution to the difficulties arising in the relationship and, when needed, sufficient openness to facing the issue in question (so it will not become a battle about who is right); and a capability of communicating one's experience in a process-compatible way, that is, in all its complexity and changeableness. As an example of the latter, Rogers describes how a therapist can communicate "boredom":

> But my feeling exists in the context of a complex and changing flow, which also needs to be communicated. I would like to share with him my distress at feeling bored and my discomfort in expressing it. As I do, I find that my boredom arises from my sense of remoteness from him and that I would like to be in closer touch with him; and even as I try to express these feelings they change. I am certainly not bored as I wait with eagerness, and perhaps a bit of apprehension, for his response. I also feel a new sensitivity to him now that I have shared this feeling which has been a barrier between us. I am far more able to hear the surprise, or perhaps the hurt, in his voice as he now finds himself speaking more genuinely because I have dared to be real with him. (1966, p. 185)

Another important aspect of congruence, besides self-knowledge, is the therapist's ego strength. Especially in interactional work, we need solid ego boundaries. Indeed, we have to be prepared to be the receiver of strong and irrational emotions without being engulfed; we have to deal constructively (i.e., without resorting to acting out) with hate and love, with the client's praise and criticism of our own person; and, in line with the principle of not going along with the client's interactional appeal, we sometimes have to firmly establish our boundaries.

Along with this, there is the link with *unconditional positive regard*. Occasional moments of confrontation are part of all interactional work. These confrontations are most likely to have a constructive effect if we can feel and communicate simultaneously a deep-seated concern for our client as a person. It is in this sense that Gendlin writes,

> But unconditional regard really meant appreciating the client as a person regardless of not liking what he is up against in himself (responding to him in his always positive struggle against whatever he is trapped in). It includes our expressing of dismay and even anger, but always in the context of both of us knowing we are seeking to meet each other warmly and honestly as people, exactly at the point at which we each are and feel. (1970, p. 549)

To be able to confront in a constructive way it is important for the therapist not to let negative feelings accumulate for too long, so as to remain sufficiently open to the client. He/she further has to let it be known clearly that his/her feelings have to do with a specific behavior of the client's, not with the client as a person. Therefore, the therapist's feedback should be as explicit and concrete as possible: how the feeling took shape and what precisely in the client's way of interacting has brought it on. Perhaps most importantly, the therapist should remain focused on the positive life tendencies behind the client's disturbing behavior and behind his/her own negative feelings, and he/she should communicate these as well. Thus, in our earlier example, Rogers communicates the inside reason for his boredom, which is his desire for more contact with the client. When we give a client feedback about a behavior that irritates us, we try to get in touch with the needs and positive intentions behind it, and include these in our discussion. Gendlin gives the following instance of this, pertaining to setting limits:

> For example, I might not let a patient touch me or grab me. I will stop the patient, but in the same words and gesture I will try to respond positively to the positive desire for closeness or physical relations. I will make personal touch with my hand as I hold the patient away from me, contact the patient's eyes, and declare that I think the physical reaching out is positive and I welcome it, even though I cannot allow it. (I know at such times that I may be partly creating this positive aspect. Perhaps this reaching is more hostile, right now, than warm. But there is warmth and health in anyone's sexual or physical need, and I can recognize that as such.) (1967, p. 397)

Interactional work demands, furthermore, a special sort of *empathy*, namely, a being in tune with what happens *between* the client and therapist, with the relational connotation contained in the client's message (see also Barrett-Lennard, 1993). Finke calls it "interaction-centered understanding" (*Interaktionsbezogenes Verstehen*). In his opinion it differs from regular empathic understanding in the sense that it not only involves empathy with the client but also the emotional resonance in the therapist of the client's interactional offer (Finke, 1994, p. 78). Hence, the therapist's and the client's frame of reference are both explicitly involved in the process. For example, a therapist might reflect, "So you always tried to be the good guy for everybody, and also here I get the feeling that receiving my approval is extremely important to you."

Important in this interpersonal exploration is that it is never limited to a behavioral analysis of the interaction as such. We find it important to follow a back-and-forth motion between obtaining a clearer picture of what happens at the interactional level, on the one hand, and the experiential basis in which this way of interacting is embedded, on the other. This means that we try to evoke the experience behind the relational issue: how, at a deeper level, does the client experience her/his way of interacting? What anxieties and desires are taking part? Which life experiences have "marked" the client in this respect? Our experience tells us that reaching this underlying experiential layer often provides a turning point in defrosting a relationship pattern that has become stuck. Within this interactional exploration work of the client's problem, interpretive interventions may be part of the "process comments"; this means clearly outlining a reaction pattern, referring to possible underlying motives, and linking up here-and-now reactions with similar reactions in present relationships or in former (family) relationships. Often, however, it is the client himself who makes the links. When the therapist does it, it is best done in an experiential way. We follow here a rule of thumb of Gendlin's that makes such interpretations end up being very close to empathic reflections or guesses about underlying feelings: "In using theories in practice, translate them into what one might feelingly find directly. Permit yourself any amount of complex reasoning privately, but make the intervention be a simple question, [say] whether the person feels something like . . . some way of feeling you can imagine he might find" (1974, p. 288).

Finally, we always have to be concerned about not imposing the interactional focus on the client, about keeping the process sufficiently *client centered*. When a client comes up with an interactional theme her-/himself, there is, of course, no problem. But when the therapist, starting from his/her own frame of reference, steers the process in the interactional direction, the problem of timing arises: Is there a chance for the client to be sufficiently receptive to my feedback about how I experience the interaction, or should other therapeutic tasks take precedence? Sometimes the relationship has not yet acquired enough security and solidity, and this should be worked on first. In moments of great vulnerability, empathic closeness is perhaps all that is needed. Sometimes the client does not (yet) recognize the interactional feedback. Sometimes the client may first need a chance to fully express her/his feelings toward the symbolic figure of the therapist, without immediately being "stopped" by a confrontation with the "reality" of how the therapist experiences it him-/herself or by an interpretation. But occasionally the therapist's experience of the interaction may be the most fruitful approach to deepening the process.

This process of mutual metacommunication should happen in a true spirit of dialogue in which the therapist shows enough openness for a possible contribution of his/her own to the interactional problem. Two rules of communication should be remembered here. The first one, to use Rogers' words, is "owning" or giving "I" messages instead of "you" messages: The therapist indicates clearly that he/she is the source of the experience and tries above all to communicate what he/she feels him-/herself, rather than making evaluative statements about the client. He/she will, for example, not say "How intrusive of you" but "When you called me for the second time this week, I felt put under pressure and as if taken possession of . . ." The second rule of communication is, in Gendlin's words, "always checking" or "openness to what comes next": After each intervention—and especially after one which originated in our own frame of reference—tuning in anew to the client's experiential track and continuing from there.

## CONCLUSION

In this chapter we turned our attention to the explicit working through of the client's interactional style in the here-and-now relationship with the therapist as an important—albeit not the only—way of approach to personality change. We discussed the nuclear ingredients of this type of interpersonal task and described how it gradually acquired a place in the evolution of client-centered/experiential psychotherapy. In the part of this chapter more explicitly devoted to practice, we discussed the idiosyncratic color that this process acquires within the experiential paradigm and considered how an interactional approach—with interventions designed to steer the process—may be embedded in the client-centered therapist's conditions of empathy, congruence and unconditional positive regard.

We hope that this description of the interactional working-through process in experiential psychotherapy will stimulate other colleagues to elaborate their views on certain aspects or modalities of this process. We believe it is a dimension of psychotherapy to which more attention ought to be paid within our paradigm. A lot of research work still awaits us before we arrive at empirically based microtheories about specific events within the realm of what Rice and Greenberg call "the interpersonal experiential learning dimension" (1990, p. 406). The growing emphasis—not only within client-centered but also within Gestalt therapy (see Hycner & Jacobs, 1995; also Gary Yontef, Chapter 4, in this volume)—on the dialogic character of the therapeutic process may well lead to an evolution in this direction.

## REFERENCES

Anchin, J. C., & Kiesler, D. J. (Eds.). (1982). *Handbook of interpersonal psychotherapy*. New York: Pergamon Press.

Andrews, J. D. W. (1991). Interpersonal challenge: The second integrative relationship factor. *Journal of Psychotherapy Integration, 1,* 265–286.

Barrett-Lennard, G. T. (1993). The phases and focus of empathy. *British Journal of Medical Psychology, 66,* 3–14.

Bateson, G. (1972). *Steps toward an ecology of mind.* New York: Ballantine.

Beier, E. G. (1966). *The silent language of psychotherapy: Social reinforcement of unconscious processes.* Chicago: Aldine.

Carkhuff, R. R. (1969). *Helping and human relations.* New York: Holt, Rinehart & Winston.

Clarkson, P. (1995). *The therapeutic relationship.* London: Whurr.

Finke, J. (1994). *Empathie und Interaktion: Methodik und Praxis der Gesprächspsychotherapie.* Stuttgart: Thieme.

Gelso, C. J., & Carter, J. A. (1994). Components of the psychotherapy relationship: Their interaction and unfolding during treatment. *Journal of Counseling Psychology, 41,* 296–306.

Gendlin, E. T. (1967). Therapeutic procedures in dealing with schizophrenics. In C. R. Rogers (Ed.), *The therapeutic relationship and its impact: A study of psychotherapy with schizophrenics* (pp. 369–400). Madison: University of Wisconsin Press.

Gendlin, E. T. (1968). The experiential response. In E. F. Hammer (Ed.), *Use of interpretation in therapy: Technique and art* (pp. 208–227). New York: Grune & Stratton.

Gendlin, E. T. (1970). A short summary and some long predictions. In J. T. Hart & T. M. Tomlinson (Eds.), *New directions in client-centered therapy* (pp. 544–562). Boston: Houghton Mifflin.

Gendlin, E. T. (1974). The role of knowledge in practice. In G. F. Farwell, N. R. Gamsky, & F. M. Coughlan (Eds.), *The counselor's handbook* (pp. 269–294). New York: Intext.

Gendlin, E. T. (1996). The client–therapist relationship. In E. T. Gendlin (Ed.), *Focusing-oriented psychotherapy: A manual of the experiential method* (pp. 283–298). New York: Guilford Press.

Horvath, A., & Greenberg, L. S. (Eds.). (1994). *The working alliance: Theory, research and practice.* New York: Wiley.

Hycner, R., & Jacobs, L. (1995). *The healing relationship in Gestalt therapy: A dialogic/self psychology approach.* Highland, NY: Gestalt Journal Press.

Kiesler, D. J. (1982). Confronting the client–therapist relationship in psychotherapy. In J. C. Anchin & D. J. Kiesler (Eds.), *Handbook of interpersonal psychotherapy* (pp. 274–295). New York: Pergamon Press.

Kiesler, D. J. (1988). *Therapeutic metacommunication.* Palo Alto, CA: Consulting Psychology Press.

Kiesler, D. J., & Van Denburg, T. F. (1993). Therapeutic impact disclosure. A last taboo in psychoanalytic theory and practice. *Clinical Psychology and Psychotherapy, 1,* 3–13.

Lazarus, A. A., & Messer, S. B. (1991). Does chaos prevail? An exchange on technical eclecticism and assimilative integration. *Journal of Psychotherapy Integration, 1,* 43–54.

Leijssen, M. (1995). *Gids voor gesprekstherapie.* Utrecht, The Netherlands: De Tijdstroom.

Leijssen, M. (1996). *Focusingprocessen in cliëntgericht-experiëntiële psychotherapie.* Unpublished doctoral dissertation, Catholic University of Leuven, Belgium.

Lietaer, G. (1992). Helping and hindering processes in client-centered/experiential psychotherapy: A content analysis of client and therapist postsession perceptions. In S. G. Toukmanian & D. L. Rennie (Eds.), *Psychotherapy process research: Paradigmatic and narrative approaches* (pp. 134–162). Newbury Park, CA: Sage.

Lietaer, G. (1993). Authenticity, congruence and transparency. In D. Brazier (Ed.), *Beyond Carl Rogers: Towards a psychotherapy for the 21st century* (pp. 17–46). London: Constable.

Lietaer, G. (1997). From non-directive to experiential: A paradigm unfolding. In B. Thorne & E. Lambers (Eds.), *Person-centred therapy: A European perspective.* London: Sage.

Lietaer, G., Dierick, P., & Neirinck, M. (1985). Inhoud en proces in experiëntiële psychotherapie: Een empirische exploratie. *Psychologica Belgica, 15,* 127–147.

Lietaer, G., Rombauts, J., & Van Balen, R. (Eds.). (1990). *Client-centered and experiential psychotherapy in the nineties.* Leuven, Belgium: Leuven University Press.

Maroda, K. J. (1991). *The power of countertranference: Innovations in analytic technique.* New York: Wiley.

Orlinsky, D. E., Grawe, K., & Parks, B. K. (1994). Process and outcome in psychotherapy: *Noch einmal.* In A. E. Bergin & S. L. Garfield (Eds.), *Handbook of psychotherapy and behavior change* (pp. 270–376). New York: Wiley.

Pfeiffer, W. (1995). Die Beziehung: Der zentrale Wirkfaktor in der Gesprächspsychotherapie. *GwG Zeitschrift, 26*(97), 27–32.

Rice, L. N. (1974). The evocative function of the therapist. In D. A. Wexler & L. N. Rice (Eds.), *Innovations in client-centered therapy* (pp. 289–311). New York: Wiley.

Rice, L. N., & Greenberg, L. S. (1990). Fundamental dimensions in experiential therapy: New directions in research. In G. Lietaer, J. Rombauts, & R. Van Balen (Eds.), *Client-centered and experiential psychotherapy in the nineties* (pp. 397–414). Leuven, Belgium: Leuven University Press.

Rogers, C. R. (1951). *Client-centered therapy.* Boston: Houghton Mifflin.

Rogers, C. R. (1961). A process equation of psychotherapy. *American Journal of Psychotherapy, 15,* 27–65.

Rogers, C. R. (1966). Client-centered therapy. In S. Arieti (Ed.), *American handbook of psychiatry* (Vol. 3, pp. 183–200). New York: Basic Books.

Rogers, C. R. (1967). A silent young man. In C. R. Rogers (Ed.), *The therapeutic relationship and its impacts: A study of psychotherapy with schizophrenics* (pp. 401–416). Madison: University of Wisconsin Press.

Rogers, C. R. (1975). Empathic: An unappreciated way of being. *The Counseling Psychologist, 5*(2), 2–10.

Sachse, R. (1997). *Persönlichkeitsstörungen: Interaktionsstile im Psychotherapieprozess.* Göttingen, Germany: Hogrefe.

Safran, J. D. (1993). Breaches in the therapeutic alliance: An arena for negotiating authentic relatedness. *Psychotherapy, 30,* 11–24.

Safran, J. D., & Segal, L. S. (1990). *Interpersonal process in cognitive therapy.* New York: Basic Books.

Shlien, J. (1987). A countertheory of transference. *Person-Centered Review, 2,* 15–49 (comments: 153–202/455–75).

Sullivan, H. S. (1953). *The interpersonal theory of psychiatry.* New York: Norton.

Szasz, T. S. (1972). *The myth of mental illness.* Zenda, WI: Paladin House.

Teyber, E. (1992). *Interpersonal process in psychotherapy.* Pacific Grove, CA: Brooks/Cole.

Tscheulin, D. (1990). Confrontation and non-confrontation as differential techniques in differential client-centered therapy. In G. Lietaer, J. Rombauts, & R. Van Balen (Eds.), *Client-centered and experiential psychotherapy in the nineties* (pp. 327–336). Leuven, Belgium: Leuven University Press.

Van Balen, R. (1990). The therapeutic relationship according to Carl Rogers: Only a climate? a dialogue? or both? In G. Lietaer, J. Rombauts, & R. Van Balen (Eds.), *Client-centered and experiential psychotherapy in the nineties* (pp. 65–86). Leuven, Belgium: Leuven University Press.

van der Linden, P., & van Kessel, W. (1991). De interactioneel-gerichte therapeut aan het werk. In H. Swildens, O. de Haas, G. Lietaer, & R. Van Balen (Eds.), *Leerboek Gesprekstherapie: De cliëntgerichte benadering* (pp. 377–393). Utrecht, The Netherlands: De Tijdstroom.

van Kessel, W. (1975). Van reflectie tot interventie. *Tijdschrift voor Psychiatrie, 17*, 342–354.

Wachtel, P. L. (1987). You can't go far in neutral: On the limits of therapeutic neutrality. In P. L. Wachtel (Ed.), *Action and insight* (pp. 176–184). New York: Guilford Press.

Watzlawick, P., Beavin, J. H., & Jackson, D. D. (1967). *Pragmatics of human communication.* New York: Norton.

Yalom, I. D. (1980). Existential isolation and psychotherapy. In I. D. Yalom (Ed.), *Existential psychotherapy* (pp. 392–415). New York: Basic Books.

Yalom, I. D. (1995). Interpersonal learning. In I. D. Yalom (Ed.), *The theory and practice of group psychotherapy* (pp. 17–46). New York: Basic Books.

# 8

***** 

# The Person as Active Agent
# in Experiential Therapy

Arthur C. Bohart
Karen Tallman

## THE CONCEPT OF THE CLIENT AS ACTIVE AGENT

Consider the following scenario. Anna comes to see you saying that she is depressed. You interview her and conclude that she meets the criteria for major depressive disorder. She is not sleeping well, has no energy, and is having trouble concentrating. Also she is eating heavily and has lost interest in sex, affecting her relationship with her boyfriend. You mention to her that one option is to refer her for medication, but you and she could decide that by the end of the session.

Anna tells you that she is feeling totally trapped. Her job is as a public defender. She has been very frustrated with the job—no one in the system, including the prosecutors and judges, seem really interested in justice or fairness. Anna says she has been thinking about leaving her job for a long time. She had wanted to go back to school and become an elementary school teacher, but just about when she had decided to leave, George, her husband, asked for a divorce. He is a successful physician and she discovered that he had started an affair. She has been divorced for about a year, and George has already married his girlfriend. The divorce was contentious, and one of the key issues was who would get custody of their 6-year-old daughter, Melissa. Anna got custody, but now she feels trapped. She feels she cannot leave her profession because she fears her husband might use her loss of income as a reason to take her back to court and try to get custody of Melissa. But she still would rather work with children or do something "meaningful." She says she pursued law because of her high-achieving family. Her older brother is a physician, her middle brother is a lawyer, and she felt pressure from her parents to do as well as her brothers did. She feels her parents would be very disappointed in her were she to give up law to become a "mere" teacher. They are already disappointed that she is "just" a public defender instead of a highly successful corporate lawyer.

As Anna talks you listen and make a few empathic reflections, such as "You're feeling very stuck" and "It is terrifying to think of losing your daughter." Anna goes on to talk more about how she had always wanted to be a teacher but just couldn't work up the courage to stand up to her parents and to tell them she didn't want to become a lawyer. She says she even married the kind of husband they wanted.

"But you know," she says, "I really do want to do something that helps people. It's important to me. But I feel trapped. I was going to quit and go back to school and become a teacher when George decided he wanted a divorce . . . That bastard! He didn't want me to quit. He didn't like the idea of giving up my income while I went back to school. We had a lot of fights about it. He said it was those fights which drove him into having an affair. But he's a real opportunist—he married one of his rich patients . . . I wonder how much my desire to be a teacher really mattered. I wonder if all that was an excuse. He certainly knew I wasn't financially ambitious—maybe he saw an opportunity with this rich patient and took it, and blamed it on me. He was never much of a father, or a husband . . . He hardly ever showed Melissa any attention. Yet he wanted custody! Why? I can't believe he really wanted her. He hardly ever visits her now . . . You know, the thought has occurred to me that the custody battle was all a big threat. Sometimes I've thought that maybe it was just a way of intimidating me into going for an easier settlement on the financial issues. He's a real manipulator, and I think I *did* go easier in the settlement in order to get custody . . . I've been worrying so much about another custody battle that I never took my thoughts on that too seriously. But I don't think he really wants custody. I've thought that before, but somehow just saying it to you makes it more real to me, and I really *do* think that. I *do* think he doesn't really want custody!"

At this point she pauses and seems lost in thought. After a few minutes of silence she says, "I think I've been worrying for nothing . . . and maybe as much as I did want to be a teacher, I'm not sure I want to now. How would I support Melissa all by myself? It was one thing when I was living with George. We could have afforded it, but I think it is different now. I couldn't afford the loss of income . . . I don't know . . . I don't like what I'm doing, but I really have to think of my daughter. She's really important to me. I have a boyfriend, and he's a good guy, but I don't want to get married again, at least not yet."

By now, Anna, who had started the session looking down, talking in a listless, energyless tone of voice, is talking in a much more reflective, active tone of voice. She is still looking down, but more as if she is thinking than as if she is depressed. She goes on: "I guess I'm beginning to feel in charge of my life now. I always felt I was living someone else's life, but now I'm suddenly feeling like my life is mine. *I'm* responsible now. I'm not living for my parents, and I'm not living for my husband. I'm living for me and my daughter. And I don't want to give that up. That's one reason I don't want to get married right away. And I guess that means I won't be able to give up the income, at least for now. If I went back to school, I'd be cheating my daughter. She's the most important thing to me. I can't do that. Maybe later. But I want a good income until she gets older."

By this time Anna is looking you in the eye, looking more energetic, and talking purposively. You notice that your time is about up, and so you bring it around to options for providing her with help. You mention again that you could refer her for medication, and you also mention that you would be happy to work with her. She says she would be happy to see you, and she schedules another appointment. Right at the moment she isn't interested in medication. As she stands up she says, "You know, I feel so much better already. Thanks so much."

Six days later, you get a call from her. She sounds much better. She says that she and her boyfriend have resumed their sex life, that she is sleeping much better, that she is concentrating much better, and that her friends at work are saying she seems so much better. She is enjoying Melissa, and she has begun to volunteer some time to work at the local battered women's shelter helping with free legal advice. She says she'd like to wait a week and see if she needs to come in. A week later she calls again to say that things are going well and that she doesn't need to come in. Talking with her over the phone, you are satisfied that she indeed is doing much better.

Yet you hardly said a word during the whole interview. How is this possible? No dysfunctional cognitions were challenged, no "shoulds" disputed, no assertion training done, no working through of guilt and dependency directed toward the parents, no couples therapy done with the boyfriend, yet Anna has gotten better in one session. Unbelievable? The above is a telescoped version of a whole session, and it is a fictionalized case, but it is modeled on one of our clients, who indeed came in presenting with major depression, and who did get better in just one session and needed no more sessions. Why? And what is surprising about Anna's case is that the therapist said virtually nothing.

How did Anna change without the therapist's help? And why did she have to come to therapy in the first place? We believe that clients have the intrinsic capacity to solve their own problems in many if not most cases. They need to come to therapy because they do not have the proper environmental support to do that in their everyday lives. Anna did not need an expert therapist to diagnose her problem and to "intervene," but she did need someone who would respectfully listen to and support her own problem-solving process—something she didn't have in her everyday life. We believe that there is a naturally occurring self-righting process (Masten, Best, & Garmazy, 1990). We are not alone in this; many strategic and solution-focused therapists (e.g., Rosenbaum, 1994; Duncan & Moynihan, 1994) also believe it. To quote Rosenbaum (1994), "our goal should be to interfere as little as possible with the client's natural process of growth" (p. 249).

This is akin to the "self-actualization" process (Rogers, 1957), but what is this process and why does it not always work so that individuals need to come to see therapists? In this chapter we hope to describe how clients are active, self-righting agents who can and do solve their own problems. Therapists are guides or aides, or sometimes nothing more than witnesses to the process. This does not minimize the usefulness of the many things therapists can do, but behind all these activities are active clients, taking whatever interventions therapists offer and integratively using them to work out their own life paths. Therapists never really make change happen in clients. Rather, they join with them. This model of the client as active, agentic, integrative problem solver is intrinsic to experiential psychotherapies.

## The Client as Active Self-Healer Model

From an experiential humanistic perspective the above scenario is possible because humans are proactive agents who generate their own psychological movement. The possibility that clients are active, creative problem solvers who can move themselves along by themselves if given the proper climate or context is an idea that does not exist in many theoretical perspectives. For them the therapist is the agent of change. The therapist is aided and abetted by the client, who must listen to the therapist, try to digest what the therapist says, follow the therapist's directions, and actively work to make the changes the therapist mandates. But it is the therapist who points out the direction the client needs to go in, and dispenses the procedures and techniques that will move the client in that direction. Clients may ultimately change themselves, but only under the expert direction of the therapist.

The idea that it is the expert therapist who is the agent of change is based on an underlying medical-like meta-model of therapy (Bohart & Tallman, 1996; Orlinsky, 1989). The influence of this medical-like way of thinking is subtle and pervasive, even when the therapy is not overtly medical but may even be educational in its nature (Bohart, O'Hara, & Leitner, 1998). The influence of this medical-like model manifests itself in the use of the *drug metaphor* (Stiles & Shapiro, 1989). Psychological interventions are thought of metaphorically as drugs, which can be administered to people and which cure disorder. They are "treatments for" conditions, just as medications are treatments for infections. They work by precipitating changes inside the organism in a mechanistic fashion. Clients have problems that they cannot solve on their own because they are stuck in their own defenses, conditioned habits, or dysfunctional schemas. Outside intervention by an expert who diagnoses these problems and applies expertly chosen techniques is what is needed. In such a medical-like model, the idea that the client could spontaneously self-right is as theoretically inexplicable as that a person could spontaneously remit from cancer without treatment. Everyone knows that such things happen, but it is assumed that they are unusual cases.

Part of the reason for this is that our culture has a great deal of difficulty accepting that people have self-generating processes inside them. As both Bakan (1996) and Gendlin (1990) have noted, most of our models, from religious ones, to traditional educational ones, to parenting ones, to psychological ones, view change as being implanted in people by outside agents. Clients change by "internalizing" the therapist, or via the therapist's extinguishing client fears, or via the therapist replacing dysfunctional cognitions with more functional ones.

Recently, based on our belief that the evidence on psychotherapy supports Rogers's (1957) contention that if clients have a supportive atmosphere they can generate all the changes themselves, we have argued that it is primarily clients who make therapy work (Bohart & Tallman, 1996). We see the client as, in essence, the *real* "therapist." Therapists are adjuncts to and facilitators of change processes that already exist in clients.

There are two senses in which the client's own self-righting processes are the active producers of change. First, clients are active *learners*. They do not passively take in "the truth" from therapists and then mechanistically implement it in their lives. Rather, they actively explore whatever "truths" are offered to them, try them on for size, try experiencing the world through them, find out if they fit, and modify them so as to do the job clients want them to do. Clients can ultimately change themselves through experientially discovering meaning in whatever the therapist gives them. Clients must discover their own meanings through the use of the procedures, just as mathematics students must go beyond mechanistic application of strategies to get a "feel for them" if they are to be able to creatively generalize their use to new problems.

The second way clients produce change is that they create new perspectives and meanings. Clients not only creatively modify recipes given them by therapists, they frequently create new recipes themselves. Clients make discoveries that were unanticipated by the therapist (e.g., Gold, 1994), use bad therapist responses creatively to grow (Tallman, Robinson, Kay, Harvey, & Bohart, 1994), creatively and productively misinterpret offhand comments by the psychologist (Corsini, 1989), and subtly shape the therapist in order to get what they want (Rennie, 1994).

## Evidence

We believe there is substantial evidence to support our contention that the client is the primary generator of change. First, it has repeatedly been found that all therapies work about the same (the "dodo bird" verdict), that differential treatments for different problems generally are not needed, and that techniques account for only a small proportion of the variance in therapeutic outcome (Bergin & Garfield, 1994; Bohart & Tallman, 1996; Duncan &

Moynihan, 1994; Lambert, 1992). Rather than technique, "nonspecific" factors such as the relationship and client variables account for the bulk of the outcome of therapy (Lambert, 1992). Of the two nonspecific factors, the client variable is the single most important, with the relationship second. These findings all make sense if we assume that the primary agent of change in therapy is the client, who is able to use whatever therapists provide for their own self-growth.

A variety of other data support the idea that the client is the major source of change. Many studies find that self-help procedures and computer-assisted therapies work about as well as professionally provided therapy (Christensen & Jacobson, 1994). Further, studies have found that talking into a tape recorder can be as effective in working through a traumatic experience as seeing a cognitive therapist (Segal & Murray, 1994) and that journaling can result in significant personal self-change (Pennebaker, 1990).

There is other evidence for the importance of client agency in therapy. In general, it is client perceptions of therapeutic events, such as of the strength of the alliance or of the therapist's empathy, which correlate with outcome (Bohart & Greenberg, 1997; Horvath, 1995). This makes sense if in fact it is the client who is using whatever the therapist has to offer to make change happen. If it were the therapist's expert application of technique that made the difference, then it should be the therapist's perceptions that correlate most highly with change.

Several writers have drawn conclusions compatible with our views. Bergin and Garfield (1994) have said, "Another important observation regarding the client variable is that it is the client more than the therapist who implements the change process. . . . Rather than argue over whether or not 'therapy works,' we could address ourselves to the question of whether or not 'the client works!' . . . As therapists have depended more on the client's resources, more change seems to occur (pp. 825–826)." Elliott and James (1989) have noted that clients are "much more planful, active and conscious in their approach to therapy than has been implied in previous research" (p. 46). Specifically, Elliott (1984) found that clients took from therapist interpretations what they wanted and needed to gain insight. Orlinsky, Grawe, and Parks (1994), based on their comprehensive review of the research, conclude that "The quality of the patient's participation in therapy stands out as the most important determinant of outcome" (p. 361).

Rennie (1990) has interviewed clients about their therapy experiences, using tape recordings of sessions to aid their recall. Rennie has shown that clients are planful and active in how they think about, react to, and process their interactions with the therapist. They evaluate therapist comments, appraise their own reactions, and "revision" (Watson & Rennie, 1994) their problems—all on their own. Clients are acutely sensitive to the therapist, work to protect the therapist's self-esteem, work *around* the therapist if necessary, try to empathically understand the therapist, and note and accept the therapist's limitations. Rennie's research supports our contentions that clients are active agents in the therapeutic interaction. They "operate on" the therapist as much as the therapist "operates on" them.

In a series of studies Howard (1996) has demonstrated the potency of personal agency to make important self-changes. Rychlak (1994) cites research demonstrating humans' capacity to think oppositionally—they do not just receive information from the environment, they work on that information, and store not only the information but how things could be otherwise. Finally, there is evidence that many individuals grow and change without any professional assistance at all (Prochaska, 1995), and that people are resilient, self-righting organisms (Masten et al., 1990). In sum, the evidence supports our contention that the client has the capacity to self-right and is the primary agent of change in psychotherapy and in life.

## How Do Clients as Active Agents Solve Problems in Therapy?

As we define it, the potential to act agentically includes the capacity to appraise one's life path in relation to present circumstances; to appraise these circumstances; to evaluate goals, beliefs, and values; to set priorities; to plan trajectories; to decide upon alternative courses of action; and then to take steps toward pursuing goals. The components of being agentic are (a) the ability to *initiate* courses of action or trajectories; (b) the ability to *appraise*, reflect, and evaluate; and (c) the ability to *create*. All of this implies a forward-looking organism whose behavior is largely guided more by its projections of where it is going or where it wants to go than by where it has been (Bohart, Humphrey, Magallanes, Guzman, Smiljanich, & Aguallo, 1993).

Experiential theorists believe that human action arises from a capacity to experience, think, plan, create, and initiate. How could a client such as Anna solve her problems herself without the therapist doing anything but listen (and occasionally empathically reflect)? Anna solved her problem because she had a chance to think about it, experience the components of it, bounce it off another person, re-present it to herself, and generate several new perspectives (e.g., on her husband's desire for custody, on her own priorities, and on who was in charge of her life). What she needed from the therapist was a "space" in which to do this work.

In the process of explaining her situation to the therapist, Anna re-presented to herself and experienced her pain over her disappointment with her career, the betrayal by her husband, and her current anguish over feeling trapped. In experiencing the relevant emotions associated with these events, she also experienced fully what these situations meant to her. She not only re-presented the problem to herself intellectually, she let herself experience the implications of the problems. As she turned her experience over in her mind, she engaged in an internal dialogue between thinking about it and entering into it. In the context of a listening other, she re-presented to herself thoughts she had previously had concerning whether or not her ex-husband really wanted custody of their daughter. As she reevaluated this, her ability to express this to another person somehow added "realness" to something she had thought to herself before. She saw things in her experience that now led her to have a firmer sense of certainty that her ex-husband wouldn't really want custody. Realizing this appeared to free her to move on to reevaluate how much *she* wanted to give up her job. It was as if as long as her attention was focused on the external threat from George, she couldn't really focus internally and figure out what she wanted. With that threat removed, she focused inside and began to realize that she didn't want to give up her well-paying job now that she had a daughter to support. She also brought in her experience of living up to others' expectations with both her parents and her husband, thought about the possibility of getting married, and juxtaposing all this, recognized that she now felt responsible for her life; it was she who had to make choices for herself and her daughter. She then decided that she wanted to stay in her job, raise her daughter, and be responsible for herself.

Anna moved from feeling chronically trapped and helpless to recognizing and "owning" her own perceptions and what she wanted in her life. The therapist facilitated this process primarily by staying out of her way, by showing that he was carefully following her and understanding her, that what she said made sense, and, through empathic responses, helped her re-present her experience and thought processes to herself. However, the active exploring, experiencing, thinking through, discovering, and integrating came from her. After she left the therapy office, she went back and tested out what she had discovered in her everyday life. After a week she reported back that she had found that she was on the right track and that she was feeling fine. She consolidated what she had discovered in therapy as she reentered her life and applied it, creatively making adjustments as she did so. One creative adjustment was that she spontaneously decided to volunteer at a battered woman's shelter, which helped supply some of the missing sense of meaning.

## How Clients Make Meaning: Conceptualizing, Experiencing, Exploring

We have previously said that thinking is at the basis of client agency. By thinking we mean a complex, integrative, synthesizing cyclical process, which includes experiencing, exploring experience, conceptualizing experience, reflecting and reviewing concepts, analysis, deduction, induction, and imagining alternative possibilities. Thinking is not intellectual, analytic, deductive concept formation alone. Such intellectual analysis is by itself impotent to help people make major life changes (Bohart, 1993). Rather, we mean by thinking something more holistic: both cognitive and experiential.

Basically the core process by which clients make meaning is a cyclical one of conceptualizing–experiencing–exploring (e.g., Kolb, 1984), and the cycle can be entered at any one of the three points. Conceptualizing can lead to exploring or experiencing. Exploring can lead to conceptualizing and experiencing, and so forth. The person explores his or her engagement in the world, articulates heretofore implicit aspects of that engagement, and develops new perspectives. There are two basic means whereby individuals make meaning: the first is through perceptual/experiential search; the second is through intellectual/conceptual analysis. These are considered in the next subsection.

## Perceptual/Experiential Search and Intellectual/Conceptual Analysis

The basic activities of intellectual, conceptual activity are the same as the basic activities of perception and are grounded in the fact that the human is an organism built to live in a world, search it for potential resources and dangers, move and navigate through it, and interact with it. Perception is an active process of searching the world to detect regularities (Gibson, 1979). Detecting a regularity can be thought of as detecting the underlying structure of something (e.g., a table), the underlying pattern or configuration in something (e.g., a work of art), or the underlying trajectory in something (e.g., where a relationship is going). A particularly important group of regularities are things that can be used by the organism to achieve its purposes ("affordances" in Gibson's term). Perception is an active/interactive process in which the organism detects regularities through continual movement and interaction with its environment, that is, through *exploration*.

Perception leads to the detection of regularities that may guide action without ever being reflected on, that is, through tacit knowing. A child, through countless interactions with her/his parents, will "know" that the parents really like and prize her/him, even if the words are never said and the child never "puts it into words" her-/himself. The child will have a wealth of complex, subtle, differentiated perceptual/experiential knowledge of human interaction and will "know" very quickly if something signals danger, love, acceptance, interest, indifference, appreciation, acceptance, and so on, at least in her/his own particular environment.

Action can be taken promptly when a person can detect regularities in an environment rapidly, that is, "without thinking." Experience in a domain can be thought of as leading to the quick and subtle detection of the structure of that particular environment, leading to smooth action. However, such smooth action is not "automated" as in traditional cognitivistic models. Rather, rapid and subtle detection of the structure of an environment allows highly spontaneous and creative improvisational action. A highly skilled, experienced basketball player is a good example. The player may encounter a configuration on the court he or she has never seen before, but because he or she is very skilled at quickly identifying the perceptual regularities in such a situation, he or she can immediately detect how this configuration is both similar and different from others he or she has encountered and can quickly and nonconsciously rapidly adjust his or her behavior. Detection of regularities is always linked up with the organism's goals and purposes; in other words, it is always in reference to something that the organism is trying to achieve, do, or be. As a result, detection of a regularity will be linked to an implicit understanding of its meaning to the organism—an implicit call to action, an emotion, a feeling, or what Gendlin (1964) calls a "felt meaning." In sum, a rich, implicit perceptual–experiential understanding in a given area of activity is at the basis of acting agentically in that area.

Humans also *reflect* (Rennie, 1994; Watson & Rennie, 1994) upon their perceptions and actions. Reflection is a kind of "meta-perceptual" activity, wherein both experiences and concepts are "paraded" before the mind and searched to detect regularities. Thinking is a form of action—a mental equivalent of exploring a terrain, turning things over in one's hand, or laying things out in front of one. Instead of searching in the world, individuals search "in their minds." Thinking, in contrast to perception, "operates" not only on perceptual images but on words and concepts. Much creative, synthetic thinking involves a dialogue between "articulate" consciousness—the typical cognitive, linguistic type of thinking—and the level of bodily felt experience (Barrett-Lennard, 1997).

As a part of being agents, humans are constantly thinking as they receive information. Humans do not simply receive information passively; rather, they actively perceive it as it comes in, rotating it, seeing how it fits with other things, analyzing it, dissecting it, searching it for new possibilities, and eventually finding ways of fitting experience together with their prior knowledge using *both* of Jean Piaget's processes of assimilation and accommodation (Cowan, 1978). Rychlak (1994) has discussed how individuals begin to generate alternative ways of looking at information as soon as they begin to receive it. Thus cognitivist models in which corrective information "impacts" on the information processing system and mechanistically alters schemas is naive and simplistic and bypasses the active, synthesizing, integrating, and differentiating activities of the agent.

## Thinking and Solving Problems

Individuals typically act agentically when confronted with problems. When the process is operating optimally, they think about the problems and try to find "solution paths" through the "problem space." They initially try to adapt solutions that have worked in the past to the present problem. First they re-present the problem to themselves mentally. They select what strikes them as the key elements and focus their attention on those. They do some kind of analysis of what the problem is. Next they try to fit a solution. Then they may imagine how that solution will play out. Or they may simply try it out. In doing this they uncover other problems. They then replay the whole scenario. They begin to "play with" variations on solutions, combine solutions, and so on, looking for the solution with the best fit. In doing this they "rotate" elements in their minds and continue to search the problem space. Elements initially in the foreground may recede into the background as they notice elements they had previously overlooked or thought not important. Yet those elements may turn out to be the stuff of creative insight and solution. For instance, in experiential therapy it is often neglected feelings, emotions, and values that come to the foreground and facilitate a shift in perspective leading to the emergence of new solutions. As they play with the elements of the problem in their minds, they shift perspectives and try out new angles on the problem. It is through doing this that they eventually may notice a new angle that provides the stuff of a solution. Once they develop a "solution map" they see how well that map fits the problem. It is as if mentally they are taking a "solution transparency" and superimposing it over the problem to see how well it fits. When it fits sufficiently well there is a "felt give" in Gendlin's (1968) sense. The process of judging if a solution fits well enough is a felt, experiential thing, and not an intellectual cogitive judgment—it is a sense of fitting—and it is when one has that felt sense of a fit between a solution model of the problem and the felt sense of the problem itself that one has an "aha" experience, one "gets it at a gut level," one "really understands it," and so on.

## Creativity

Humans do not merely passively apply old concepts to new information. Rather, they creatively generate new concepts, or new variations on old concepts, all the time (Glucksburg & Keysar, 1990). This can be in the form of metaphorical extensions of old concepts to cover new circumstances that are similar but not identical to old circumstances. Concepts are endlessly created and re-created. Concepts are *tools* used and generated by individuals to solve problems that they encounter in their life spaces. They are not "fixed schemas" that form the structure of mind and mechanistically filter and construct information, and produce responses. Rather than being the structure *of* mind, they are things used *by* the mind or by the organism.

Creativity is a constant and ongoing part of everyday life (Ward, Finke, & Smith, 1995). As Epstein (1991), a radical behaviorist, has observed, "The behavior of organisms has many firsts, so many, in fact, that it's not clear that there are any seconds. . . . When you look closely enough, behavior that appears to have been repeated proves to be novel in some fashion" (p. 362). Neisser (1967) notes that, in contrast to the idea that we repetitively apply old learnings to new situations, in fact variation in our behavior is the rule. Thus, there is an ongoing, imperceptible process of continual change and novelty in human behavior. Creativity is often in the form of small triumphs, or small variations, rather than large ones. As individuals struggle to find paths out of problem areas, they spontaneously generate new maps which can help find ways out. These maps may be variations on old maps ("first-order solutions" in Watzlawick's [1987] term) or entirely new maps ("second-order solutions" in Watzlawick's [1987] term).

Creativity is facilitated by an open, nonjudgmental atmosphere that encourages novelty and exploration (Sternberg & Davidson, 1995). Creativity also needs some structure to operate on (Finke, 1995). Structures that facilitate creativity are ambiguous yet have some underlying sense of meaningfulness, are novel, and allow for different uses (Finke, 1995). However, the form cannot be too ambiguous. There must be some constraints. It could be said that good therapy situations provide just such structure. In particular, the tasks of experiential therapies seem to fulfill these requirements.

## Experiencing

When exploring a problem, individuals need to be able to experientially explore as well as conceptually explore. They need to be able to experience the meaning of the problem to them, directly or vicariously experience new ways of being and behaving vis-à-vis the problem, and experientially re-present problem situations to themselves. If they only engage in an abstract intellectual analysis, no change will take place (Bohart, 1993). Experiencing without thinking will not help, nor will thinking without experiencing. Concrete images of experiences in the problem situation need to be accessed, re-presented, and reexperienced. One must be, in some sense, experientially present in the problem situation or complex. Clients can "enter in" to their experience of problem situations and complexes through various role play and enactment exercises, through the use of imagery, or through vivid discussion wherein they attempt to capture the flavor of their experience in words and symbols.

While in the moment of the problem individuals were too busy acting and experiencing to step back and see what was going on, in the therapist's office they can both experience and meta-cognitively reflect upon the experience. This allows them to begin to "reprocess" it. The "problem space" becomes clearer—the relationships become clearer, and their priorities begin to stand out. Gaining some distance and seeing things in context, they begin to feel more in charge of the situation and the sense of threat diminishes. They begin to feel calmer and more relieved. They are more in a position to begin to think proactively about what they want to do next.

Bohart (1993) has argued that typical cognitivist models of human knowing do not adequately account for experiencing. We are a cognitivistic culture, and we tend to reduce all human knowing to *cognition as conceptual thinking*. Cognitive therapies tend to assume that experience is constructed out of little sentences that run around in our heads at an automatic level. However, experiencing is much more "seamless" than that. The sense of immediacy and full-bodied presence I have when I am fully involved in having a deep conversation with someone, sharing an intense romantic moment, or even acutely hating myself does not arise from my saying a whole lot of little sentences to myself very quickly at an automatic, nonconscious level. Experience is not constructed out of sentences. Rather, sentences, thoughts, concepts, etc., arise *from* experience: they are attempts to capture and conceptualize what is known more fundamentally in a nonverbal, nonconceptual sense (Gendlin, 1964; Lakoff, 1987). They can, however, feed back into and inform experience, either through shifting attentional focus or through triggering experiential images and feelings.

Experience is more fundamentally perceptual and recognitional than conceptual. Perception is immediate. Things are given to us "directly" in perception. They are "recognized," and the experience of recognition is different than that of conceptualization. While at a philosophical level we may wish to argue that all experience, even immediate experience, is "constructed by the mind," nonetheless at the phenomenological level there is a clear difference between knowing that has an immediate, "present" quality and knowing that is mediated by thinking and conceptualization.

## Experiential Understanding

It is when we *recognize* (i.e, directly experience) relationships that we "really understand" them. True insight is perceptual and experiential (Bohart & Associates, 1996; Sternberg & Davidson, 1995). When one recognizes relationships between two things, one attains an understanding of it at a deeper and more profound level than when one merely has an intellectual grasp of it. One has a fine-tuned *felt sense* (Gendlin, 1996) of the relationships involved. This allows one to operate in an agentic fashion *from* such understanding. When one has attained this level of understanding, one is able to operate from "within" that understanding in a creative, generative way. It can be said that when one has attained such a level of understanding one has "indwelled" (Polyani, 1967) or "inhabited" it.

An example of this comes from a research study in which actors were interviewed about their process of mastering a part. Typical cognitivist theories locate creativity in "top-down" or "controlled" processing. Experiential theory assumes that creativity comes from an experiential, or "gut-level," understanding. Top-down, conceptual processes are then enlisted to articulate, hone, and carry forward what is first sensed experientially. In this study, it was found that actors felt most mechanistic and least creative when they were acting in a top-down fashion, that is, out of an intellectually generated understanding of the part. They felt most able to be truly spontaneous and creative in terms of the part when they had acquired a gut-level understanding, when they had "inhabited" the part, or when they had "become" the part (Bohart & Associates, 1996; Loesch, Hamilton, Seferian, Rush, & Bohart, 1994). Similarly, artists of various kinds were interviewed about their creative process. They reported that the experience of gestating a creative idea was a felt, experiential, gut-level, or perceptual phenomenon. It was *not* conceptual. Conceptual aspects came later as the individual worked to turn the initial insight or inspiration into a full-fledged work of art.

Experiential understanding is attained through action, interaction, trying something on for size, seeing how something feels, walking the path, and so on. Thus it is not understanding that can simply be told to someone. One must discover it for oneself. Given this, therapy becomes the provision of the opportunity for *experiential self-discovery*, that is, discovery by the self of new knowledge through experiential encounter.

### Experiential Presence

Experiential theories are the only theories to deal with concepts like "immediacy," "being fully present," "being fully there," "being in contact," and "truly meeting another person." These are all full-bodied perceptual–experiential states and not primarily cognitive, conceptual states. None of these concepts easily map into cognitive theories. Yet experientially most people know the difference between moments when they felt "fully present" or "fully into something" versus moments when they felt removed, distanced, and so on.

The moments when we are being most effectively agentic are often those that could be best described as moments of "immediacy," of "full presence," and of "full contact." We are more likely to feel coordinated, "all of a piece," "integrated," and working smoothly. This does not mean events necessarily are going smoothly. We may be working quite hard to master a difficult situation. But there is a sense of being fully "there" in the situation (Csikszentmihalyi, 1990). Dweck and Leggett (1988) have found that people work most productively when they are "mastery oriented." Their attention is fully absorbed into the task rather than on evaluation of themselves. At such moments they are more open to feedback, learn from mistakes, are nondefensive, and think creatively.

Tallman (1996) has argued that such an absorbed, open working state characterizes what others have referred to as good in-session client behavior. Measures of "high levels of experiencing" on the Experiencing Scale (Mathieu-Coughlan & Klein, 1984) and focused or emotional vocal quality (Rice & Kerr, 1986) may be correlates of this state. In regard to this, the turning point on the Experiencing Scale from ineffective to effective client behavior is where the person moves from distanced describing and analyzing to "inhabiting" and being fully present in what he/she is talking about.

## CLIENT AGENCY AND PSYCHOTHERAPY

Now that we have presented our model of how people can actively and agentically experience and think through their problems we can ask this question: Why do clients come to therapy? Basically our answer is that clients come to therapy when their self-generated problem-solving efforts do not work and may even be making things worse. Why does this happen? There are probably many reasons, but we focus on two. First, experiential theories have assumed that clients have learned not to trust their own experience. Instead, they have learned to rely on the rules and precepts of others. When suddenly they face life problems that these precepts do not handle comfortably, clients do not know how to think and experience themselves out of the spot they are in. Experiential therapists help by providing empathic support for clients' self-healing processes, as well as specific experiential exercises to more productively mobilize these processes. Our second answer is that many clients do not have the supportive kind of "work space" they need in their everyday lives to engage in productive self-healing. Clients need time, safety, and support. If they are feeling too overloaded by stress, or too threatened and defensive, they adopt a conservative risk-avoidance strategy of relying on old problem-solving techniques, even if these strategies are not only not working but perhaps making things worse. Their thinking is not free and creative, but rather ruminative and obsessive. In everyday life individuals may not be able to psychologically set aside the threats and the stressors sufficiently to "clear a space" (Gendlin, 1996) to engage freely in the productive thinking process. Many do not have empathic individuals who will listen to them and not interrupt with premature advice either. As a result, individuals are not able to productively use their own self-healing capacities, and instead may become mired in a downward spiral as they try over and over to get out of the trap they are in.

## What Does Therapy Provide?

With the example of Anna in mind, we propose a model of how clients utilize therapy. We suggest five basic things therapy provides for clients.

*First*, clients may use therapy as a structured, safe space within which to think. Anna did not have such a space. She did not have an empathic, supportive listener who would provide her an hour of undivided attention and simply *listen* to her think aloud. In addition, Anna's life was hectic and chaotic. She had a child to care for and a job to attend to. Even when she had moments to herself, she did not have "psychological time." Subjectively she felt pressure to make a decision, and that pressure resulted in her ruminating about her problem over and over again. In therapy, she was able to take a deep breath, step back, and begin to see things in a broader perspective.

The therapist's role in this first function of therapy is most basically that of simple "witnessing" of the client's process. Clients, through their own verbal expression (e.g., Clark, 1993), can lay their problems out, re-present them to themselves, explore them, experience them, and think them through. It is the provision of this time and space that is the single most important resource a therapist has to offer. There is something about "laying the problem out" that seems to help. It is as if the client must get the problem "outside herself" in order to look at it. It is as if she can get "above it all" and notice patterns and relationships she had been missing. This can occur in journaling, but expressing the problem to a therapist can add something. There is evidence that there is more personal involvement in spoken than in written language (Clark, 1993). Therefore we speculate that the act of expressing the problem to another person makes what is expressed more vivid and more experiential. It "comes alive" more and adds a kind of real- ness to it.

The *second* major function of therapy is that some clients use it as an opportunity for interpersonal exploration and learning. Here the clients' attention is much more on the interaction with the therapist. While Anna was concerned with what the therapist thought, for the most part her atten- tion was focused inward, on her own unfolding and evolving thought pro- cess. However, some clients are very concerned with what the therapist thinks. For them therapy is much more of an interpersonal encounter and "test" situation. Will the therapist like them? Will the therapist accept them? This will be especially true where they are vitally concerned with the question "Am I OK?" Having an empathic therapist understand them and validate them provides them with an opportunity to test out their perceptions of interper- sonal worth, as well as practice some of their interpersonal skills. Disclosing painful and shameful things to the therapist facilitates the client's having the courage to "own" and accept these things publicly.

The *third* function the therapist can supply is to provide material for client thinking. This can come in the form of provocative questions, inter- pretations, empathic conjectures, deep empathic reflections, advice, reframes, or self-disclosures. The important thing is that these are only useful if clients actively incorporate them into their own thinking process. None of these will be useful if the client passively adopts the information.

The *fourth* function of the therapist, for clients who want and need it, is to provide *structured exercises* for exploratory thinking. Such exercises function as *tools* to help the client explore and synthesize new meaning. They include the whole set of exercises in the experiential therapies but also in- clude exercises in other therapies. The important thing is that all techniques are ultimately structured opportunities for clients' creative learning processes, not mechanistic techniques that "extinguish emotions," restructure cogni- tions, or train good assertion habits.

The *fifth* thing therapists can do is teach *specific skills*. This includes communication skills training, problem solving training, managing one's emotions, combatting dysfunctional cognitions, thinking rationally, dream analysis, focusing, relaxation, and a whole host of other skills. Again, these skills only become useful to clients when they make them their own through their own exploration.

In sum, therapists help by joining the process of the client and by offer- ing things the client can use in making meaning in terms of his or her own life space. The therapist is not unlike a good, empathic home decorator, who comes in, listens to what the client wants, and helps the client figure out how to achieve it. Varying degrees of activity on the part of the home decorator will be needed depending on what the client wants/needs.

## Being an Active Agent in Experiential Therapies

In experiential therapies humans are seen as acting agentically all the time. Psychological problems are problems of agency: individuals are acting agentically, but not in effective ways. Yet they have the potential to act effectively, whether it is called a thrust toward self-actualization (Rogers, 1961), deep experiencing potential (Mahrer, 1996), the capacity to think more intelligently and critically (Van Balen, 1990; Zimring, 1990), the ability to generate new process steps through experiential focusing (Gendlin, 1990, 1996), the potential to stand on their own two feet, to take responsibility for themselves, and to be in contact with the moment to solve problems at the contact boundary (Gestalt therapy), or the capacity to act authentically, to face up to anxiety, and to take risks (existential therapy).

Clients' behavior is agentic even if dysfunctional. They are ongoing processes moving down the road, even if they do not experience themselves as such, and even if they are not consciously and deliberately planning their moves. Their "moves" as they travel may lead to blind alleys, or get them into even more hot water, but they are trying to move down the road as they see it. They may be, for instance, stuck in one place on their road, almost like a vehicle spinning its wheels in the mud, but they are still trying to advance. Even depressives are usually struggling, albeit ineffectively, to get out of their depression—dysfunctional cognitions could paradoxically be seen as efforts to extricate themselves—efforts that backfire. Severely dysfunctional clients, who may not really know how to productively use their internal resources (Gendlin, 1964), are still struggling agentically to proceed with life.

The fact that clients are acting agentically does not mean that we can blame them when therapy does not go well. They are not *choosing* their negative outcomes. A particularly pernicious idea, fostered by some early existential and Gestalt therapists, as well as by some psychodynamic theorists, is that individuals are "unconsciously" choosing to be miserable and dysfunctional. In contrast, we believe, along with Watzlawick (1987) and others, that individuals are acting to try to promote their lives, but how they're doing it is dysfunctional and paradoxically backfires and either keeps them stuck or makes things worse. Thus an individual becomes highly self-critical, believing that self-criticism (i.e., "being honest with oneself") will lead to more effective behavior. Instead it is self-paralyzing, leading to further rounds of self-criticism.

This view of agency contrasts with other approaches. At the theory level many approaches assume that clients are fundamentally impaired in their ability to be agentic and it is the job of the therapist to restore this. Object relations theory holds that client problems go back to impaired agency from early childhood due to a separation–individuation failure. The therapist provides the insights and the experiences the client needs to individuate so that the client can become an agent. Cognitive and behavior therapies assume that clients lack the skills to be agentic. It is the job of the therapist to assess the deficiency and then provide the corrective training techniques. In essence, the formal theories of psychoanalysis, cognitive, and behavioral therapies have no central construct of client agency as a variable mediating change in therapy.

## Agency and Experiential Psychotherapy

Experiential therapies try to promote effective agency on the part of the client. They do this by encouraging their experiential involvement in exploring their problems. This occurs by (1) vividly reevoking experience (Mahrer, 1996; Rice & Saperia, 1984); (2) engaging in exercises that allow experiential exploration, such as two-chair or empty-chair work (Greenberg, Rice, & Elliott, 1993); (3) responding in an empathic, experiential manner (Bozarth, 1997; Gendlin, 1968; Greenberg et al., 1993); (4) turning clients inward to their own experiencing (Gendlin, 1996); or (5) using guided imagery (Mahrer, 1996). These lead clients to be able to process their own experience, think through their problems, and discover new, creatively, personally meaningful solutions that fit their life spaces. Watson, Greenberg, and Goldman (1996) have suggested that therapy promotes accessing of emotions, symbolizing feelings, and then the reflexive self-examination of experience.

We now turn to a closer examination of how specific experiential psychotherapies facilitate effective agency.

In classical client-centered therapy (Rogers, 1957) the client's agentic exploration is *the* operative therapeutic ingredient. The therapist provides a good working atmosphere in which the client's intrinsic capacity for growth can operate. The therapist does nothing but accompany the client on this journey of self-evolution, responding empathically to the client's agency (Brodley, 1996). This kind of relationship provides the client the freedom to move into a state of high internal openness to experiencing, become mastery oriented (Tallman, 1996), and creatively sort through problems and make decisions. Compatible with this, Zimring (1990) has found the processes of client-centered therapy facilitate clear thinking.

Recent experiential approaches (Gendlin, 1996; Greenberg et al., 1993; Mahrer, 1996) are more systematic than client-centered therapy. Therapists provide more specific guidance. In process-experiential therapy (Greenberg et al., 1993), for instance, when clients exhibit specific "markers" it is assumed they are posed to work on and resolve particular "tasks." Therapists specify procedures that are presumed to help clients work through those tasks. However, it is the client who does the work and who comes up with the resolution. Thus the procedures suggested by the therapist are really tools that promote clients' own agentic task resolution. These procedures provide structured experiences that allow clients to engage in the conceptualizing–experiencing–exploring process previously described. In particular they create the opportunity for clients to exercise their capacity for free intelligence, to get out of cycles of ruminative thinking and to think and experience in the kind of dialogic way which is useful.

For instance, in the two-chair exercise (Greenberg et al., 1993) the client role plays the two sides of an intrapersonal split: the self-critical side, and the self-defending, experiential side. The two sides of the issue are separated. The client has the chance to stand back, compare and contrast the two sides, and to thoughtfully inhabit each side to spell out its implicit logic. The procedure facilitates intelligent, creative, resourceful thinking about the conflict. Similarly, the empty chair procedure helps clients gain a meta-cognitive perspective on feelings of unfinished business with a significant other. The person is able to move back from a ruminative over-focus on the injuries they have suffered, and to gain a broader, more balanced perspective on themselves and their lives. They then can make more productive choices for themselves.

We next examine the problematic reaction point procedure (Rice & Saperia, 1984) in more detail. We illustrate how agency and experiencing could play a role in the generation of these kinds of problems and in their resolution.

## OUR AGENTIC, EXPERIENTIAL MODEL
## OF THE PROBLEMATIC REACTION POINT PROCEDURE

*How a Problematic Reaction Occurs.*   Individuals in everyday life often operate out of their tacit knowledge of a situation, represented in an implicit felt experiential sense of what is going on, because they do not have time to cognitively think and reflect. Thus they may at times be acting agentically out of this implicit sense but may behave in ways that their more cognitive, reflective selves find inexplicable or confusing. Problematic reaction points are situations where people have done something or reacted in some way they find confusing or incomprehensible. Upon reflection on the issue, they may agentically try to understand the problem of how they have behaved. They might adopt a reflective, metacognitive, third person perspective. They may try to intellectually analyze why they reacted as they did (Gendlin, 1964), or they may engage in evaluative self-criticism (Rice & Saperia, 1984). They may "search" the problem space from this third person perspective, trying to understand their own behavior.

However, this frequently does not work. One reason is that whatever they come to via this procedure is intellectual, analytic, and deductive. It is not *recognitional* and grounded in their actual experience. They have not accessed their own implicit experiential reasons for acting as they did. They may conclude that they acted in such and such a manner because of such and such a reason; but, as a distanced, intellectual deduction, this conclusion does not have the felt immediacy of a "gut-level" recognition. They are not "inhabiting" their own experience, and thus have difficulty in agentically operating to change.

*The Therapeutic Procedure.*   In the problematic reaction point procedure clients are asked to vividly imagine the situation and to "reinhabit" how they were experiencing when they reacted as they did. They are actually asked to "see through their own eyes" instead of adopting a "third person perspective." "Walking in their own shoes," so to speak, they are now able to search the problem space from a much more intimate perspective while still metacognitively reflecting upon themselves. They experientially follow the steps that led up to their reaction. They uncover the implicit reason for their response (the "meaning bridge"). This is recognized, not just conceptualized. They now experientially understand what led them to react as they did. Being in the experiential presence of the problem as they were construing it in that moment, they now experience themselves as having some control, as being able to do otherwise. They may build a cognitive, conceptual model of why they reacted as they did, but this model is based on direct experiential recognition. A sense of agency is restored. They no longer feel so "out of control." The therapist's role throughout this procedure is that of guide.

## CONCLUSIONS

Echoing Bergin and Garfield (1994), we believe that as therapists respect clients' agency and rely on client's active intelligence and resources more, the therapists will be more effective. Such reliance is an explicit theoretical part of experiential therapies. Establishing a truly collaborative relationship, being willing to go where the client wants to go, utilizing the client's frame of reference (Bohart & Greenberg, 1997; Duncan & Moynihan, 1994), trusting client process, facilitating client creativity, and—most of all—realizing that one is dialoguing with another creative intelligence is the best way to promote change.

## REFERENCES

Bakan, D. (1996). Origination, self-determination, and psychology. *Journal of Humanistic Psychology, 36*, 9–20.

Barrett-Lennard, G. T. (1997). The recovery of empathy: Toward others and self. In A. C. Bohart & L. S. Greenberg (Eds.), *Empathy reconsidered: New directions in psychotherapy* (pp. 103–121). Washington, DC: American Psychological Association.

Bergin, A. E., & Garfield, S. L. (1994). Overview, trends, and future issues. In A. E. Bergin & S. L. Garfield (Eds.), *Handbook of psychotherapy and behavior change* (4th ed., pp. 821–830). New York: Wiley.

Bohart, A. C. (1993). Experiencing: The basis of psychotherapy. *Journal of Psychotherapy Integration, 3*, 51–67.

Bohart, A. C., & Associates. (1996). Experiencing, knowing, and change. In R. Hutterer, G. Pawlowsky, P. F. Schmid, & R. Stipsits (Eds.), *Client-centered and experiential psychotherapy: A paradigm in motion* (pp. 190–212). Vienna: Lang.

Bohart, A. C., & Greenberg, L. S. (1997). Empathy in psychotherapy: An introductory overview. In A. Bohart & L. S. Greenberg (Eds.), *Empathy reconsidered: New directions in psychotherapy* (pp. 3–31). Washington, DC: American Psychological Association.

Bohart, A. C., Humphrey, A., Magallanes, M., Guzman, R., Smiljanich, K., & Aguallo, S. (1993). Emphasizing the future in empathy responses. *Journal of Humanistic Psychology, 33,* 12–29.

Bohart, A. C., O'Hara, M., & Leitner, L. (1998). Empirically violated treatments: Disenfranchisement of humanistic and other approaches. *Psychotherapy Research, 8,* 141–157.

Bohart, A. C., & Tallman, K. (1996). The active client: Therapy as self-help. *Journal of Humanistic Psychology, 36,* 7–30

Bozarth, J. D. (1997). Empathy from the framework of client-centered theory and the Rogerian hypothesis. In A. Bohart & L. S. Greenberg (Eds.), *Empathy reconsidered: New directions in psychotherapy* (pp. 81–102). Washington, DC: American Psychological Association.

Brodley, B. T. (1996). Empathic understanding and feelings in client-centered therapy. *The Person-Centered Journal, 3,* 22–30.

Christensen, A., & Jacobson, N. S. (1994). Who (or what) can do psychotherapy? The status and challenge of nonprofessional therapies. *Psychological Science, 5,* 8–14.

Clark, L. (1993). Stress and the cognitive-conversational benefits of social interaction. *Journal of Social and Clinical Psychology, 12,* 25–55.

Corsini, R. (1989). Introduction. In R. Corsini & D. Wedding (Eds.), *Current psychotherapies* (4th ed., pp. 1–18). Itasca, IL: F. E. Peacock.

Cowan, P. (1978). *Piaget: With feeling.* New York: Holt, Rinehart & Winston.

Csikszentmihalyi, M. (1990). *Flow: The psychology of optimal experience.* New York: Harper & Row.

Duncan, B. L., & Moynihan, D. W. (1994). Applying outcome research: Intentional utilization of the client's frame of reference. *Psychotherapy, 31,* 294–301.

Dweck, C. S., & Leggett, E. L. (1988). A social-cognitive approach to motivation and personality. *Psychological Review, 95,* 256–273.

Elliott, R. (1984). A discovery-oriented approach to significant change events in psychotherapy: Interpersonal process recall and comprehensive process analysis. In L. N. Rice & L. S. Greenberg (Eds.), *Patterns of change* (pp. 249–286). New York: Guilford Press.

Elliott, R., & James, E. (1989). Varieties of client experience in psychotherapy: An analysis of the literature. *Clinical Psychology Review, 9,* 443–467.

Epstein, R. (1991). Skinner, creativity, and the problem of spontaneous behavior. *Psychological Science, 2,* 362–370.

Finke, R. A. (1995). Creative insight and preinventive forms. In R. J. Sternberg & J. E. Davidson (Eds.), *The nature of insight* (pp. 255–280). Cambridge, MA: MIT Press.

Gendlin, E. T. (1964). A theory of personality change. In P. Worchel & D. Byrne (Eds.), *Personality change.* New York: Wiley.

Gendlin, E. T. (1968). The experiential response. In E. Hammer (Ed.), *Use of interpretation in treatment.* New York: Grune & Stratton.

Gendlin, E. T. (1990). The small steps of the therapy process: How they come and how to help them come. In G. Lietaer, J. Rombauts, & R. Van Balen (Eds.),

*Client-centered and experiential psychotherapy in the nineties* (pp. 205–224). Leuven, Belgium: Leuven University Press.

Gendlin, E. T. (1996). *Focusing-oriented psychotherapy: A manual of the experiential method*. New York: Guilford Press.

Gibson, J. J. (1979). *The ecological approach to visual perception*. Boston: Houghton Mifflin.

Glucksberg, S., & Keysar, B. (1990). Understanding metaphorical comparisons: Beyond similarity. *Psychological Review*, 97, 3–18.

Gold, J. R. (1994). When the patient does the integrating: Lessons for theory and practice. *Journal of Psychotherapy Integration*, 4, 133–158.

Greenberg, L. S., Rice, L. N., & Elliott, R. (1993). *Facilitating emotional change: The moment-by-moment process*. New York: Guilford Press.

Horvath, A. O. (1995). The therapeutic relationship: From transference to alliance. *In Session*, 1, 7–17.

Howard, G. S. (1996). *Understanding human nature: An owner's manual*. Notre Dame, IN: Academic Publications.

Kolb, D. A. (1984). *Experiential learning*. Englewood Cliffs, NJ: Prentice-Hall.

Lakoff, G. (1987). *Women, fire, and dangerous things*. Chicago: University of Chicago Press.

Lambert, M. J. (1992). Psychotherapy outcome research. In J. C. Norcross & M. R. Goldfried (Eds.), *Handbook of psychotherapy integration* (pp. 94–129). New York: Basic Books.

Loesch, M., Hamilton, H., Seferian, L., Rush, S., & Bohart, A. C. (1994, August). *Intellectual versus experiential knowledge: Creative artists and actors learning roles*. Paper presented at the annual meeting of the American Psychological Association, Los Angeles.

Mahrer, A. R. (1996). *The complete guide to experiential psychotherapy*. New York: Wiley.

Masten, A. S., Best, K. M., & Garmazy, N. (1990). Resilience and development: Contribution from the study of children who overcome adversity. *Development and Psychopathology*, 2, 425–444.

Mathieu-Coughlan, P., & Klein, M. H. (1984). Experiential psychotherapy: Key events in client-centered interaction. In L. N. Rice & L. S. Greenberg (Eds.), *Patterns of change* (pp. 194–212). New York: Guilford Press.

Neisser, U. (1967). *Cognitive psychology*. New York: Appleton-Century-Crofts.

Orlinsky, D. E. (1989). Researchers' images of psychotherapy: Their origins and influence on research. *Clinical Psychology Review*, 9, 413–442.

Orlinsky, D. E., Grawe, K., & Parks, B. K. (1994). Process and outcome in psychotherapy: *Noch einmal*. In A. E. Bergin & S. L. Garfield (Eds.), *Handbook of psychotherapy and behavior change* (4th ed., pp. 270–376). New York: Wiley.

Pennebaker, J. W. (1990). *Opening up: The healing power of confiding in others*. New York: Morrow.

Polyani, M. (1967). *The tacit dimension*. New York: Anchor.

Prochaska, J. O. (1995). An eclectic and integrative approach: Transtheoretical therapy. In A. Gurman & S. Messer (Eds.), *Essential psychotherapies* (pp. 403–440). New York: Guilford Press.

Rennie, D. L. (1990). Toward a representation of the client's experience of the psychotherapy hour. In G. Lietaer, J. Rombauts, & R. Van Balen (Eds.), *Client-*

*centered and experiential therapy in the nineties* (pp. 155–172). Leuven, Belgium: Leuven University Press.

Rennie, D. (1994). Storytelling in psychotherapy. *Psychotherapy, 31*, 234–243.

Rice, L. N., & Kerr, G. P. (1986). Measures of client and therapist vocal quality. In L. S. Greenberg & W. M. Pinsof (Eds.), *The psychotherapy process: A research handbook* (pp. 73–106). New York: Guilford Press.

Rice, L. N., & Saperia, E. P. (1984). Task analysis of the resolution of problematic reactions. In L. N. Rice & L. S. Greenberg (Eds.), *Patterns of change* (pp. 29–66). New York: Guilford Press.

Rogers, C. R. (1957). The necessary and sufficient conditions of therapeutic personality change. *Journal of Consulting Psychology, 21*, 95–103.

Rogers, C. R. (1961). *On becoming a person.* Boston: Houghton Mifflin.

Rosenbaum, R. (1994). Single-session therapies: Intrinsic integration? *Journal of Psychotherapy Integration, 4*, 229–252.

Rychlak, J. F. (1994). *Logical learning theory.* Lincoln: University of Nebraska Press.

Segal, D. L., & Murray, E. J. (1994). Emotional processing in cognitive therapy and vocal expression of feeling. *Journal of Social and Clinical Psychology, 13*, 189–206.

Sternberg, R. J., & Davidson, J. E. (Eds.). (1995). *The nature of insight.* Cambridge, MA: MIT Press.

Stiles, W. B., & Shapiro, D. A. (1989). Abuse of the drug metaphor in psychotherapy process-outcome research. *Clinical Psychology Review, 9*, 521–544.

Tallman, K. (1996). *The state of mind theory: Goal orientation concepts applied to clinical psychology.* Unpublished master's thesis, California State University, Dominguez Hills.

Tallman, K., Robinson, E., Kay, D., Harvey, S., & Bohart, A. C. (1994, August). *Experiential and nonexperiential Rogerian therapy: An analogue study.* Paper presented at the annual meeting of the American Psychological Association, Los Angeles.

Van Balen, R. (1990). The therapeutic relationship according to Carl Rogers: Only a climate? a dialogue? or both? In G. Lietaer, J. Rombauts, & R. Van Balen (Eds.), *Client-centered and experiential psychotherapy in the nineties* (pp. 65–86). Leuven, Belgium: Leuven University Press.

Ward, T. B., Finke, R. A., & Smith, S. M. (1995). *Creativity and the mind.* New York: Plenum.

Watson, J. C., Greenberg, L. S., & Goldman, R. (1996). Change processes in experiential therapy. In R. Hutterer, G. Pawlowsky, P. F. Schmid, & R. Stipsits (Eds.), *Client-centered and experiential psychotherapy: A paradigm in motion* (pp. 35–46). Vienna: Lang.

Watson, J. C., & Rennie, D. L. (1994). Qualitative analysis of clients' subjective experience of significant moments during the exploration of problematic reactions. *Journal of Counseling Psychology, 41*, 500–509.

Watzlawick, P. (1987). "If you desire to see, learn how to act." In J. K. Zeig (Ed.), *The evolution of psychotherapy* (pp. 91–100). New York: Brunner/Mazel.

Zimring, F. (1990). Cognitive processes as a cause of psychotherapeutic change: Self-initiated processes. In G. Lietaer, J. Rombauts, & R. Van Balen (Eds.), *Client-centered and experiential psychotherapy in the nineties* (pp. 361–380). Leuven, Belgium: Leuven University Press.

# 9

*****

# How Can Impressive In-Session Changes Become Impressive Postsession Changes?

## Alvin R. Mahrer

*In this chapter* I would like to identify two rather particular kinds of impressive in-session changes and then show how a therapist and a person (patient, client) can help these two impressive in-session changes continue out into the postsession extratherapy world.

## WHAT ARE THE TWO TARGETED KINDS OF IMPRESSIVE IN-SESSION CHANGES?

The focus is on two very particular kinds of impressive in-session changes. The reason for focusing on these two kinds of changes and on their explicit meaning comes from a particular experiential theory or model of human beings and psychotherapy (Mahrer, 1989, 1996). In the same way, the proposed ways of enabling these particular in-session changes to become postsession changes also come from that particular experiential theory or model. Because so much hinges on the explicit theory or model of human beings and psychotherapy, it is important first to touch on the touchy question of whether there is one experiential psychotherapy or perhaps many.

### Is There One Experiential Psychotherapy or Perhaps Many?

You can make a case for a single, organized, identifiable experiential psy-chotherapy. If you take this position, it is understandable to allow for some in-house variability while still preserving the identity of an overall experiential psychotherapy. On the other hand, it is also understandable that the effort to have a single overall experiential psychotherapy can easily pressure alien experiential psychotherapies to conform to the dominant ways of thinking or to risk exclusion and alienation.

You can also make a case for many experiential psychotherapies, some of which fundamentally differ from one another. The term "experiential psychotherapy" was perhaps first used in a substantive way to identify the approach of Carl A. Whitaker, John Warkentin, Thomas P. Malone, and Richard E. Felder (Malone, Whitaker, Warkentin, & Felder, 1961; Whitaker, Felder, Malone, & Warkentin, 1962; Whitaker & Malone, 1953, 1969). Since then, there have been about two dozen psychotherapies that formally designate themselves as experiential psychotherapy, and upwards of an additional two dozen that semiofficially call themselves experiential psychotherapies (Mahrer & Fairweather, 1993).

Making a case for one or many experiential psychotherapies depends in part on how each approach answers questions such as these: What is the conceptualization of the structure and contents of personality? What is the conceptualization of the foundation or deeper level of personality? What accounts for personal pain, anguish, suffering? What is the conceptualization of what a person is capable of becoming, of optimal functioning? What are the principles for determining the valued psychotherapeutic objectives and goals for the individual person? What are the valued determinants of psychotherapeutic change? What does the therapist do to help bring about psychotherapeutic change? What constitute useful therapeutic data, and how does the therapist best elicit whatever the therapist selects as useful therapeutic data?

If we take a careful look at all the approaches that are formally or informally designated as experiential, and if we examine their answers to these kinds of questions, a case can be made that (1) there is probably a fair number of fundamentally different approaches designated as experiential psychotherapies, and (2) there is probably as great a variability among designated experiential psychotherapies as exists between these and many other psychotherapies.

The spirit underlying this chapter is a little bit of both cases. I appreciate the effort to identify a single kind of experiential psychotherapy, and yet I tend to see my particular experiential psychotherapy (Mahrer, 1989, 1996) as perhaps relatively distinctive from most others, starting from its position on most of the above questions.

More practically, it is this particular experiential conceptualization that provides explicit meaning to the two kinds of impressive in-session changes.

## What Is the Explicit Meaning of an In-Session Qualitative Change in the Person?

Almost any conceptualization can have its own meaning of a "qualitative change" in the person. I am referring to a rather particular meaning of what this is, and it is this particular meaning that is understood as the impressive change to be continued out into the extratherapy world through the methods described later.

In this model (Figure 9.1), the person is conceptualized in terms of "potentials for experiencing." These are very particularized kinds of experiencings that are available in this particular person. As the building blocks of personality, each potential for experiencing is to be carefully described as it is in this particular person. For example, in one person an operating potential (OP1, Figure 9.1) may be described as the experiencing of loss, loneliness, aloneness, isolation. Another potential may consist of the experiencing of being pinned down, invaded, torn apart. It is important to describe each potential carefully to capture the explicit nature of the particular experiencing in this particular person.

Some potentials for experiencing are more closely tied to the way the person behaves, acts, constructs, and is in the personal world in which the person exists, functions, and operates. These are understood as the person's operating potentials, indicated as OP1, OP2, and OP3 at the left in Figure 9.1. A person's operating potentials constitute the more or less conscious, aware identity or self.

Some potentials for experiencing are deeper, much less connected to the way the person behaves, acts, functions, or operates in the external world. These are referred to as deeper and basic potentials, identified as DP4, DP5, DP6 and BP7, BP8, BP9, respectively, at the left in Figure 9.1. Deeper and basic potentials are understood as outside the ordinary range of the operating person's understanding, knowledge, consciousness, awareness.

Relationships of operating potentials toward deeper potentials are, in this model, uniformly and aggressively negative, unfriendly, distancing, disintegrative. This state of affairs is indicated by the negative signs in the relationships between operating potentials and deeper potentials (Figure 9.1). Relationships among operating potentials may be positive, friendly, welcoming, integrative. These are indicated by the positive sign in the relation between OP1 and OP2 at the left in the figure. Or, relationships between operating potentials may be negative, unfriendly, disintegrative, indicated by the negative signs in relations between OP1 and OP3, and between OP3 and OP2 in the figure.

What is the explicit meaning of this first in-session impressive change? As indicated on the right in the figure, (1) what had been sealed off, kept down inside the person, is now a part of the operating, functioning person or self or domain. A deeper potential (DP5, at the left in the figure) is now an operating potential (OP5, at the right in the figure). In addition, (2) relationships between operating potentials have moved in the direction of greater positive, friendly, welcoming, integrative relationships. This is indicated by the increase of positive signs in relations among operating potentials at the right in the figure. Even further, (3) an operating potential in the former person (OP1, at the left in the figure) is now much less present or may even be gone. This is indicated by the dotted circle around OP1 at the right in the figure.

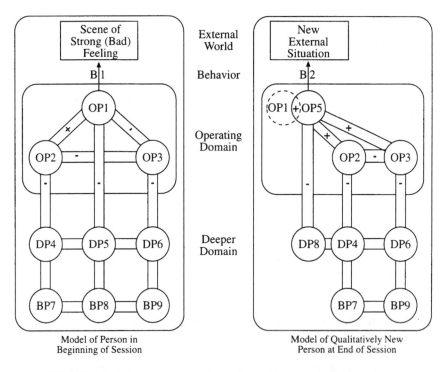

FIGURE 9.1. Model of person in the beginning and at end of session.

In the terms of this model of personality, here is the explicit meaning of the first in-session impressive change. Here is an impressively qualitative change in who and what this person has become, a deep-seated change in the way the new person thinks, acts, comes across, feels, experiences. Especially if you look at the operating, functioning domain, here is a qualitatively new person. In more general terms, here is a much more integrated and actualized new person. In still more general terms, this is the explicit meaning of a "qualitatively new person." But this is just one of the two in-session impressive changes.

## What Is the Explicit Meaning of Being Free of Situations of Bad Feeling?

The second impressive in-session change is that the qualitatively new person is essentially free of particular painful life situations and the hurtful bad feelings that occur in those situations. Quite practically, those particular painful life situations are no longer a part of the person's world, and as they wash out of the person's world, what also washes away are the hurtful bad feelings that the person had in those situations.

What is the explicit meaning of this second impressive change? On the left in Figure 9.1, the person (OP1) behaves (B1) in appropriate ways to construct and build very particular kinds of painful scenes and situations in which the person has hurtful bad feelings. Why is it that the person has these painful scenes and situations, and has such bad feelings in these particular scenes and situations? As understood in this model, the explanation or cause lies mainly in the particular nature of the operating potential (OP1), and also in its negative, disintegrative relationship with its deeper potential (DP5). The net result is, for example, that a person may have quite bad feelings as she/ he is undergoing a painful sense of loss, aloneness, isolation, sitting by her-/ himself in the living room, hearing all the others happily chattering and laugh- ing as they are eating in the dining room.

The impressive change is portrayed and accounted for at the right in Figure 9.1. Quite specifically, in the qualitatively new person's world, the old scene or situation of bad feelings is gone. The qualitatively new person's world is essentially free of the old person's scene or situation of bad feeling, and also of the bad feelings that occur in that scene or situation. Compared with the state of affairs indicated at the left in the figure, the main causes are essentially gone. That is, (1) the former operating potential is no longer present, indicated by the dotted circle around OP1 at the right in the figure; (2) instead of negative relations between OP1 and DP5, there are now posi- tive relations between the new OP5 and OP1.

The practical result is that the qualitatively new person is now essen- tially free of the old person's scene or situation of painful bad feelings, and also of the painful bad feelings that occur in that kind of scene or situation.

I hope it is clear why it is so important to have explicit meanings of the two impressive in-session changes that are loosely referred to as a qualita- tive change in the person and being free of situations of bad feeling.

One more point needs clarification. In this model of psychotherapy, each session starts by trying to identify a scene or situation of strong feeling that is front and center for this person in this session. Each session provides the person with an opportunity to attain these two impressive in-session changes. In other words, each session is understood as its own minitherapy, whether this is the only session or there are subsequent sessions.

## HOW ARE THE IMPRESSIVE CHANGES BROUGHT ABOUT IN THE SESSION?

Each session goes through three steps in helping to bring about the impres- sive in-session changes. Before we discuss how to help impressive in-session changes become impressive postsession changes, it is important to have a picture of how these impressive changes are brought about in the first place. The three in-session steps are considered sequentially in the following subsections.

## First Step: A Scene of Strong Feeling Is Identified and a Deeper Potential for Experiencing Is Accessed, Discovered, and Opened Up

In each session the first step is that the person identifies some scene of very strong feeling, enters into living and being in the scene, locates the precise moment when the feeling is so strong; what is accessed, discovered, opened up is a deeper potential for experiencing, an inner potential that had been kept down, sealed off, hidden. Here are two examples of scenes of strong feeling and the deeper potentials for experiencing that were accessed by careful probing down into each scene of strong feeling:

With one patient, an older woman, the scene of strong feeling is when she is sitting alone in the living room of her home, a little drunk, crying lightly. She is clutching the cap of her husband who died suddenly, of a heart attack, nearly 3 years ago. Intensely hurtful feelings are occurring in the surface experiencing of profound loss, loneliness, aloneness, slipping into herself, intense gloominess, and isolation. The deeper potential that is opened up, newly discovered, accessed, is the inner deeper experiencing of being free, independent, liberated, free of constraints and restrictive control.

With the second patient, a middle-aged man, the scene of strong feeling is when he is filled with painful feelings accompanying the experiencing of being pinned, invaded, torn apart, as his wealthy cousin, the head of the firm where he works, is accusing him of being a lifelong loser, scared to take risks, and being a wimp who is pushed around by his wife and adolescent daughters. Sealed off and hidden by the operating potential is a deeper potential for experiencing powerful sexuality, complete sexual arousal, a wallowing in wholesale eroticism.

For both patients, the scenes of strong feeling were quite recent and the feelings were quite painful. Identifying these scenes of strong painful feeling is important because one of the postsession impressive changes is that these patients will be enabled to be reasonably free of such bad-feeling scenes and situations.

For both patients, the deeper potentials for experiencing were indeed deep inside, hidden, not what the patients experienced in their ordinary daily lives. Accessing these deeper potentials for experiencing is important because they are to become integral parts of who and what the qualitatively new persons can be in their impressive postsession changes.

## Second Step: The Deeper Potential for Experiencing Is Welcomed, Appreciated, and Loved

The second in-session step is that the person relates to the deeper potential in a way that is welcoming, appreciating, loving. The relationship now becomes "integrative." Up to now, in this session, relationships with the deeper potential have typically been hateful, fearful, distancing, separating, fraught with bad feelings, disintegrative.

The change is that the widowed woman now welcomes and appreciates the deeper, inner potential for experiencing a sense of freedom, independence, liberation, being unconstrained and uncontrolled. The impressive change is that the middle-aged man now relates warmly and lovingly to the newfound deeper potential for experiencing powerful sexuality, complete sexual arousal, wallowing in wholesale eroticism.

This second step necessarily follows from the first because accessing and discovering the deeper potential for experiencing provides an opportunity to welcome and appreciate whatever deeper potential for experiencing has been discovered and opened up. This second step is also important because it opens the door to the third step.

## Third Step: The Person Undergoes a Radical Shift into Being the Qualitatively New Person in the Context of Past Scenes and Situations

The third step is that the person undergoes a radical shift out of being the ordinary, continuing person and into being the qualitatively new person who *is* the deeper potential. This is almost always a massive change, probably the first time that the person has become a whole new person who *is* the deeper potential.

She has shifted drastically into being the qualitatively new person who is free, independent, liberated, unconstrained, uncontrolled. He is now being the whole new person who *is* the absolute sheer experiencing of powerful sexuality, complete sexual arousal, and wallowing in wholesale eroticism. They are being these qualitatively new persons in the context of past scenes and situations, some of which are relatively recent, some of which are from very early in life. We find three or five or more scenes from their past, and they have plenty of opportunities to be the qualitatively new persons in the context of these past scenes and situations.

She revels in fully being the qualitatively new person when she is lying in the crib, letting the feces flow; when she is in second grade, telling the class about her older brother's new bicycle; when she is an adolescent who should be practicing the piano before the lesson tomorrow; when she is sitting in the library near the fellow to whom she is so attracted; when she was reviewing the notes for the important committee meeting at work.

We find a number of scenes and situations in which he can undergo the qualitative shift into being the whole new person who experiences powerful sexuality, complete sexual arousal, wallowing in wholesale eroticism. In some of these scenes, there may have been a slight glow of this experiencing. In other past scenes, there was not a whisper; indeed, this particular kind of experiencing was nowhere to be seen—would have been conspicuously inappropriate.

Yet the main point is that both persons are now bathing in being qualitatively new persons, fully and enjoyably, in the protective and safe contexts of past scenes and situations. At the same time, she is simply no longer the former person who lives in a world of drunken, crying loss, aloneness, loneliness, intense gloom and isolation, sitting alone and clutching the cap of her dead husband. He is no longer the person who lives in a world in which elevated key figures take it upon themselves to judge him in aggressively nasty ways and he feels painfully pinned, invaded, torn apart. Instead, both persons are fully and happily being qualitatively new persons, wound around the deeper potentials for experiencing. The impressive change that can become the impressive postsession change is the wholesome being of the qualitatively new person.

These are the first three steps that are to occur in each session. They are the important steps that culminate in the fourth and final step in each session. At the end of the third step, the person is being the qualitatively new person, and this new person is essentially free of the scenes of bad feeling that were there for the old person in the beginning of the session. The purpose of the fourth and final step is to prepare the qualitatively new person to be in the imminent postsession new world. But first we must be clear about the importance of postsession change in this model.

## HOW AND WHY IS POSTSESSION CHANGE SO IMPORTANT?

How and why is it so important that impressive postsession changes become impressive extratherapy changes?

### Postsession Change Is the Bottom Line, the Outcome

One answer, a rather common answer, is that postsession changes are important because postsession changes are important. That is, psychotherapy is supposed to help bring about changes in the extratherapy world. The goal, the payoff of psychotherapy, is that the person be different in the extratherapy world. This is why the payoff changes in the extratherapy world are called "outcomes." Psychotherapy can be judged as successful and effective if it results in the desired outcomes in the extratherapy world.

According to this way of looking at postsession change, the end result of successful therapy is that the woman is no longer depressed and withdrawn, drunk and alone, wallowing in the disbelief of the death of her husband. The outcome of effective treatment is that the middle-aged man is no longer the unassertive wimp, the person who is so tense and torn apart when others confront him with what he is like. The extratherapy world is the arena in which the changes are to occur.

Postsession and posttreatment changes are so important because the very worth of psychotherapy, its success and effectiveness, starts and ends with welcomed and desired changes in the extratherapy real world. This is the accepted common answer. From this perspective such an answer is eminently sensible. What other answer could there be?

## Postsession Change Is a Means toward Achieving Personal Change

Now let us shift to a different perspective. In the above common perspective therapeutic change is important because it leads to, brings about, causes extratherapy change, and extratherapy change is the valued end result, the important outcome, the bottom-line payoff. In an alternative perspective, the tables are turned. Extratherapy change is important because it leads to, helps bring about, is a requisite step toward the achievement of personal change! Actually being the new person in the postsession extratherapy world is necessary for the person to be the qualitatively new person, and for this whole new person to live in a new world that is essentially free of the scenes and situations of bad feeling.

If the person is truly going to become a qualitatively new person, in-session work is essential. But it is not sufficient. If the person is going to be a person who is free of the bad-feeling scenes and of the bad feelings, in-session work is essential. But it is not sufficient. What makes personal change sufficient is actual experience in the postsession real world. What happens in the postsession real world is a means, an avenue, and the bottom-line consequent payoff or final outcome is that the person becomes a qualitatively new person who is free of the bad-feeling scenes and the bad feelings.

We are now ready to answer the target question of this chapter: When the person has achieved a radical change into being the qualitatively new person, what can the therapist do to help the impressive in-session changes become impressive postsession changes? The balance of this chapter describes a way to accomplish this final step of the session.

## WHAT CAN THE THERAPIST DO TO HELP IMPRESSIVE IN-SESSION CHANGES BECOME IMPRESSIVE POSTSESSION CHANGES?

There is a point in the session where the person actually is being the qualitatively new person. It is right here that the therapist and the new person face at least two wonderful possibilities. One is that this qualitatively new person can be the one who leaves the office and lives in the postsession extratherapy world. Wouldn't it be wonderful if this qualitatively new person stayed present? The second is that this new world is essentially free of those scenes of bad feeling that had been in the old person's world. Wouldn't that be wonderful? But how? What can the therapist and person do to help ensure that these impressive in-session changes can become impressive postsession changes?

For therapists outside this experiential approach, the broader question may be this: At the point in the session where the person has achieved an impressive change, what can the therapist do to help the impressive in-session change become an impressive postsession change?

There are five things to do, and they should occur in the following order:

## First, Think of a Number of Prospective Scenes and Behaviors for Being the Qualitatively New Person in Playful Unreality

The first task is for the two of you to find several prospective scenes and situations in which the new person can be, exist, live. These can occur right after the session is over, or in the next few days or so, rather than weeks or months from now. You ought also to think of a number of behaviors that the new person can carry out, ways for the new person to undergo the new experiencing.

What is most important is that no ceiling be placed on how and where the new person can live and be. Set reality aside. Set all serious constraints aside. In order to enable the new person to live and to be, what is galvanized is sheer fantasy, unreality, burlesque, craziness, caricature, outrageousness, silliness, hilarity, zaniness.

The working question is, for each of the above patients: How and where can she have the wonderful experiencing of being free, independent, liberated, free of constraints and restrictive control? How and where can he have the wonderful experiencing of powerful sexuality, complete sexual arousal, wallowing in wholesale eroticism?

Answering this question is made easier when, as she/he should be, the person who is here right now is the qualitatively new person. Then the two of you can have productive fun thinking of how and where to be this qualitatively new person in the postsession world.

### Here Are Ways to Get Prospective Scenes

You can generate prospective scenes from scenes already used in the session. In the beginning of the session, what was central to the fellow was when his cousin, the head of the firm, was accusing him of being a lifelong wimp, a loser. So look ahead to forthcoming times when someone is accusing him of being something rotten. He thinks right away of how his cousin, before the meeting tomorrow, will instruct him to not mention anything about what the consultant said last week to the patient. "And I'll do what he wants! Damn!"

There are also lots of prospective scenes that could be generated from the earlier life scenes that were found and used earlier in the session. She had recollected lying in a crib and just letting the feces flow. Looking ahead to the next days or so, when and where could she be in something like a crib, "something that encloses you, all around you"? She finds a situation: "Yes, a bath. A big old bathtub. Sure! God, I haven't just luxuriated in a big warm bath for years . . . Since I was a kid, I think." What about the earlier scene when she was an adolescent who should have been practicing for the piano lesson tomorrow? Both of you now look ahead to "something you should be preparing for, getting ready for." She finds a scene: "I'm supposed to give a talk Wednesday. I should be getting notes together. I'm always prepared . . ."

In addition to getting prospective scenes from earlier life scenes already used in the session, you can get prospective scenes by starting from the deeper potential that was accessed. Send that special inner experiencing out into the next few days or so, and see what prospective scenes can be generated.

One way to accomplish this is to imagine this whole new person, undergoing this whole new experiencing, in ways that are utterly unrealistic, fanciful, zany, outrageous. What scenes are generated when you imagine the fellow experiencing powerful sexuality, complete sexual arousal, a wallowing in wholesale eroticism? Scenes emerge of his being in his office, writhing on the floor, slithering with sexual arousal, with loud erotic moans and groans.

Another way is to imagine the qualitatively new person in all of those absolutely mundane little daily prospective scenes that just about everyone goes through. See the new person being fully free, independent, liberated, free of constraints and restrictive control as she is awakening and getting out of bed in the morning. See her making breakfast. See the way she walks along the street. See the look on her face as she talks on the phone to her sister tomorrow.

Still another way of generating scenes is to picture the kinds of optimal scenes in this qualitatively new person's absolutely ideal world, ideally designed for this inner experiencing. Through this lens, being free, independent, liberated yields a world of having her own apartment, of traveling where she wants and when she wants, of being free of the constraints of going to work and dealing with her grown-up children, of just taking off in her convertible sports car.

Another way is to picture forthcoming scenes in which it would be unthinkable, impossible, awful, absolutely inappropriate, outrageous, disastrous, for this fellow to be undergoing powerful sexuality, complete sexual arousal, a wallowing in wholesale eroticism. "In church, right in the middle of a sermon . . . and when my wife's parents come over for dinner, with my daughters and everyone . . . ! The worst place? At work! I'd be history! In the middle of a board meeting, and I suddenly . . . That's it! It's all over! Yipes!!"

Or you can look to forthcoming times and places where she would probably have a little glow of this inner experiencing of being free, independent, liberated, free of constraints and restrictive control. She'll likely feel it a little anyhow, but when and where? "I thought of when I drink. But that's not it. Not really. But I get it a little when I read. I like reading at night sometimes, a good book. Historical fiction. Yeah, I will get that feeling a little, then."

## Here Are Ways to Get Prospective Behaviors

How can you come up with new and useful ways for the qualitatively new person to behave, act, be, in the postsession world? One way is to use behaviors that the person already used in the session. In working with earlier life scenes, she threw herself into doing things that would provide a blast of being free, independent, liberated, free of constraints and restrictive control. For example, earlier in the session she was a baby, lying in the crib, and she just reveled in letting the feces flow. She enjoyed going through this right here in the session, so maybe she just might behave in this unrestrained, fun-filled way in the next few days. Instead of practicing the piano, she had fun getting her friend from next door and riding their bicycles out in the country, singing and laughing. She did this in the session. She could do this tomorrow. His earlier scene involved watching a pornographic video with some friends. In *being* the deeper potential, he patted his huge erection, slithered and writhed around the floor, and went into a whole state of powerful sexual arousal. Maybe he could carry out these new behaviors in the next few days. New behaviors can come from those actually used in the session. But this is only one way to get prospective new behaviors.

A second way to produce prospective behaviors is by literally being the whole new person, the inner deeper experiencing, in prospective scenes, and seeing what sorts of new behaviors are produced. You can do this within scenes that are rather realistic, doable, and practical. Or you can invent behaviors by having the scenes be wild, outlandish, zany, fanciful, silly, risky, dangerous, impractical, impossible, unrealistic. For example, he knows that his cousin, before the meeting tomorrow, will instruct him to not mention anything about what the cousin said last week to the patient. Now imagine the way the patient would behave if he were the whole new person exuding powerful sexuality, complete sexual arousal, a wallowing in wholesale eroticism, and the context is sheer silliness, outlandishness. Go ahead. Picture what happens. This is what the therapist does. Take the mundane little scene of her walking from the place where she parks her car to her arriving at work. Now picture the way she would walk if she were undergoing the wholesale experiencing of being free, independent, liberated, free of restraints and restrictive controls. You are generating whole new behaviors, and this is what the therapist does.

You have been able to think of, to picture, a number of prospective behaviors and scenes for these two persons to be the qualitatively new persons in wholesale, playful unreality. Now it is to happen.

## Second, Be the Qualitatively New Person (a) Fully, (b) with Wonderful Feelings, and (c) in a Spirit of Playful Unreality

The qualitatively new person is to live and be, as much as possible, in scenes from the next few days or so. Essentially, the qualitatively new person is to get a taste, a sample, of what it is like to be this whole new person in the extratherapy world.

But, to make things safe, the context is playful unreality. Make it exceedingly clear that this is not for real. Instead, the atmosphere is one of sheer nonsense, silliness, outrageousness, caricature. Make it clear that the aim is just to gain a sense of what it could be like to be this whole new person out in the extratherapy world. Make it clear that the person need not be this way for real. The therapist lays all the cards out on the table so that the person knows what to do and what is to be accomplished and why it is helpful to do it all in playful unreality.

Furthermore, the therapist explains and shows the person how to do this as fully as possible, so that there are bodily sensations just about all over the body, top to bottom, inside and out. The key is intensity and saturation. This is to ensure that the qualitatively new person is fully present, rather than here just a little bit or just moderately. Finally, the new person is to be here enough and in the right ways to be filled with feelings that are simply wonderful.

### *Be the Qualitatively New Person in Prospective Scenes*

Given these instructions, she throws herself into the wholesale experiencing of being free, independent, liberated, free of constraints and restrictive control. She starts by declaring her independence to the kids, cutting all the clinging bonds that kept them tightly wrapped around her, giving them the booze, and distributing the material things that belonged to her husband, except the few things she wanted for herself. She had fun pleading for her daughter's bicycle and then calling up her friend and going on spontaneous, free, long rides together, even on a trip around the island where they lived. Instead of preparing for the talk this coming Wednesday, she reveled in her first bath since she was an adolescent, a luxuriating bubble bath, singing raucously and listening to some great music. She was having a wonderful time being this whole new person, but, of course, in a context of playful unreality.

For the fellow, the qualitatively new person included the experiencing of powerful sexuality, complete sexual arousal, a wallowing in wholesale eroticism. His wife's parents were coming over the next Sunday for dinner, so he played out what it might be like to receive them in his robe, with a massive erection, envelop them in a magical swirl of erotic sexuality, lead them to the guest room for a predinner orgy, and then slither to the bedroom where he and his wife would open new heights of delicious sexuality. At the board meeting on Monday, he played out having everyone drink love potions, take off their clothes, watch pornographic videos, cover each other's bodies in oil, and simply ooze sexual arousal. Board meetings would never be the same.

If the bodily sensations are over most of the body and if the feelings are wonderful, it helps to move on to some other prospective scenes, some other ways of being the whole new person. If bodily sensations are rather limited to one part of the body and they are only mildly pleasant, one can modify what is done slightly, or throw oneself further into being and doing it, until bodily sensations are over most of the body and the feelings are delightful.

In any case, the aim is for the person to be the qualitatively new person, fully and with wonderful feelings, and in the context of prospective scenes from the next few days or so. But the spirit is one of robust playful unreality to help make it easier to fully be the whole new person.

## Be the Qualitatively New Person in Prospective Scenes of Bad Feeling

It can be helpful if the qualitatively new person can get a taste of what it can be like to be this new person in forthcoming scenes of bad feeling just like the ones that were front and center for the old person in the beginning of the session. Almost always, those bad-feelinged scenes are going to happen soon. Here is an opportunity for the qualitatively new person to see what it is like to be in that scene. Another option is for the qualitatively new person to join the old person in the scene of bad feeling. Here is a chance for the qualitatively new person to watch, be with, talk to, the old person who has such bad feelings in those scenes. In any case, the qualitatively new person is invited to fully live and be in the same scenes of bad feeling when they happen in the imminent future. Make sure the context is one of playful, outrageous unreality.

You may even invite or challenge the qualitatively new person to have the bad feelings in the forthcoming scene. "All right, here is the big test. You are sitting, all alone, in the living room of the house. Right? You are drunk. Go ahead. Be drunk. Cry. Lightly. Clutch the cap of your husband who died of a heart attack 3 years ago. Go ahead and feel rotten, gloomy, lonely, isolated, alone. Do it and feel awful. Can you do it?" Almost always, the new person cannot be in the scene the same way, and with the same old bad feelings. She says, "Uh . . . I can't! I feel too good!" You say, "Oh, come on. Give it a try!" The new person is almost unable to be in the same old scene in the same bad-feelinged way.

You may invite the qualitatively new person to be there and to relate to that forlorn, unhappy old person: "So if you are here with her, you know, maybe sitting next to her, and she is crying, missing him terribly, you'd probably do something. Go ahead. Be with her. Talk to her." As the whole new person she says, "You poor kid! Come on! Be with me! I'm taking you to a whole new apartment. Let's sell this place. We're free! There's a whole new life. I'm going to show you how to live! You can miss him. Sure you can. But you can do things with me. Come on! You've got a whole new life to live and . . . I know it sounds awful, but . . . we're free! We can do what we want! Come on! (*She is giggling.*)"

Put the qualitatively new person in the forthcoming prospective scene of bad feeling. Let the new person have a chance to live and be in this imminent scene. "He's going to start in on you again, right? Sure. Can you see the sucker, the wealthy cousin? And he is again accusing you. 'You're a lifelong loser. Admit it! You are a wimp who's scared of taking risks. You're pushed around by your wife and your daughters! You wimp!' It's going to happen soon. Right? And all that you are feeling is sex. Nice throbbing sex. So you . . . What?" He starts yelling, "It's time for sex!! God, I feel sexy! Before it's too late, let's find some gorgeous ladies and spend a whole day with bodies, touching and naked and doing what we can do, all of us! Wait! I want to go away with Ann (*his wife*). No kids, just us. Off to a great motel, in Vegas. So just shut up, and I'll see you in a week. I'm going!!! Wow! Yeah! Beautiful erotic sex! Whew!"

Within the context of utterly unrealistic playfulness, the person is being the whole new person in forthcoming scenes. Now it is time to get serious, to get realistic.

## Third, Be the Qualitatively New Person in More Realistic Scenes

She has had a number of chances to be the whole new person, and in scenes from tomorrow and the next few days or so, although always in a context of utterly playful unreality. Now it is time to get serious. Where and when is she ready and willing to be this whole new person for real and in the real extratherapy world? Sometimes we can move from playful unreality to more serious reality, using very much the same kinds of scenes. Other times it is more helpful to find some new and different scenes if we are looking for when and where she can really be this whole new person. You say, "Maybe we can get a little serious now. Why not really be this way? Why not really enjoy feeling free, independent, liberated, free of constraints? It can feel great. But where? Let's get serious. Are you thinking of how you can get this feeling, be this way, today, tomorrow, in the next few days? What do you think?"

She is still dripping with the delight of selling the house, getting her own apartment, and passing out the booze to her grown-up children, whom she would love to ease out of the house. "I'd love to get them together and have a family cabinet meeting. I'm the boss, CEO. And yes, I am announcing that I am going to find a great apartment for myself. All for me. Just to do whatever I want. No more burdens of a big house!"

We are ready to try it out. Just to see how it feels. "All right. So let's see. Go ahead. Try it out. For real now. I'm picturing it's going to happen after dinner. Right? No?" She is drawn toward looking for an apartment. "My friend Karen. She's got a great apartment. Plenty of light. A fireplace. It's just what I wanted. I'm going to go looking with her. I've seen buildings near Randall Avenue. Lovely buildings, apartments. Let's go there. You've always talked about it. Yes, let's look. And, yes, I am going to tell the kids. But I have to round them up. Dinner's bad. They're not home much. Wednesday night meeting. The three of us. Hello darlings. I am setting you free. You spend most of your time with your boyfriends anyhow. Move in. I'll give you the money from the estate. It's yours. Your share. Move out. We all are. Get on with your lives. I am! Yes!!"

The fellow has thrown himself into several forthcoming playfully unrealistic scenes of having a full sense of powerful sexuality, complete sexual arousal, a wallowing in wholesale eroticism. "Now it is time to get more serious, more. Where can you really have this wonderful feeling, like in the next few days or so? You thinking of some place already? No?" He is. "I wake up, middle of the night. I have a . . . I must have had a sex dream cause I am feeling just sex. You know what? I'm going to . . ." The therapist encourages him to try it out. "Let's just see what it's like. Make it real. OK, so what do you do?" He lives in this scene. It is real. He is moaning, breathing fast yet deep. Wanting his wife. Touching her. Together. They are like one person, entwining and lightly touching, arousing, wholly thrown into newfound sexual being together, pleasure and arousal. He is undergoing this ecstatic experiencing languorously, slowly, yet with a saturated charge of tingling eroticism.

## Fourth, Rehearse and Refine the New Way of Being and Behaving in the Scene until It Feels Right

They have tried out the new way of being and behaving in the new scenes, and done so within a context of reality, of actually being this new way. Now they have a chance to rehearse it further, to refine and shape everything until it feels just right. They may even decide not to be this way, either in this particular new scene or perhaps not at all.

After trying out the new way of being and behaving, the person and therapist check their bodies. What are the sensations like? Are they only moderately pleasant, or perhaps neutral or even somewhat unpleasant? On the basis of the bodily sensations, of literally seeing how it feels, you can keep rehearsing and refining and checking bodily sensations until the bodily sensations are very good and over most of the body. If bodily sensations are neutral or even unpleasant, and are confined to some small part of the body, it is probably sensible not to carry out that particular way of being and behaving. You might try some different way of being and behaving or even give it up for this session.

In addition, trying out the new way of being and behaving gives both the therapist and the person a chance to invite other parts of the person to respond and react, to have their say, to voice their worries and objections. Whether the new way of being and behaving seems to feel right or not, now is the time to bring up all sorts of constraints, worries, and negative reactions. If you look at Figure 9.1, you are giving OP1, OP2, and OP3 plenty of opportunity to raise every objection imaginable. Bring up all sorts of reality constraints. As therapist, give voice to every kind of worry and objection and constraint that every part of the person might have. He would ruin his life. All the important people in her world would hate her. He just can't be like that. She should consider the feelings of others. Being this new way is bad, dangerous, immoral, disastrous, uncivilized, crazy. Make sure that the therapist and patient voice the absolutely oppositional objections from every part of the person.

The process is one of trying out the new way of being and behaving in a context of increasing reality. This allows you to keep rehearsing and refining, guided by the nature and the extent of bodily sensations.

He has just finished trying out what it can be like to undergo a new sense of powerful sexuality, a wallowing in wholesale eroticism, with his wife, in the middle of the night. "All right. Now check your body. Where do you feel things in your body, and what is it like? What is happening in your body, and where?" Actually, there is a kind of mild tension all over his chest. No, the bodily sensations are not good. The bodily sensations are roughly the same in the therapist. We are not done.

This new person would just love to be this way with his wife, Ann, but perhaps only when they talk about this more together. "We really don't spend much time together. But I want her so much. Touching. I want to talk with her. I think I want to tell her how I feel. She's so lovely . . ." He rehearses what it can be like to go for walks with her, to be alone together, to tell her just how he feels, to hold her and touch her. He tries out what this can be like, walking together in the park near where they live. When he checks out the bodily sensations, there are sexual tinglings all over his body, a kind of throbbing sensation inside and a light sexual tingling from head to toe. Yes, this feels wonderful.

We deliberately raise all sorts of objections. What would Ann think? It's liable to get out of control. Maybe you are a sexual maniac. You are a loser, a wimp. It won't work. Maybe Ann likes to push you around, so how might she feel if you change? Maybe it won't work out? What's going to happen at work? He even brings up possible sexual feelings toward his wealthy cousin's wife, and laughs about getting aroused when the four of them are together. All of these constraints and objections bounce off of him, and he is in buoyant good spirits as he dances with each of them. He has found a way of being and behaving that feels right.

She finished giving the speech to her grown up children, announcing that she is going to move out of the house and will look for an apartment for herself. When she checks her body, it feels good, with a kind of pleasant lightness in her head. Would she like to modify it a little? Yes, she would. She tries out what it is like to be even more free, independent, liberated, free of constraints—and, this time, pouring all the booze down the drain with them and inviting them to come with her to find an apartment. "If you want to join me, fine. If not, fine. I want to start tomorrow. There's a great apartment house near where Karen lives, and yes, this means you are free too. I loved being married, but now's the time for me to live my own life. It's been a long time. And you can come visit. By the way, it's going to take a lot of work to sell this big old place. I can do it myself, but I sure could use help!"

Checking the bodily sensations, she felt all sorts of energy in her upper body. "And my feet are shaking! And they're freezing! I think I'm excited! Damn, it feels good!" When we turned to every sort of objection we could find, we both mentioned her kids. "They'll flip! Gotta stay home with Mom. They're babies! They'll hate you! They'll all come live with you in the apartment! You'll be even worse! More crying. More booze. You'll be alone!" She was laughing as she dismissed or countered the reality constraints and objections. "They are more mature than I am . . . and if not, what the hell, they'll have enough to live on, and they are working. So suffer a little. It's not so bad. I feel good. This is nice!"

We have arrived at a rather concrete way of being and behaving as this new person. We have tried it out, and it is accompanied with good bodily sensations. We have also raised all sorts of reality constraints, allowed various parts of the person to have their voices and objections. Now it is time to see if the new person is ready and eager to be this new way for real.

### Fifth, Be Ready, Determined, and Committed to Carry Out the Postsession Change

Whether or not the new person actually carries this out in the postsession world is up to her/him. So far, the person seems to be able to carry it out, has rehearsed and is pleasantly satisfied with being this new person, and may even be eager to be this new way in the real world. The final little nudge comes from the person's own self-determination and self-commitment. "You can be this way, you seem to like being this way, it seems that everything agrees it would be good to be this way. So what about it? Do you truly want to do it? Will you?"

In some approaches, and with some kinds of postsession changes, it may be that merely requesting the person to carry it out may be enough (e.g., Brady, 1972; Goldfried & Davison, 1976; Kanfer & Grimm, 1980; Mahrer, Nordin, & Miller, 1995; Nelson & Borkovic, 1989; Papajohn, 1982; Prochaska & DiClemente, 1982). But there are circumstances when such a simple request may not be enough, and when it seems important for the person to be quite determined and committed to carrying out the postsession change (Bandura & Adams, 1977; Goldfried, 1982; Haley, 1984;

Linehan, 1993; Mahrer, 1996; Mahrer, Gagnon, Fairweather, Boulet, & Herring, 1994; Montgomery & Montgomery, 1975; Prochaska & DiClemente, 1982; Tosi & Henderson, 1983).

Give the person a chance to be determined, to be committed, to truly intend to be this new person in this particular way, doing this particular thing, and in this particular scene. The session's work is done if and when the new person says something along the lines of, "Yes! . . . I am going to do it . . . I will do it . . . Yes!"

It may be that the new person will only be and behave in this one scene and in this one way. It may be that the new person will go on to be and behave in lots of ways and in lots of scenes. It may be that this session has transformed the old person into a whole new person who is going to be here from now on. It may be that the new person shows up only in being and behaving in this one isolated way and in this one defined scene. No matter how extensive is the change, the commitment is to be this new way in this defined scene.

The woman is ready to commit herself to being this free, independent, liberated person who is free of constraints and restrictive controls as she arranges to pour all the booze down the drain with her kids and invite them to join with her in finding her wonderful apartment. "Yes! I am! I want to do it! Yes, I do!" Here is the final flourish of self-commitment to undergo this new way of being and behaving in this concrete way and in this concrete situation.

The man is bubbling with eagerness to go for a walk in the park with his wife, fueled by this exciting sense of powerful sexuality, complete sexual arousal, a wallowing in wholesale eroticism. There is a flowering of sexual feelings as he is with her, a knife-edged awareness of her body and his as they walk along, a tingling erotic sense as he listens to her voice, as he lightly touches her, as he allows the strong sexual feelings to have their say. He is so ready to do this that he can barely restrain himself. "I want to do this tonight. Or tomorrow. Any time! Oh I want to do things differently with her. I want to talk with her. Whew!"

You ask if they really are ready to do it, if they truly feel committed to be this way, to do it. They are. You are pleased. They are pleased, and they are quite ready and determined to be this whole new way in this specific new way. The session's work is done.

## HOW CAN THE THERAPIST FIND OUT
## IF THE IMPRESSIVE IN-SESSION CHANGES
## ACTUALLY BECAME IMPRESSIVE
## POSTSESSION CHANGES?

The opening of the next session usually gives you a chance to see if the impressive postsession changes actually occurred. Each session opens with the therapist showing the person how to identify scenes of strong feeling. These are the starting places for each session. Conveniently, such "scenes of strong feeling" can include scenes related to the homework, for example. "Maybe the two of you went for a great walk, and there was a wonderful feeling of powerful sexuality, complete sexual arousal, a wallowing in wholesale eroticism as there was touching and talking and being together. Or maybe it was terrible, bad, awful . . .".

A second way is to see who shows up for the subsequent session. Is she now the qualitatively new person, the person who is free, independent, liberated, free of constraints and restrictive control?

A third way is to include in the opening kinds of scenes of strong feeling the same bad-feelinged scenes that were there at the beginning of the last session: "Times when there is a bad feeling of loneliness, being so alone, gloomy and all isolated. You're drunk, all by yourself in the living room, and you're holding his favorite cap. Feels terrible. Or some other time when you have that same miserable feeling of racking loneliness, that all-consuming aloneness, that gloomy isolation." You may begin the next session with the middle-aged fellow with this scene: "You have this same painful feeling of being pinned, invaded, torn apart. Maybe it happened when your wealthy cousin just accused you of being a loser. Or maybe that same awful feeling happened somewhere else, but it is here, and it feels so bad . . ."

The standard way of opening each session gives the person a fair chance to let the therapist know if the impressive in-session changes actually occurred as impressive postsession changes. Sometimes it is sadly clear that little or nothing happened when the same old person shows up in both the beginning of the present session and in the previous session. It is even more sadly clear when the same old person is unhappily concerned with just about the same bad-feeling scene as in the previous session.

## SO WHAT HAPPENED? DID THE IMPRESSIVE IN-SESSION CHANGES BECOME IMPRESSIVE POSTSESSION CHANGES?

Both patients did their homework. Both carried out the new way of being and behaving, or something rather close. In the beginning of the next session, he tells about what happened a few days ago. He found himself picturing his wife's face, and he sketched her face, something he had done when they were going together before their marriage. He felt more alive, and sentimental. Although he was not especially sexually aroused as he sketched her face, he was so concentrated on the lift of her cheek and capturing a precious look on her face that his eyes became watery. He called her, wanted to tell her that he loved her, but she wasn't home. That night, he must have had a different look on his face. She grinned and asked what happened. He and she moved into touching each other, and there was a slowly accumulating erotic feeling as they enjoyed each other's bodies in ways that had not occurred before. Something changed between them. They became truly best friends. And their love making was different, more shared, more mutual, and much more like entering into another world of erotic sexuality.

He did not mention any incidents with his wealthy cousin, but, after several more sessions, he mentioned having taken another job. Were there any feelings of being pinned down, invaded, torn apart, being pushed around? He acknowledged having some such feelings, but only mildly, and they were no longer the focus of session work. Not in the subsequent session, nor in later sessions.

She carried out her homework to the letter. When she assembled her two grown-up daughters and informed them of her intention to sell the house, they were overjoyed and kept laughing about whether she was truly drunk or high or somehow different. Instead of pouring the booze down the drain, they made a ceremony out of smashing the bottles against a tree, and after they went back into the house, they all went for a bicycle ride. She did sell the house, rather quickly. And the newfound sense of freedom, independence, being free of constraints seemed to bubble up in so many little ways—just in ordinary mundane little ways such as chatting with strangers, laughing more easily, and initiating little things to do with friends. She still had stretches of reminiscing about her husband, but it was more of a feeling of warm melancholy than the old state of profound loss, jabbing loneliness, and frozen isolation.

## CONCLUSIONS

1. Many therapists would like impressive in-session changes to continue out into the person's postsession world. The most common reason is that the way the person is in the postsession world is the only game in town, the way to tell if the session was any good, the whole purpose of the therapy. Another reason is that impressive in-session changes in who and what the person is can be deepened and solidified when the impressive in-session changes also occur in the actual postsession world. In this experiential psychotherapy, both reasons hold, with the edge to the latter reason.

2. This chapter focused on two impressive in-session changes: (a) The person becomes a qualitatively new person; there is a deep-seated change in who and what the new person is. (b) The new person is essentially free of the situations or scenes of bad feeling that were so painful and troublesome for the old person.

3. In order to achieve these impressive in-session changes, each session should proceed through the following steps:

- First, the therapist and person are to identify some scene of strong feeling, and they are to use that scene of strong feeling to access, open up, discover something deeper inside the person, a deeper potential for experiencing.

- Second, the person is to welcome, to appreciate, to love that deeper potential for experiencing.
- Third, the person is to undergo a radical change into actually being a qualitatively new person in the context of past scenes and situations.

4. In order for these impressive in-session changes to become impressive postsession changes, a sequence of steps should be followed:

- The person is literally to "be" the qualitatively new person in a variety of prospective scenes, and is to do so with feelings that are full and exceedingly pleasant and in a context of exaggeratedly playful unreality.
- Shifting to a more reality-grounded context, the new person is to go back and forth between rehearsing and refining–modifying the new way of being and behaving in a defined prospective scene until it feels fitting and right.
- The new person is to be reasonably committed to actually carrying out the new way of being in the defined prospective scene.

## REFERENCES

Bandura, A., & Adams, N. E. (1977). Analysis of self-efficacy theory of behavior change. *Cognitive Therapy and Research*, 1, 287–310.

Brady, J. P. (1972). Systematic desensitization. In W. S. Agras (Ed.), *Behavior modification: Principles and clinical applications* (pp. 127–153). Boston: Little, Brown.

Goldfried, M. R. (1982). Resistance and clinical behavior therapy. In P. L. Wachtel (Ed.), *Resistance: Psychodynamic and behavioral approaches* (pp. 95–113). New York: Plenum.

Goldfried, M. R., & Davison, G. C. (1976). *Clinical behavior therapy*. New York: Holt, Rinehart & Winston.

Haley, J. (1984). *Ordeal therapy: Unusual ways to change behavior*. San Francisco: Jossey-Bass.

Kanfer, F. H., & Grimm, L. G. (1980). Managing clinical change: A process model of therapy. *Behavior Modification*, 4, 419–444.

Linehan, M. M. (1993). *Cognitive-behavioral treatment of borderline personality disorder*. New York: Guilford Press.

Mahrer, A. R. (1989). *Experiencing: A humanistic theory of psychology and psychiatry*. Ottawa, Ontario, Canada: University of Ottawa Press.

Mahrer, A. R. (1996). *The complete guide to experiential psychotherapy*. New York: Wiley.

Mahrer, A. R., & Fairweather, D. R. (1993). What is "experiencing"?: A critical review of meanings and applications in psychotherapy. *The Humanistic Psychologist*, 21, 2–25.

Mahrer, A. R., Gagnon, R., Fairweather, D. R., Boulet, D. B., & Herring, C. B. (1994). Client commitment and resolve to carry out postsession behaviors. *Journal of Counseling Psychology*, 41, 407–414.

Mahrer, A. R., Nordin, S., & Miller, L. S. (1995). If a client has this kind of problem, prescribe that kind of post-session behavior. *Psychotherapy, 32,* 194–203.

Malone, T. P., Whitaker, C. A., Warkentin, J., & Felder, R. A. (1961). Rational and nonrational psychotherapy. *American Journal of Psychotherapy, 15,* 212–220.

Montgomery, A. G., & Montgomery, D. J. (1975). *Facilitating treatment adherence.* New York: Plenum.

Nelson, R. A., & Borkovec, T. D. (1989). Relationship of client participation to psychotherapy. *Journal of Behavior Therapy and Experimental Psychiatry, 20,* 155–162.

Papajohn, J. C. (1982). *Intensive behavior therapy.* New York: Pergamon Press.

Prochaska, J. O., & DiClemente, C. C. (1982). Transtheoretical therapy: Toward a more integrated model of change. *Psychotherapy: Theory, Research and Practice, 19,* 276–288.

Tosi, D. J., & Henderson, G. W. (1983). Rational stage-directed therapy: A cognitive experiential system using hypnosis, imagery, cognitive restructuring, and developmental staging. *Journal of Rational Emotive Therapy, 1,* 15–19.

Whitaker, C. A., Felder, R. E., Malone, T. P., & Warkentin, J. (1962). First-stage techniques in the experiential psychotherapy of chronic schizophrenic patients. In J. H. Masserman (Ed.), *Current psychiatric therapies* (Vol. 2, pp. 218–257). New York: Grune & Stratton.

Whitaker, C. A., & Malone, T. P. (1953). *The roots of psychotherapy.* New York: Blakiston.

Whitaker, C. A., & Malone, T. P. (1969). Experiential or nonrational psychotherapy. In W. Sahakian (Ed.), *Psychotherapy and counseling: Studies in technique* (pp. 416–431). Chicago: Rand McNally.

# III

*****

# DIFFERENTIAL TREATMENT APPLICATIONS

# 10

\*\*\*\*\*

# Process-Experiential
# Therapy of Depression

Leslie S. Greenberg
Jeanne C. Watson
Rhonda Goldman

*Clinical depression is characterized* by feelings of discouragement, feeling sad, blue, down, and depleted. Depression involves an accentuation in the intensity and duration of these everyday experiences. The syndrome is defined by the fact that these mood disturbances endure over weeks. In depression it is as though once people go down they simply stay down. Resilience has been lost. The world turns gray and a sense of isolation sets in. Sometimes the depressed feeling is the prolongation of sadness of a loss or a defeat that lingers, seemingly for ever. At other times depression involves a qualitatively different experience. It is experienced as embodied anguish and physical deadness. The sense of one's body is different. A heaviness sets in and one feels immensely burdened, moving one's limbs with difficulty; one is suffocated by a shroud of pain, and all seems hopeless.

Depression according to DSM-IV (American Psychiatric Association, 1994) is recognizable by nine features: depressed mood for most of the day, for more days than not; loss of pleasure in most activities; significant weight change; disturbed sleep; psychomotor agitation or retardation; fatigue or loss of energy; feelings of worthlessness or guilt; trouble concentrating or making decisions; and thoughts of death and suicide. If at least five of these features have been present during a 2-week period, including either depressed mood or loss of interest or pleasure, a person satisfies criteria for a major depressive episode. In therapy, depressed clients, in response to empathic understanding of their depressed state and exploration of its generators, often begin to say things such as "I always feel like the failure of my marriage was my fault"; "Even though I'm objectively doing OK I still say to myself, 'You're no good, what's the use of trying'"; "I just feel I'm not quite good enough"; "I'm afraid to start another relationship. I'll just lose myself again"; or "I can't live without her. Everything just seems hollow."

Depression is a complex biopsychosocial phenomena. No single cause can be isolated. In this chapter we will discuss our brief treatment of moderately depressed individuals whose functional impairment was not so great as to keep them at home under the covers, unable to get out of bed and go to work. Our clients functioned in their world, parented, worked, or went to school, although often with difficulty, and always with little or no satisfaction. Although all our clients met criteria for major depressive disorder, they varied markedly. Some were highly self-critical and felt like failures. Others were disappointed in relationship, felt abandoned, and were sad and angry. Others felt empty, confused, and aimless. Yet others were highly afraid and anxious as well as hopeless. Some were highly avoidant; others worried obsessively. Some were openly fragile; others, highly guarded. Some were concrete and rational in their style of thinking and talking, whereas others were very associative and internally focused. Despite these differences they were all depressed, and as we worked with them certain subgroup commonalities did emerge.

In treatment we found that clients tended to focus either on problematic self–self relations, such as self criticalness, loss of control or status, and identity issues, or on self–other relationship issues, such as unresolved loss or anger, or issues of abandonment, isolation and loss of connectedness. In all, there was a type of closing down or withdrawing at the emotional level and a sense of weakness or disempowerment—a sense of a defeated self. In their striving for perfection many of the self-critical types chastised and bullied themselves into passive submissiveness. In the search for intimacy and connection the more dependent types forfeited expressing what they felt and prevented who they were from emerging in relationships. Notions of what it was to be a competent professional, a good parent, or a good wife or husband often prevented them from expressing parts of themselves and kept them trapped or invalidated. They often felt deeply discouraged and expressed a high degree of negativity and disgust and contempt toward themselves. In others deep feelings of insecurity, most often related to loss of relationships, left them feeling as though they could not survive without the connection or as though that connection was too dangerous.

Our therapy of depression seemed to work by accessing and confirming people's ability to survive. It helped them contact an emotionally based will to live, and this reempowered the self. The ability to connect was promoted by accessing primary biologically adaptive feelings and needs. As people accessed their primary emotions and needs and these were validated by their therapists, they gained a sense of self-worth. Moreover, access to their emotions gave people information about their reactions to situations and organized them to act to attain the adaptive goals that emotions set as organismic priorities. Once they symbolized their feelings and needs in awareness they were able to reflect on themselves and their worlds and create new meaning. They integrated their "heads" and their "hearts" to cope more adaptively. Being confirmed as authentic sources of experience by their therapists' empathic responsiveness and continual focus on their internal experience led them to take themsleves seriously and be more empathic to themselves.

## DIFFERENTIAL TREATMENT PERSPECTIVES

Depressed individuals are not a homogeneous group. Depression symptoms are the result of a variety of generating processes, and specific people have specific generating processes or underlying determinants of the disorder. Each individual's depression needs to be understood in its own terms. A person's depression may be produced by a variety of determinants such as loss, self-criticisms, meaninglessness, role disruptions, trauma, prior abuse, isolation, or powerlessness.

Is there then any merit in focusing on a specific treatment for this particular type of distress, given that depression involves different determinants and that other disorders such as anxiety or addiction may involve the same or similar determinants? One might in addition question the need for a differential treatment of depression, given that a therapeutic relationship characterized by attitudes of positive regard and genuine concern, as well as a form of responding that is empathic and experience centered, is helpful for different types of problems and diagnostic groups.

Although many depressed clients have multiple forms of distress and present with dual diagnoses, including either anxiety disorders or personality disorders, there are certain common features in working with depressive malaise and its generators that do seem to merit a specific form of experiential treatment of depression. At an initial level all depressed clients in successful therapy move from hopelessness to hopefulness, from demobilization to mobilization, and from feeling sad and blue to again feeling the more positive emotions of interest and excitement. Working with depressed clients requires special sensitivity to these and other issues.

We have in addition observed both in practice and research contexts that, during treatment of depressed people, *specific types* of in-session problem states or markers of underlying determinants come up more often or with greater significance, and these are embedded within specific types of depressive themes. More specifically we found that self-critical splits, embedded within themes of failure and lack of self-esteem, and a variety of types of lingering unresolved feelings or unfinished business with significant others, embedded within themes of dependence and loss, characterize the in-session issues that formed the focus of our treatments of depression. We hope in this chapter to convey some of the specific elements of an experiential treatment of depression that help contribute specific change processes over and above those promoted by the empathic, confirming relationship.

Before this, however, we will outline a theoretical model of the depressogenic process that has emerged from both our study of depression and our theoretical reflections on emotion and cognition in the process of change (Greenberg & Watson, 1998; Watson & Greenberg, 1996; Watson, Greenberg, & Goldman, 1996; Greenberg & Pascual-Leone, 1995; Greenberg & Paivio, 1997).

## A PROCESS-EXPERIENTIAL MODEL OF DEPRESSION

Our model of depression suggests that it is the activation of core emotion linked depressogenic schemes that is crucial in producing depressed self-organizations (Greenberg & Paivio, 1997). In our view depression results when a person feels disempowered and the self's ability to organize experience in its usual more hopeful, positive manner is lost.

We thus propose that psychogenic depression, at the most general level, is related to the evocation of a set of emotion schemes that constitute a core weak/bad self. An *emotion scheme*, as we have defined the term elsewhere (Greenberg, Rice, & Elliott, 1993, pp. 66–67; Greenberg & Paivio, 1997), is a response-producing internal organization that synthesizes a variety of levels and types of information including sensorimotor, emotion memory, and conceptual-level information. In contrast to a *cognitive schema* this is a structure that includes a large component of nonverbal and affective experience. It represents an integration of each person's biology and experience in that it is the product of the synthesis of a representation of his/her own emotional experience in situations with a representation of the evoking situational cues and with subsequent learned beliefs or rules governing that experience. It is in the final analysis a synthesis of affect, cognition, motivation, and action and when evoked produces an integrated experience that gives us our sense of things and of ourselves.

This view of emotion scheme activation is offered as an alternative to current empirically tested, interpersonal and cognitive views, that hypothesize that either role disruptions and interpersonal isolation, or negative thoughts and beliefs are the key determinants of depression (Beck, Rush, Shaw, & Emery, 1979; Klerman, Weissman, Rounsaville, & Chevron, 1984). Although these all often may be precursorsors or maintainers of depression, we propose a different central determinant (cf. Teasdale, 1996; Teasdale & Barnard, 1993).

In relation to a cognitive view of depression it is important to recognize that it is often impossible to identify negative automatic thoughts preceding bad moods and that in many clinical instances changes in negative thoughts do not lead to changes in feeling. Further, it is important to note that, on different occasions, the same negative thought often has very different effects, sometimes producing bad feelings and at other times having little or no effect. Thoughts that arise from purely conceptual processing do not produce bad feelings. They simply "bounce off" a secure or competent sense of oneself rather than activate depressive experience. Thus, although thought can and does influence experience, it is not a sufficient or major cause of depression (Greenberg & Paivio, 1997). In relation to an interpersonal view, role disruptions or severe losses, even when suffered in isolation, do not necessarily precipitate depression. Although interpersonal support and loss effect mood, they do not themselves produce enduring mood disturbance. This implies that it is not the thought or the loss itself but the affective significance of the experience that evokes emotion schematic memories. What seems important in generating depression and constitutes a vulnerability to it is that current emotional reactions evoke emotional memories of prior loss or perceived failures (Greenberg & Paivio, 1997). Although failure, isolation, and loss of status or connectedness may precipitate depression, ultimately it is the self's emotional response to these experiences that is important. Depression is thus an emotional disorder of the self.

Based on our clinical observation, it appears that depression occurs if a person's emotionally based, powerless, hopeless, weak/bad self-organization is triggered. This is more than a negative view of self, others, and the world, or loss, or relational ruptures. Rather, what has been activated is a deeply insecure sense of self, encoded from life's experience as weak unprotected and unable to cope on one's own, or an encoded sense of self as worthless, bad, incompetent, and inadequate. If people's life experiences of loss and abandonment have left them with a weak sense of self, they remain vulnerable to interpersonal loss and abandonment and suffer from dependence-type depressions (Blatt & Mouradas, 1992). If they suffered from invalidation and have not formed a competent sense of self, a self-critical self-organization can be evoked by threats to competence, and this results in a self-critical depression. These forms of self-criticalness and anxious dependence often are highly intertwined.

Depression is thus an emotionally based inability to respond to life with baseline interest, excitement, and other contact-oriented emotions because of the evocation of a powerless self-organization. The powerless, weak/bad organization, although it is a recurrent, possible self-organization and therefore possesses some degree of structuralization, does not predominate in the person's everyday functioning and is not necessarily accessible under normal circumstances. Other forms of self-organization develop and help the person function in the world.

The presence of a powerless, weak/bad self-organization constitutes an experiential vulnerability to depression. If this, once activated, is not overcome, the person sinks into depression. In addition, in self-critical depressions it appears that it is the intensity of contemptuous affect accompanying the negative view of self that is the crucial variable in invoking the bad sense of self, not the negative view itself. This is not a view that anger turned inward produces depression, but rather that it is the contempt or disgust to-

ward the self that accompanies the negative view of the self that is depressogenic. This self-contempt also often appears in dependence depressions where
people are scornful of themselves for being so pathetically needy and weak.
In addition to the contempt it is the intensity of the self's affective response
to the threatened dissolution of the self that is important in both types of
depression. It is the nonresilient reaction of panic and powerlessness that leads
to the emotional collapse of the self.

In our model the core depressogenic weak/bad self-scheme is activated
by a current emotional experience of loss or failure. It is the whole integrated
emotional meaning of an event, rather than thoughts alone, that govern
depressive functioning. When people suffer a loss or failure they feel sad and
disappointed or angry and powerless; it is this experience that acts as a major
trigger of a more core experience of self as deeply inadequate or insecure. It
is the emotion-cued evocation of related emotion memories, as well as tacit
organizations of experience of prior vulnerabilities, that begins the process
of defeat setting in. The self now is no longer organized in terms of strengths
and resources, but rather around a sense of powerlessness inadequacy and
insecurity. Resilience is lost and the person experiences him-/herself as powerless, and weak or bad.

Smith (1996) recently demonstrated that depressed subjects showed an
elevated proportion of negative emotion memories of the more distant past.
This indicated that their memories were not as much about the recent life
stress that precipitated the depression but more about painful earlier life
experience. This finding supports the idea that it is the evocation of emotion
schematic memory that is important in producing depressive experience. Thus
it is the emotional response to loss and failure that activates a core maladaptive emotion scheme of powerlessness. This in conjunction with introjected
negative evaluations and contempt such as "You're worthless" produces an
enduring weak/bad sense of self. The experience of powerlessness, of feeling
weak or bad, often occurs tacitly and is unsymbolized. What is conscious is
the more secondary emotional response of hopelessness, the enduring depression, and the resulting lethargy and inactivity.

The process of depression also involves an escalatory process of secondary self-criticism—for being depressed. The person chastises the self for being
depressed, and "coaches" the self, more and more coercively and disparag-
ingly, on how to "snap out of it." This, in turn, produces further emotional
experience of failure or unworthiness, which further evokes the core maladaptive emotion schemes related to failure and loss.

Treatment then involves accessing the core weak/bad sense of self in order
to bring it into contact with other emotionally based, biologically adaptive
resources in the personality. Once the core maladaptive emotion schemes are
accessed, primary emotions and needs and healthy resources are focused on
and this brings adaptive strivings to the fore. These then act to restructure
the maladaptive schemes, combat the negative cognitions and self-contempt,

access self-soothing capacities, and provide an inner sense of direction and a greater sense of personal power (Greenberg & Paivio, 1997).

For example, Jan, a client suffering from a major depressive episode whose treatment will be described more fully at the end of this chapter, came into therapy saying she could no longer cope, that she was continually tearful and was unable to get herself going. She chastised herself harshly for being so weak. The therapist empathized with her sense of hopelessness but continued to focus on her more primary sadness and vulnerability, and therapy soon progressed beyond this level of secondary bad feeling. The central focus became her sense of failure generating the hopelessness. She felt as though she had failed—failed to be a perfect wife, sister, daughter, and mother. Through exploring her feelings concerning this issue, she began to talk about how trapped and helpless she felt. Attending to and accessing this experience opened up her powerless, weak/bad schematic complex for exploration. She talked about how she had always tried to appease her parents and be a good little girl but that she never felt good enough. She began to feel sad, and this evoked feelings of only being acceptable if she was a good girl or a superwoman. She explored how she had lived her life to please her parents and everybody else and how tired she was of trying to live up to these expectations. She wept for herself, for how hard it had been, and for how guilty she had felt for not living up to the expectations of perfect wife, mother, daughter, and salesperson. Once this core maladaptive self-organization was symbolized and explored, and her grief was experienced and expressed, focusing on her adaptive anger at her family for expecting too much of her helped her to set boundaries and feel entitled to do this. Her self-organization began to shift. Her assertion of her self, based on feeling entitled to her unmet needs for acceptance, was an important antidote to depression. Having mobilized her sense of agency, and feeling confirmed by the therapist, she reassessed her culpability in leaving her children with a husband who had been abusing her.She accepted that she had had limited options at the time. This helped her resolve her guilt about abandoning her children and failing in her first marriage. She had condemned herself and felt that her parents also condemned her for this. By helping her grieve for her losses, acknowledge her anger at her parents and sister, mobilize her needs for autonomy, and hold her ex-husband accountable for his important part in their failed marriage, she was able to accept the choices she had made. She forgave herself and was able for the first time to accept, at an emotional level, her children's forgiveness of her for having left them. Once she felt more accepting of herself and her needs, she began to confront her issues with her current husband that had probably precipitated her depression. She realized she had tried to be superwoman in this marriage in order to gain her second husband's love, to appease him and not fail again. She had remained quiet because she was "afraid to rock the boat." She decided that "I have to learn to say no at times because I have to put myself first and do what's good for me. I can't be liked by everybody." At the end of therapy it was a major shift for her to say, "It's OK for me to ask for help. I don't have to be super-woman—people won't think less of me if I can't manage. It has been important for me to give myself permission to be human".

Her core emotion scheme had changed. Now she was less perfectionistic and less vulnerable to depression. Minifailures or small setbacks were less likely to evoke emotional memories of the distant past, unresolved guilt, or a deep sense of failure. Now disappointment was more likely to lead to the process of feeling disappointed, expressing it, and reaching out to others or moving on rather than precipitating a downward spiral into depression. Her scores at termination of treatment on the Beck Depression Inventory and other instruments indicated full recovery and increase in self-esteem and reduction in interpersonal problems that were maintained to 18-month follow-up.

## THE PROCESS-EXPERIENTIAL APPROACH
## TO TREATMENT OF DEPRESSION

Our approach to treatment involves two major principles: establishing a relationship and the promotion of therapeutic work (Greenberg et al., 1993). The three relationship principles involve empathic attunement, creation of a therapeutic bond, and collaboration on treatment tasks and goals. The task principles involve facilitating, experiential processing, growth and choice, and task completion. Our approach is thus both relationally and task oriented, involving both an empathic responsive aspect and a process-directive, task-oriented aspect. The task aspect, however, never takes precedence over the relational aspect. Thus the personhood of the client is never made subservient to the task or goal. The principles reflect a collaborative style in which there is a dynamic tension between following and leading. A form of synchrony occurs where the experience of leading and following disappears in a collaborative flowing together, as in good dancing or improvisational jazz.

In the treatment of depression, empathy and interpersonal support give the depressed person an opportunity to focus on internal experience. The therapist's consistent empathic attunement to clients' experience helps them turn inward to focus on their own experience and confirms them as authentic sources of experience. This empowers clients and help them find their own voices. In this interpersonal environment clients begin to attend to and symbolize feelings and needs, and this helps them clarify what is problematic and to establish what their own goals truly are. In this process clients organize and reorganize personal meanings to form more and more coherent views of themselves and their circumstances.

As the treatment progresses the relational aspect is integrated with a more process-directive form of treatment in which the client's experience is evoked in order to make it more accessible to reorganization. Markers of clients problematic experiential states are recognized as they emerge. They are viewed as opportunities for particular kinds of interventions designed to facilitate particular types of exploration processes that are most suited to these states. This form of task-oriented treatment helps clients engage in those modes of exploration most likely to help resolve the particular experiential problem state they are in at the moment.

## Alliance Development and Formulation in the Treatment of Depression

We found that the development of a collaborative focus on the generators of the depression was of particular importance in the early stage of treatment (Watson & Greenberg, 1995, 1996). Those clients with whom a thematic focus on some depression-generating concern was not collaboratively established did not benefit nearly as much from treatment as those with whom an early focus was clearly established. Early alliance work of this nature involved implicit or explicit agreement on the overall goals of treatment and clients' involvement in the therapeutic processes and tasks used to achieve these (Weerasekera, Linder, Greenberg, & Watson, 1998).

Developing a collaborative alliance with a focus on generators of depression often took up to five sessions, although the focus could easily develop in the second or third session. The focus on a theme emerged by a co-constructive process in which the therapist followed the client's lead and consistently attended to the most salient and poignant material, thereby helping create a focus. Once a focus was established it gave clients a sense of hope. Particularly important early on was helping clients engage in the major task of experiential therapy to move to a focus on internal experience such that they were talking about their own experience and psychological difficulties rather than blaming others, talking about symptoms, or blaming themselves for having depression and being weak or lazy. Once they moved to an internal focus and established themselves as agents in the construction of their own experience, they no longer experienced themselves purely as victims but also as authors of their experience. They thereby become more empowered and engaged in the task of self-exploration.

Establishing such self-foci as "I feel inadequate as a mother and wife" or "I feel like a failure" early on in treatment gave both clients and therapists a sense of direction. Without identifying issues such as these as important generators of the depression, clients remained focused on recounting their depressive symptoms or unfortunate circumstances. They focused outward, blamed others or circumstances, and felt hopeless. Another set of self-foci related to lack of personal clarity, confusion, and/or apathy. A client might say, "I have so many thoughts and feelings I don't know what I feel, I just feel so confused" or "I just get so overwhelmed." These types of experiences served to create a focus of becoming more aware of one's feelings and needs. Other more interpersonal foci such as "My husband is an inveterate gambler and I can't cope any longer" or "I don't know if I can meet his expectations,or want to" or "My wife left me and I feel so discarded" all focused on dealing with problematic relationship issues. These focused most often on intimate partners.

## Process Diagnosis

### Styles of Processing

In our approach therapists make tacit moment-by-moment assessments of client's states and processes that guide their responses. Assessment of different types of clients' momentary processing lead to different momentary interventions that facilitate different types of exploratory processes. Process diagnoses of this type, in our treatment of depression, involve discriminating such things as whether the client is processing predominantly in an internal experiential manner or in a conceptual and externally focused manner. For example, at a particular point in a session, a momentary assessment that indicated that a client was processing experience in an abstract, conceptual manner led the therapist to reflect into the client's underlying feelings, focusing the person inward on a bodily felt experience of what the client was talking about. When, however, clients were already processing productively at an internal level, therapists decided how best to differentially facilitate optimal experiential exploration at that moment. They may, for example, have attempted to differentiate a global feeling of sadness into a sense of feeling drained and discouraged, or intensify a muted expression by asking the person to repeat a key phrase.

Therapists also distinguished between primary, secondary, and instrumental emotional responses (Greenberg & Safran, 1987; Greenberg et al., 1993). Primary emotions are here-and-now, immediate, direct responses to situations. Examples of the major primary adaptive emotions in the treatment of depression were sadness in relation to loss and anger in response to violation. Secondary emotions are reactive responses to more primary emotions or thoughts. They often obscure the primary generating process. In depression secondary sadness, for example, is often expressed when the primary feeling is anger. Depressed clients often cried plaintively when their primary emotion was anger, whereas others were agitated and angry when ther primary feeling was sadness. Instrumental emotions are those expressions that are expressed to achieve an aim such as, in depression, expressing hopelessness in efforts to elicit comfort or expressing anger to intimidate (Greenberg & Safran, 1989; Greenberg & Paivio, 1997). The primary goal in differentiating types of emotional response was to enhance therapists' ability to help clients access primary organismic emotional responses that had not been acknowledged. The therapist evaluated the nature of ongoing emotional expressions based on such nonverbal cues as vividness of language use, vocal quality, and facial and bodily expression, as well as on an understanding of biologically based emotional responses that occur in reaction to violation, threat, and frustration of goal attainment. For example, a person while looking sad may have expressed anger in a high-pitched airy tone, with a ranting quality (secondary feelings). The therapist, sensing that this is secondary to the more primary sadness and hurt, might say, "I hear that you feel very angry right now, and I imagine that inside you are also feeling quite hurt."

It is important to note that these types of process diagnoses, rather than occuring by explicitly thinking about the clients process, often take place tacitly. Therapists' responses occur spontaneously and seamlessly most of the time, like the automated skill of playing the piano. The process diagnoses guiding the moment-by-moment process only become explicit when the therapist experiences some difficulty or complexity that leads to thought or when they are made explicit in the training/learning context.

Therapists also work to facilitate different modes of client engagement depending on what the momentary formulation suggests is best to achieve at this moment. The therapist might choose to use any of the following four global modes of processing to facilitate the client's access to emotional experience (Greenberg et al., 1993): *Attending* involves making contact with basic sensory information about the self and external reality, from which further meaning can be constructed. *Experiential search* involves focusing on idiosyncratic inner experience and beginning to symbolize it in words. *Active expression*, involves clients expressing their experience in words or actions. This gives clients an opportunity to experiment with what it is they feel and to claim from this what fits as their own. *Interpersonal contact* with therapists helps clients feel safe and promotes new experiences, often serving to disconfirm dysfunctional beliefs about self and others.

## Marker Identification

A further major form of process diagnosis involves identifying markers of problematic experiential states. These markers signal not only that a person is in a particular state such as in conflict, or puzzling over a particular reaction that she/he had in a specific situation, but also that the person is amenable at this time to interventions designed to help facilitate resolution of that particular problem (Rice & Greenberg, 1984).

The four main affective problem markers that we have found useful in the treatment of depression are described below:

1. *Problematic reactions.* These are expressed through puzzlement about emotional or behavioral responses to particular situations. These markers indicate a clients readiness to reenter and reexperience the moment of reaction. Two main types of problematic reaction arose in the treatment of de-

pression One was related to inexplicable shifts into depression. These did not occur as often as expected, as many clinically depressed clients have a continuous sense of depression. The seçond type related more to puzzling about one's interpersonal reactions, say, why one felt so betrayed by a seemingly innocuous action of a professor. These were more related to identity issues related to the person's depression, such as low self-esteem or problems with intimacy or assertion, than to specific depressive symptoms,

2. *An absent or unclear felt sense indicating that the person was on the surface of, or feeling confused and unable to get a clear sense of, his/ her experience.* This marker indicates a readiness to attend to and symbolize internal experience. Markers of this type that most often arose were related to feelings of emptiness or confusion. For example, one client would come into a session saying that he felt that his work as an artist was meaningless and he felt aimless, whereas another client often reported feeling alienated and isolated, hence unable to feel connected to her boyfriend. Focusing at these moments helped clients contact a felt sense of the problem and explore it.

3. *Conflict splits in which one aspect of the self is critical or coercive toward another.* This marker indicates a current felt sense of struggle and a readiness for the two sides to make contact. In depression this marker related most directly to the self-critical determinants of depression in which the person's harsh criticism was highly depressogenic. Another form of split relevant to the therapy of depression involves the interruption and suppression by one part of the self of emotional experience and expression.

4. *Unfinished business.* This involved a lingering unresolved feeling toward a significant other. This marker indicated an opportunity to express previously interrupted feelings to a significant other and mobilize unmet needs. In depression this marker related to basic issues of separation, loss, or unresolved interpersonal issues.

Note that it is often only through a continuing empathic focus on the client's subjective experience that markers such as these arise in the session as signals of different types of current affective–cognitive schematic processing problems. Having identified a marker and intervened differentially by facilitating a particular task, the therapist is guided in further process diagnosis, both explicitly and tacitly, by a preexisting map of how such tasks tend to unfold. Such maps represent optimal problem-solving processes in particular experiential contexts. In this process the therapist attends, as fully as possible, to the client's momentary experience and responds so as to facilitate experiential exploration of a next step. This continues through to some recognizable point of resolution of the current problematic state. The stages involved in the resolution of these affective tasks have been intensively analyzed and modeled. These models also offer specific guidance to therapists on how to make appropriate momentary process diagnoses in the context of the task (Greenberg et al., 1993).

## Intervention

As with process diagnosis we think of intervention in terms both of moment-by-moment responding and of larger affective tasks at specific problem markers. Momentary responding can take a number of different forms depending on the intention behind the response. We have discriminated three major overall classes of intentional responses, in process-experiential therapy: (1) empathic understanding; (2) empathic exploration; and (3) process directions. *Empathic understanding* is carried out through various responses and seeks to communicate that the therapist understands the client's message. *Empathic exploration* responses are designed to facilitate client exploration. These responses take a number of different forms, including exploratory reflections, exploratory questions, and empathic conjectures. *Process directions* are directive in process but not in content. The therapist does not give advice but rather will suggest that the client try certain ways of exploring within the session.

## MAJOR THERAPEUTIC TASKS IN DEPRESSION

Identification of one of the previously described markers indicates an opportunity for the introduction of a specific task. Examples of tasks from the York Depression Project are given below.

In a fourth session of a therapy in which self-criticalness had been established as an important theme, a self-evaluative marker, "I'm just not good enough," arose. The therapist asked the client to put the evaluative side of himself in one chair and to make the other side feel like a failure. When an internalized self-critic was accessed, the therapist facilitated the expression of some of the contempt or harshness of the critic, for example, "You make me sick." Once the harshness of the critic had been accessed, the therapist facilitated the dialogue by encouraging the expression of more specific criticisms ("You do not work hard enough. You are stupid.") This work with the critic continued until such time as the underlying maladaptive emotion scheme of failure and inadequacy was accessed in the experiencing self. At this stage, guided by the emerging process, the therapist made another process diagnosis that it would be helpful to facilitate the expression of underlying feelings and therefore asked the person to express feeling reactions to the critic in the other chair ("I feel worthless when you say that—I feel like a nothing"). The therapist continued to make such process diagnoses throughout the dialogue, facilitating the appropriate type of expression at the appropriate moment.

At a comparable point in a similar dialogue two sessions later, when the client's primary adaptive feelings of sadness at the pain of his suffering at the hands of his critic was accessed, the therapist encouraged an assertion toward the critic of the needs for support related to this emotion. Once the needs for support and recognition, on the one hand, and the values and standards (those of wishing to be a valuable and productive contributor) underlying the criticisms, on the other, were put in dialectical opposition, the therapist continued to facilitate any emerging shifts in the critic to promote softening into a more accepting stance. All these steps helped the client integrate the opposing aspects of self (Greenberg et al., 1993).

In a therapy in which a client midway in treatment expressed sadness after remembering that her father missed her fifth birthday, the therapist asked the client to imagine her father in an empty chair and express her feelings to him. The client's insecurity in close relationships already had been established as a focus in understanding her feelings of anxiety and her depression. In the imaginary dialogue feelings of blame and complaint were differentiated into expressions of pure sadness and pure anger by process directives such as "Tell him what you resent" and "What's it like inside when you say that?" Early in life she had learned to interrupt the experience and expression of these intense feelings toward this significant figure in her life. When her feelings of sadness had been accessed, deeper exploration reminded her of other experiences of feeling abandoned and neglected by her father. The therapist made a process diagnosis that the intensification of this expression to her father in the empty chair might help evoke her core maladaptive, emotion scheme. Asking her to tell her father repeatedly how much she missed him facilitated the emergence of her emotional memories of feeling neglected and abandoned, and her childhood feelings of being unlovable. After promoting the full expression of, first her primary anger at her father's neglect and then her sadness at the loss, the therapist facilitated an expression of her unmet needs for love and recognition. According to the model of resolution of an unfinished business dialogue (Greenberg et al., 1993), this task ended with her affirming herself and understading him. She recognized that her father had tried to give her affection but that his own problems had prevented him from providing what she had needed.

A marker of a problematic reaction of a client reporting a puzzling outburst of anger toward his wife indicated that evocative unfolding would be productive. Initially, the therapist vividly evoked the scene in which the reaction occurred, and then in line with the model of resolution of problematic reactions (Greenberg et al., 1993) he helped the client determine the salient element in the situation that triggered the reaction (e.g., his wife's scornful look). Next, the therapist helped the client further explore his reaction of anger and attend to other associated feelings such as hurt and vulnerability. When these feelings had been sufficiently explored and differentiated, the client began to broaden his scope of understanding. At this point, the client moved from his idiosyncratic construal of the situation—of his wife as scornfully diminishing and himself as humiliatingly small—to his own feelings of diminishment when criticized. In this example, the client understood how his perception of being criticized involved intense felings of being wiped out and totally worthless, and that these feelings had originated in his relationship with his critical father (Greenberg et al., 1993; Watson & Rennie, 1994). This helped the client and therapist establish the feelings of diminishment and annihilation as an important focus of treatment.

In the case of the emergence of unclear felt sense markers therapists gave clients focusing instructions to help them explore what was occurring (see Gendlin, 1996, for details of this process). First the client would be helped to 'clear a space' for the exploration, then to focus on a bodily felt sense directly and to let words come from that which seemed most important or central at that moment. Continued focusing work involved shifting between symbol and referent and was promoted until a felt shift occurred. At times this led to the emergence of another client marker and the focus shifted, often to self-critical or unfinished business work.

## RESEARCH

We compared the effectiveness of process-experiential psychotherapy with one of its components, client-centered psychotherapy, in the treatment of thirty-four adults suffering from major depression (Greenberg & Watson, 1998). The client-centered treatment emphasized the establishment and maintenance of the Rogerian relationship conditions and empathic responding. The experiential treatment consisted of the client-centered conditions, in addition to the use of specific process-directive interventions at client markers. Both treatments were effective in reducing depressive symptomatology at termination and at 6-month follow-up. The active-intervention experiential treatment, however, had superior effects at midtreatment on depression and at termination on the total level of symptoms, self-esteem, and reduction of interpersonal problems. The addition to the relational conditions of specific active interventions at appropriate points in the treatment of depression appeared to hasten and enhance improvement.

In a study of the in-session processes in these treatments it was found that there were distinct differences in the types of client processes that were facilitated by the two treatments (Watson & Greenbeg, 1996). In the experiential tasks clients were observed to be engaged in differentiating their inner experience and using this to resolve issues in more personally meaningful ways than in the client-centered treatment. The process-experiential clients had deeper levels of experiencing, more productive vocal quality and expressive stance, and greater problem resolution than did the client-centered group. Two-chair and empty-chair dialogues clearly gave clients greater access to their inner experience and facilitated greater resolution of the specific cognitive–affective problems on which they were working. Systematic evocative unfolding did not result in demonstrably different in-session process than did the client-centered treatment in this study. This result may be explained partly by the low number of sessions in which clients explored problematic reactions, thereby limiting the power of the analysis to show significant differences. Focusing interventions were not investigated in the process study.

This study indicated that overall clients in process-experiential therapy more than in client-centered therapy were expressing their emotions during the session and trying to express their inner needs and desires, and were more internally focused and able to examine carefully and reflect on their experience so as to resolve their problems in personally meaningful ways.

An important additional objective of the process study was to explore possible links between clients' in-session problem resolution, postsession change, and final therapy outcome. This link was demonstrated in part. We found that sustained resolution over more than one session on the tasks related to outcome at termination and 6- and 18-month follow-up and that, regardless of the type of treatment, clients' reports at postsession of feeling resolved about the specific problems and tasks worked on in the session were related to change on the Beck Depression Inventory at termination and at 6-month follow-up.

## CASE EXAMPLE

Jan, the client mentioned earlier, was a 44-year-old woman who entered therapy feeling depressed. Her difficulty in functioning well at work as well as increasing bouts of tearfulness precipitated her seeking treatment. She had been screened for her appropriateness for short-term therapy of depression (16–20 sessions). She displayed a number of somatic symptoms including indigestion and hives. Currently involved in her second marriage, she felt that the communication had broken down and the marriage was "on the rocks." She said she had left home at the age of 16 and recalled feeling overburdened with responsibility in her family of origin, feeling underappreciated and emotionally neglected. She soon entered her first marriage in which she was emotionally and physically abused. After 6 years she left this marriage, leaving behind her two sons. She feared that taking them with her might endanger all of them. She carried a great deal of grief over her decision to leave her sons with their father, in spite of presently being on good terms with them.

In the first few sessions, the therapist was primarily concerned with establishing a therapeutic bond by means of empathic understanding. As the therapist responded to Jan's "central meanings" of needing to be a "superwoman" and the most poignant feelings underlying her hurt, the client began to move away from a description of her symptoms and her sense of loss of control, and focus more and more on her internal vulnerability and her difficulty accepting it. The client's growing awareness and symbolization of her internal experience will be illustrated by an excerpt from her first session.

In the following segment from the first session, Jan describes what became one of the central themes of her therapy (momentary therapist interventions are specified within brackets in places throughout the transcripts):

CLIENT: I guess over the years I have this image of myself as superwoman, to be able to do everything, hold down a full-time job, do the cleaning, cook gourmet meals, do all the housework, drive my family around, be there for them when they need me.

THERAPIST: So that's why you are here then, to try to understand, you are aware of a lot of feelings, a lot happening in your life, you work very hard for everybody, you are there for your whole family, you are the one who should be working hard, sounds like a lot. [Confirming response]

CLIENT: Well, I guess I put myself in that role, and maybe I'm not happy in it anymore and I don't know how to get out of it.

THERAPIST: Well I guess that's our job in here to explore together . . . but I guess it says a lot about how much you have really suffered, sounds like your body and your emotional world inside, everything has been really hurting . . . [Establishing focus, empathic understanding]

CLIENT: Well, part of me says give into it, and a part of me says there are people who are worse off than yourself.

THERAPIST: So because you haven't had to endure all the horrible stuff some people have . . . sounds like that is the same part that says you should be able to do everything, your work, your husband's work . . .

In the following few sessions, the therapist continues to follow the client's internal track, listening for what is most emotionally meaningful and poignant, and focusing on underlying determinants that could be causing her current suffering. In the fourth session, Jan reports feeling resentful toward her husband, and censoring her desire to be more open with him for fear of him laughing at her or changing the subject. The therapist implements an unfinished business task to enable the client to express her feelings to her husband in the empty chair:

CLIENT: I actually wanted to discuss it with my husband, how I felt, but I couldn't make myself do it, I can't talk to him yet about what's going on in here

THERAPIST: You would like to be able to open up, but it's kind of tough. I'm wondering if we could bring him in here, and you could talk to him, and we could help you with this kind of block or whatever it is you feel kind of apprehensive about. [Structuring the task]

As the dialogue progresses, the client expresses anger over feeling shut down and lingering resentment over not feeling like her husband's top priority. The therapeutic work she does with her husband reveals a split between a part of herself that wants to be open and a part that does not want to be vulnerable. She begins to have a dialogue between two parts of herself when she sees that one part of her is actually prohibiting herself from being vulnerable with him and expressing her feelings:

CLIENT: I feel this feeling coming over me of wanting to be in complete control, I feel she (*the controlling part*) is very strong and independent . . . I guess I have fought all my life to be independent and not be wishy-washy.

Later in the session, she realizes—

CLIENT: How can I be upset because somebody doesn't give me the things I want when I don't allow him to.

In session 6, Jan reports a recent family conflict over a Christmas dinner that her parents have canceled because of conflicts with Ann, their youngest daughter. Jan feels hurt and unappreciated, particularly by her mother—again a marker of unfinished business—this time with her mother. The therapist suggests having a dialogue with her mother in the empty chair:

THERAPIST: What do you see, what does she look like? [Evoking the presence of the significant other]

CLIENT: I don't see a happy women, she's always got a scowl on her face.

THERAPIST: What's happening to you? [Accessing client's initial feelings in response to significant other]

CLIENT: I feel like I'm going to break down and cry (*starts to cry*).

THERAPIST: Just let the tears come. What are you feeling right now, can you tell her? [Promoting expression of primary/adaptive feelings to significant other]

CLIENT: It hurts to see you so unhappy, it rubs off and it makes me unhappy too. I guess it hurts that I am second best, I guess because I am the oldest one I'm supposed to be responsible for everyone, so my feelings get pushed aside.

The dialogue helps Jan to consolidate an important theme throughout therapy: her feelings of being unappreciated and her need for approval, particularly from her mother. Later in the dialogue—

THERAPIST: What do you want from her? [facilitating expression of unmet need to significant other]

CLIENT: I'd like you to acknowledge that I'm as lovable as Ann (*tears*).

THERAPIST: Let it come, let those tears come. Tell her how much you are feeling now, can you speak from those tears and tell her how hurt you are. [Facilitating full expression of primary adaptive emotion to significant other]

CLIENT: I've been carrying this around for years and it's finally dawned on me, I've been trying for so many years to make you happy and do everything, but no matter what I do it's never enough.

The following segment describes significant episodes later in therapy in relation to two of the major themes of Jan's therapy: her need to be strong, perfect, and infallible, and her relationship with her mother. In session 10, Jan reported a current conflict with her husband in which she felt afraid to reveal her fears and wishes in relation to their financial situation. She did not want to confront him because she was afraid she would lose emotional control, break down, and cry. She felt that she should be strong and independent, and resolve the problem within herself. The therapist recognized this as a marker for a two-chair dialogue and suggested putting the different aspects of herself into two separate chairs. The dialogue reveals one side as a "strong" part of herself that feels the other part is weak for needing people:

THERAPIST: Tell her what you feel toward her. [Promoting awareness of self-criticisms]

CLIENT: You should be less needy, you are weak.

The other part feels afraid. She feels she wants her husband's approval and does not want to hurt him. A shift in the dialogue occurs after the client has accessed her primary sadness about how alone she feels in the marriage and the therapist encourages the client to express her needs:

THERAPIST: What do you want from her (*to the critic*)? [Encouraging expression of need]

CLIENT: I want to feel I am OK. I want to be more like her, to feel more confident.

THERAPIST: [Noticing a shift in her posture and face] What are you feeling now? [Facilitating negotiation]

CLIENT: I feel that the two sides have suddenly merged. It is as if the stronger person came over here and sat with me and said you're OK.

Later in the dialogue, consolidating the integration, she says to her critic in the other chair:

CLIENT: I'm not so scared anymore to confront the issues. I feel like stronger and like you are going to protect me.

In session 9, Jan talks about her guilt about leaving her two sons with her ex-husband, worrying that she "messed up their lives." She has a dialogue both with her abusive ex-husband and with her sons. Despite feeling that her son has forgiven her, she feels unable to forgive herself. In session 11, she works through her guilt in an empty-chair dialogue in which she confronts her mother's extreme disapproval of her decision:

CLIENT: Mom, I don't think we're ever going to see eye to eye because you see it in a different light.

THERAPIST: Can you tell her how you feel? [Differentiating feelings to the significant other]

CLIENT: I feel that I've lived my life to please everybody else, and it's been very hard and I don't want to do it anymore, and maybe we should agree that your life has been hard and you will never understand how difficult it has been for me.

THERAPIST: Is there anything you want from her? [Facilitating expression of unfulfilled needs and expectations in regard to the other]

CLIENT: Don't expect so much from me anymore, 'cause I don't think I'm going to be able to deliver it.

THERAPIST: How do you feel saying that?

CLIENT: I don't feel so guilty anymore, that I can't jump every time they want something . . . It's been a real burden trying to live up to what everybody else thought of me, and it's made me very sad.

In session 13, Jan reports feeling more self-confident, in charge of her life, and able to make changes. She continues to report positive feelings for the duration of therapy. In session 14, she reports standing up to her mother, not letting her push her around, and feeling more self-confidence in asserting her needs. In session 15, she takes responsibility for trying to be "superwoman," and not allowing others to help her:

CLIENT: I put myself in the position of trying to protect and serve everybody . . . I always felt I could be superwoman, that I could handle two full-time jobs, do all the housework.

THERAPIST: You were never going to show any vulnerability. [Exploratory reflection]

CLIENT: Yeah, I never asked for help.

Later in the session, she reports an awareness that she was the one devaluing her own feelings:

CLIENT: I felt like such a whiner, complaining and crying, but it was me discrediting my emotions . . . My feelings do count, they are legitimate, sometimes they may be foolish but that's OK.

In session 16, she continues to portray a much more confident, self-valuing stance:

CLIENT: It's useless to think that way, and it's OK not to be liked by everybody, that's all right. I can't kill myself trying to please everybody. If I don't start looking after myself nobody is going to do it for me.

Jan thus resolved the conflict between the more dominant "superwoman" voice in her personality and the weaker voice expressing her more human emotions and needs. Resolution occurred, with the different parts integrating into a more self-supportive internal organization.

## CONCLUSION

The demonstration of the efficacy of two forms of experiential therapy of depression, client-centered and process-experiential, is an important demonstration for critics and proponents alike that experiential therapy is potentially as effective as other empirically validated treatments of depression. The findings that, in a brief treatment, adding more specific, marker-guided, process-directive interventions to the relationship conditions quickens and broadens the effects of the relational conditions alone will we hope encourage all experientially oriented therapists to include the tested interventions in their treatments.

## REFERENCES

American Psychiatric Association. (1994). *Diagnostic and statistical manual of mental disorders* (4th ed.). Washington, DC: APA Books.

Beck, A. T., Rush, J., Shaw, B., & Emery, G. (1979). *Cognitive therapy of depression.* New York: Guilford Press.

Blatt, S., & Maroudas, C. (1992). Convergences among psychoanalytic and cognitive-behavioral theories of depression. *Psychoanalytic Psychology, 9*(2), 157–190.

Gendlin, E. T. (1996). *Focusing-oriented psychotherapy: A manual of the experiential method.* New York: Guilford Press.

Greenberg, L. S., & Paivio, S. (1997). *Working with emotions.* New York: Guilford Press.

Greenberg, L. S., & Pascual-Leone, J. (1995). A dialectical constructivist approach to experiential change. In R. Neimeyer & M. Mahoney (Eds.), *Constructivism in psychotherapy.* Washington, DC: American Psychological Associates Press.

Greenberg, L. S., Rice, L. N., & Elliott, R. (1993). *Facilitating emotional change: The moment-by-moment process.* New York: Guilford Press.

Greenberg, L. S., & Safran, J. D. (1987). *Emotion in psychotherapy: Affect, cognition, and the process of change.* New York: Guilford Press.

Greenberg, L. S., & Safran, J. D. (1989). Emotion in psychotherapy. *American Psychologist, 44,* 19–29.

Greenberg, L. S., & Watson, J. C. (1998). Experiential therapy of depression: Differential effects of client-centered relationship conditions and process experiential interventions. *Psychotherapy Research, 8*(2), 210–224.

Klerman, G. L., Weissman, M. M., Rounsaville, B. J., & Chevron, E. S. (1984). *Interpersonal psychotherapy of depression.* New York: Basic Books.

Rice, L. N., & Greenberg, L. S. (1984). *Patterns of change: Intensive analysis of psychotherapeutic process.* New York: Guilford Press.

Smith, T. (1996, August). *Severe life stress, major depression, and emotion-related negative memory.* Paper presented at the International Society for Research in Emotion, Toronto, Canada.

Teasdale, J. (1996). Clinically relevant theory. In P. Salkovskis (Ed.), *Frontiers of cognitive therapy.* New York: Guilford Press.

Teasdale, J., & Barnard, J. (1993). *Affect, cognition, and change.* Hillsdale, NJ: Erlbaum.

Watson, J. C., & Greenberg, L. S. (1995). Alliance ruptures and repairs in experiential therapy. *In Session: Psychotherapy in Practice, 1*(1), 19–32.

Watson, J. C., & Greenberg, L. S. (1996). Pathways to change in the psychotherapy of depression: Relating process to session change and outcome. *Psychotherapy, 33*(2), 262–274 [Special issue on outcome research].

Watson, J. C., Greenberg, L. S., & Goldman, R. (1996). Change processes in experiential therapy. In R. Hutterer, G. Pawlowsky, P. Schmid, & R. Stipsitz (Eds.), *Client-centered and experiential psychotherapy: A paradigm in motion.* Vienna, Austria: Peter Lang.

Watson, J. C., & Rennie, D. (1994). Qualitative analysis of clients' subjective experience of significant moments during the exploration of problematic reactions. *Journal of Counselling Psychology, 41,* 500–509.

Weeresekera, P., Linder, B., Greenberg, L. S., & Watson, J. C. (1998). *The alliance across treatment in experiential therapy.* Manuscript submitted.

# 11

**\*\*\*\*\***

# Process-Experiential Therapy for Posttraumatic Stress Difficulties

Robert Elliott
Kenneth L. Davis
Emil Slatick

*For an experiential* therapist working with a client who has been through a traumatic event, the starting point is understanding how drastically the client's perceived world has been transformed by the trauma. A criminal or sexual assault or a natural or human disaster divides the client's life into three phenomenological "moments"—before, during, and after the traumatic event (Wertz, 1985). In the client's experience, each of these moments is at the same time a "world," consisting of particular views of self, other people, and the world at large. Thus, we begin this chapter with a general description of these three "world-moments," building on the phenomenological research of Fischer and Wertz (1979; also Wertz, 1985):

    1. Before the trauma, the person experiences the *previctimization world* as safe. While this world contains the possibility of victimization, this possibility is experienced in the abstract. Instead, the person feels whole, powerful, and immune from harm, or at least adequately protected by a surrounding community of helpful others and routine precautions, as he or she lives narratives of ordinariness and progress toward carrying out "life projects" (e.g., completing school, raising a family).

    2. In the moment of the trauma, the *victimization world* emerges. The previous sense of safety and agency is lost, and, in terror, the person discov-

ers that he or she has suddenly become the prey of a malevolent other or an uncaring impersonal force (e.g., earthquake, fire). This overpowering other or force typically threatens to end the person's continued existence; this threat leaves the person helpless, terror stricken, and vulnerable. Alternatively, the trauma may consist of being forced to stand by as a horrified witness while another person faces threatened or actual death or grave injury. In either case, the person feels cut off and isolated from the community of helpful or well-intentioned others (friends, neighbors, spouse, parents). During this moment, time sometimes seems to slow or stop as the victim attempts to stave off death. This moment later comes to be seen as central in the person's life, splitting his or her life narrative into discontinuous "before" and "after" stories.

3. Afterwards, in the *postvictimization world*, the person lives constantly in active anticipation of further victimization. He or she lives this possibility through a wide range of difficulties: the body is more anxious and easily startled; the senses are exquisitely tuned to any impending danger; sleep is disrupted by repeated nightmares of recurrent victimization; the future comes to be seen as all too brief or limited; the person's hopes for attaining happiness or success are put on hold, and the person is stuck in a passive narrative of continuing to exist with a damaged life/self while waiting either for something to change or for another, perhaps final, victimization. In order to escape this pervasive intrusion of the victimization world into the person's postvictimization existence, the person attempts to avoid thoughts, feelings or memories related to the victimization, often withdrawing from routine activities or using various substances to dull the emotional pain. Nevertheless, the reality of the victimization experience continually reasserts itself, leaving the person torn and confused.

Process-experiential therapy with posttraumatic stress difficulties (PTSD) begins with an interest in the client's individual, unique experience of these three world-moments, informed by a sensitivity to the general forms and specific varieties that this experience may take. As client and therapist explore these and other sets of emotionally tinged perceptions and beliefs ("emotion schemes"), a number of key therapeutic tasks routinely emerge, for example, unfinished business (i.e., lingering bad feelings toward unhelpful others or the perpetrator; Greenberg, Rice, & Elliott, 1993). Formation of a positive working alliance between the client and therapist is critical, even more so than with other types of psychological difficulty, because the victimized clients typically experience repeated disappointments or even revictimizations at the hands of legal authorities and medical and mental health professionals. If the therapist can establish him-/herself as a helpful representative of the client's community, then therapeutic work can move forward and particular therapeutic tasks can be addressed (e.g., using empty-chair work). Reconnecting with a helpful other, making meaning out of the trauma, confronting the hidden vulnerability, facing (in imagination) the unhelpful others or even the perpetrator, or discovering and overcoming the underlying divisions in the self—any or all of these may help the client begin to reconstruct his or her victimization-haunted life-world into one in which he or she once again feels able to pursue important life projects.

In this chapter, we present a process-experiential conceptualization of the nature of PTSD, together with an outline of the therapeutic intervention strategies utilized to help the client overcome these difficulties. In our presentation we will speak of posttraumatic stress "difficulties" rather than "disorder." For the victimized individual, the word "difficulties" better captures the sense of being caught up in continuing problems stemming from the victimization. Although these difficulties affect the person's body, undoubtedly including aspects of his or her brain function, PTSD is not a "disease," but rather an existentially based state of profound uneasiness about self, others, and the world.

It is vital for therapists to appreciate and respect the many different forms of trauma and posttraumatic difficulty. To begin with, different types of traumatic event present different problems for each person: For example, the terror of a single victimization by a malevolent stranger differs greatly from the horror of witnessing the violent death of a loved one. In turn, both of these differ significantly from the grinding awfulness of repeated victimization by a hostile, controlling parent figure or from the sudden shock of a nonintentional victimization due to an accident or natural disaster. In addition, although all victimizations are in some sense ongoing, there is an enormous difference between a victimization that is definitively over (e.g., due to the perpetrator's death) and a victimization that is ongoing (e.g., drawnout legal involvement with the perpetrator). More important, "objective" differences in the circumstances of the victimization have relatively little to do with the meaning made by the person. Thus, the same trauma may result in a full set of PTSD in one person but not in another.

Finally, traumatic events give rise to a wide variety of difficulties not limited to the reexperiencing, avoiding, and hypersensitivity problem clusters listed in DSM-IV (American Psychiatric Association, 1994). Distrust of others, difficult relationships, disrupted sense of self, depression, intense anger, impulsive behavior, substance misuse, and self-destructive or even suicidal acts comprise aspects of a more complex, broader "disorder of extreme stress" (DES; Herman, 1992; Zlotnick et al., 1996), which overlaps substantially with borderline personality "disorder." Clearly, the wide range of PTSD and related treatment issues defies our ability to address them all in a single chapter. We urge therapists not to adopt a "one size fits all" attitude in dealing with particular clients' PTSD.

## A PROCESS-EXPERIENTIAL THEORY OF PTSD

The conceptual model of PTSD presented in this chapter consists of two major components, an emotional processing conflict model and a trauma-related emotion schemes model. These models describe aspects of PTSD that have been largely neglected by the dominant conditioning models (e.g., Blake, Abueg, & Woodward, 1993). These characterizations are intended to provide heuristic devices to increase therapist empathic sensitivity to important, common features of victimization experiences.

## PTSD as Emotional Processing Conflict

DSM-IV lists organizes PTSD symptoms into three clusters: reexperiencing, avoiding/distancing, and hyperarousal (American Psychiatric Association, 1994). We believe that this classification has considerable phenomenological validity and needs to be accounted for by any theory of PTSD. In the following, we present our understanding of the underlying, conflicting self-processes that give rise to each type of difficulty.

### Reexperiencing the Trauma

A key assumption of humanistic–experiential therapies is that there is a basic human need for growth and mastery. One important facet of this growth tendency is a need to resolve and master important painful or interrupted emotional experiences. More specifically, the process-experiential approach (Greenberg et al., 1993) assumes that emotions are biologically adaptive processes that integrate rapid, automatic processing of environmental information with appropriate action tendencies and emotional expression. This process gives rise to reexperiencing difficulties, such as intrusive thoughts and images, flashbacks, and nightmares. In other words, these problems are *not* seen as caused by a passive "overgeneralization" as a result of traumatic conditioning. Instead, the reexperiencing difficulties are viewed as expressions of an underlying organismic need to finish some unfinished aspect of the trauma (e.g., to understand why it happened, who was responsible, or how a reoccurrence can be prevented).

Sometimes, the person is at least partially aware of his or her desire to dwell on the painful experiences and deliberately reflects or ruminates on aspects of the trauma. Often, however, because of the painfulness of the trauma, reexperiencing is avoided and interrupted. When interrupted, this desire for completion is likely to express itself in sudden or ego-alien forms, such as flashbacks, unwanted images, and recurrent trauma-related nightmares. Furthermore, when the person's adaptive emotional processes are interrupted, he or she remains in a state of incompletion (referred to as "unfinished emotional business"); under these conditions, the reexperiencing difficulties express the part of the self that is attempting to cope by resolving the unresolved aspects of the trauma. Finally, the reexperiencing aspect of the self may also be explicitly engaged in protecting the person from repeated victimization by constantly reminding him or her of possible danger, "lest you forget."

## Avoiding Pain/Danger

To varying degrees, persons suffering from trauma-related difficulties also try to avoid the feelings, ideas, and activities related to the trauma. Often, these attempts are deliberate, as when the person tries to distract him-/herself. However, avoiding painful experiences may also become automatic, taking the form of dissociation, emotional numbing, and interpersonal detachment. From a process-experiential perspective, this tendency is seen as a function of the person's biological need to protect the self from pain (which signals danger), as well as to conserve resources when injured. In many instances, the individual seeks to avoid his or her painful experience by using a variety of legal and illegal substances that numb or distract him or her from emotional pain. The part of the self that expresses these avoiding processes often adopts an explicitly protective stance in which the reexperiencing processes are viewed as a threat to the person's physical or mental integrity.

The person with unresolved traumas thus continues to experience a conflict between two competing self-organizations: (1) a reexperiencing part of the self, which repeatedly returns to the victimization world of the traumatic event; and (2) an avoiding part of the self, which tries to interrupt the reexperiencing, in a sense attempting to return to the *pre*victimization world. As already noted, in its simplest form this conflict is between the need to avoid pain and the need to resolve the painful experience through completion of interrupted action or expression. This conflict generates the characteristic alternation in PTSD between reexperiencing and distancing (Horowitz, 1986). The result is a continuing state of internal tension between the two action tendencies. It is essential that the therapist recognize and respect both growth-oriented reexperiencing and safety-oriented avoiding aspects of self (Maslow, 1968). However, because this conflict often lies outside the client's immediate frame of reference, it may be difficult to work with directly in therapy.

## Hyperarousal: Continuing Fearful Vulnerability and Conflict

The third set of common posttraumatic difficulties involves signs of heightened arousal, including insomnia, irritability, concentration problems, hypervigilance, exaggerated startle responses, physical reactivity, and a sense of a foreshortened future. Most centrally, these difficulties indicate a continued living in the victimization world; they express a sense of self as vulnerable to further harm at any moment. In addition, these "hyperarousal" difficulties often indicate a continuing state of conflict between the competing needs for reexperiencing/completion and avoidance of pain.

### Common Trauma-Related Emotion Schemes

As a convenient shorthand, emotion schemes can be referred to in terms of either their organizing emotion (in PTSD, typically fear or anxiety) and object (world, others, self). The emotion schemes described here are so common in PTSD that knowledge of them can give therapists greater empathic sensitivity to their traumatized clients' experiences. As noted earlier, therapists should use these concepts to listen to clients but should never impose them.

From a process-experiential perspective, PTSD involves competing sets of emotion schemes. One set of emotion schemes (which can be referred to as "ordinariness") are characteristic of the previctimization world and create difficulties because the traumatic event cannot be assimilated to them. The other set of emotion schemes ("fearful vulnerability") is activated during the trauma and accurately represents the victimization world of the traumatic event itself (see Table 11.1). These emotion schemes center around the emotion of fear and associated perceptions (e.g., dangerousness) and action tendencies (e.g., flight, avoidance).

When a person is victimized he or she experiences a profound challenge to a set of key emotion schemes, referred to as "cherished beliefs" (Clarke, 1989). These cherished beliefs and their trauma-related alternative emotion schemes involve self, others, and the world, and have been described vividly by Wertz (1985) and Fischer and Wertz (1979) in their work on criminal victimization, as well as by Janoff-Bulman (1992) (see Table 11.1). These include the following:

1. *The unsafe world.* Before their victimization, most people assume a baseline "safe world" scheme in which their physical and social environment is seen as essentially benign. After the victimization, this emotion scheme is

**TABLE 11.1. Common Previctimization and Trauma-Related Emotion Schemes**

| Previctimization world | Victimization world |
|---|---|
| "Ordinariness" (cherished beliefs challenged by trauma) | "Fearful vulnerability" (trauma-related emotion schemes) |
| *. . . about the world* | |
| 1. Safe: predictable, controllable | 1. Dangerous: unpredictable, uncontrollable |
| *. . . about others* | |
| 2. Neutral: uninvolved with me, harmless | 2. Malevolent: predatory, powerful |
| 3. Helpful: present, caring, effective | 3. Unhelpful: absent, uncaring, ineffectual |
| *. . . about self* | |
| 4. Invulnerable: special, powerful, whole, "that can't happen to me" | 4. Vulnerable: weak, damaged, blameworthy |

replaced with a highly generalized sense of the world as fundamentally un-safe, both dangerous and unpredictable.

2. *The malevolent other.* Traumas involving criminal victimization or sexual abuse (vs. disasters or accidents) are fundamentally interpersonal. Interpersonal violence or violation activates an emotion scheme of a power-ful, malevolent, detrimental, predatory "perpetrator." After victimization, this malevolent other is seen as potentially present in a wide variety of others who would formerly have been viewed as innocuous or even helpful.

3. *Unhelpful others.* Victimization also disrupts the person's belief that others provide an enveloping community that can be depended upon to pro-vide offer protection, assistance, and concern. Helpful others (friends, fam-ily, legal authorities, mental health professionals) were unable to prevent the victimization in the first place, then were experienced as absent or unavail-able during the victimization, and finally were seen as ineffectual or uncar-ing after the victimization.

4. *Vulnerable self.* Finally, emotion schemes or "cherished beliefs" about personal power, self-efficacy, invulnerability, goodness, or "special-ness" (Yalom, 1980) are challenged by the trauma (e.g., "If I'm careful, nothing bad will happen to me"). Typically, the person struggles against giving up the earlier beliefs; at the same time, he or she adopts an alter-native self-organization in which the self is experienced as weak, helpless, fragmented, vulnerable, and sometimes even deserving of further, future victimizations.

The exact nature and combination of the challenged cherished beliefs with newer, trauma-related emotion schemes varies with each person and with the nature of the victimization experience. For example, recent trau-mas can interact in idiosyncratic ways with traumas from earlier in the person's life. One client was pleased with how she had been able to bring about an end to her stepfather's earlier molestation of her, but that only emphasized how powerless she was to stop the perpetrator in her primary victimization experience from attempting to murder her. For the therapist, the important thing is to understand the unique forms the emotion schemes take with each client.

## Common Emotional Processing Difficulties

In addition to the cherished and trauma-related emotion schemes described, the person commonly experiences a number of related difficulties in the manner in which he or she processes experience.

First, much of the traumatized person's schematic processing is highly automatic, in part because threats to physical integrity activate the primary appraisal system, which is rapid and preverbal (i.e., experienced bodily) in nature (Zajonc, 1980); this makes these emotion schemes difficult for the person to access and change.

Second, the emotional distancing strategies used by the person interrupt full schematic processing through generalized emotional numbing or through dissociation of specific trauma memories.

Third, the trauma disrupts the person's narrative processing (Wigren, 1994). The victimization itself creates a massive discontinuity in the person's life narrative and meaning-making processes (Clarke, 1989, 1991), breaking the previously unitary life narrative into two separate stories: The previctimization narrative is an interrupted story that typically deals with progress toward accomplishment of life projects (e.g., career) within the ordinariness of everyday life. The postvictimization narrative, on the other hand, is a variant form of "illness" or "recovery" narrative, taken up with the struggle to survive, to reestablish a normal existence, and to restart derailed life projects. In addition, the trauma narrative itself is likely to contain "narrative defects" (Wigren, 1994) in the form of memory gaps and explanatory discontinuities. The result is that the person's trauma narrative neither holds together as a story in itself nor fits with the interrupted previctimization story.

## Treatment Implications

This analysis of the role of emotion schemes and experiential processing in PTSD has a number of implications for treatment. The therapist can use the analysis of types of trauma-related emotion schemes to enhance his or her empathic sensitivity to those key aspects of the client's experience. At the same time, it is a good idea to prepare oneself for the client's having a difficult time accessing highly automatic, trauma-driven schematic processing. It is therefore useful to listen for in-session evidence that distancing processes are interrupting emotions and memories related to the trauma. The therapist can then help the client attend to these interrupting processes. Finally, it is important to help the client to tell (and retell) the three relevant stories—the traumatic event, the previctimization life, and the postvictimization life—in order to facilitate the recovery of missing story elements (memories or explanatory links) and to help create continuities within and between stories.

## A Note on Work with Disorder of Extreme Stress (DES)

As noted, clients with long-term sexual abuse or multiple victimizations experience trauma on top of preexisting trauma-related emotion schemes. We are struck by how these clients lack easily accessible nontrauma emotion schemes. Instead, the person has often developed a chronic "damaged self" scheme, which may contain nongrowth elements such as "If I'm emotionally distant or cold, I'll be less vulnerable to sexual predators." A subsequent victimization may validate these components, reinforcing the person's underlying sense of damagedness and vulnerability, as well as the lack of adequate protection and support from others. This damaged self often leads to increased vigilance to the point of emotional paralysis or, in contrast, to an increase in risky, "what-does-it-matter-anyway?" behavior, such as sexual promiscuity. In addition, for many repeatedly victimized clients, the moment of the most recent victimization melts into the person's previous traumas.

## PROCESS-EXPERIENTIAL THERAPY FOR CLIENTS WITH PTSD
### Overcoming Victimization: A General View of the Change Process

In their phenomenological investigation of the experience of criminal victimization, Fischer and Wertz (1979) described three changes that must occur in order for an interpersonal victimization experience to be successfully resolved:

1. *Reempowering the self.* In order to overcome a one-time victimization, the person must regain a sense of his or her own ability to make meaningful choices and to return to important life projects that were derailed by the victimization. Regardless of the degree of previous victimization, the reempowerment process may take a number of forms in process-experiential therapy: First, it is important for the therapist to help the client clarify the nature of the interrupted life project in the initial session and to underscore the client's interest in overcoming the interruption. Second, throughout therapy, the therapist also empathically selects emergent, self-assertive experience and offers the client choices about the therapeutic process, emphasizing the client's agency wherever possible. Third, the therapist helps the client explore and express emotions. Helping the client to work with his or her anger is especially important, because the adaptive action tendency that accompanies anger is assertive self-protection in the face of potential violation.

2. *Providing the presence of a caring other.* Helpful, caring, empathic others provide an alternative, "corrective emotional experience" to negative images of others as uncaring, ineffectual, or malevolent. This is usually the first task of therapy, and it often takes a number of sessions for the traumatized client to develop trust that the therapist genuinely understands and cares. Indeed, helping the client feel safe enough to reveal his/her deep sense of vulnerability may be the key change process in the process-experiential treatment of PTSD.

3. *Reestablishing world as partially trustworthy.* Finally, the environment must show over a period of time that it is at least partially trustworthy, so that extreme vigilance is no longer needed. As Wertz (1985) points out, the postvictimization world can never be as safe as the previctimization world, but some safety must be reestablished in order for the person to return to a tolerable life and to continue with important life projects. In an experiential therapy, safety or trustworthiness is first established in the thera-

peutic relationship. However, it is essential that clients be able to face their environments and to discover that their vigilance can be relaxed, at least under the appropriate circumstances. At the same time, it is vital that it be the *client* who decides when and where to begin to trust aspects of his/her world.

We have found that it can be helpful for the client, early in therapy, to be helped to identify a real or imagined "safe place" as a kind of "base" from which to explore the victimization experience. For one client this took the form of an imaginary, totally walled-off room in which to hide, whereas for another client the safe place was an actual location, a favorite sunny clearing in a local park. Gendlin's "clearing a space" method (1996), can be used to help the client establish such a safe place.

## Treatment Principles as They Apply to PTSD

Greenberg and colleagues (1993) have described six treatment principles that provide the overall guidelines for process-experiential therapy. The first three involve facilitating a therapeutic relationship, while the last three involve helping the client to engage in work on specific therapeutic tasks (see Greenberg et al., 1993, for more details:)

1. *Empathic attunement.* The therapist attempts to enter and stay with the client's internal frame of reference.
2. *Therapeutic bond.* The therapist communicates his or her empathy for the client within a genuine, prizing relationship.
3. *Task collaboration.* The therapist facilitates the client's involvement in the goals and tasks of therapy, and is personally involved as well.
4. *Experiential processing.* The therapist facilitates the client processes that are likely to be optimal for the particular moment in therapy.
5. *Growth/choice.* The therapist fosters the client's growth and self-determination.
6. *Task completion/focus.* The therapist facilitates the client's completion of key therapeutic tasks.

## Major Therapeutic Tasks with Trauma-Related Difficulties

Process-experiential therapy for PTSD integrates a variety of different experiential tasks, drawn from client-centered, Gestalt, and existential therapy traditions. These tasks all include three elements: a *marker* signaling the client's immediate state of readiness to work on a particular issue or experiential task; a *task intervention* sequence of therapist and client task-relevant actions; and a desired *resolution* or end state. We find it useful to divide process-experiential tasks for trauma-related difficulties into three groupings (Elliott et al., 1996), based on the predominant client "modes of engagement" (Greenberg et al., 1993) called for by the task (see Table 11.2).

**TABLE 11.2. Process-Experiential Tasks and Corresponding Posttraumatic Experience**

| Task intervention/marker | Relevant posttraumatic Experience |
|---|---|
| *Experiential search tasks* | |
| *Empathic exploration* of trauma-related experiences | Undifferentiated nature of trauma-related experiences |
| *Facilitating retelling* of trauma-related stories (victimization, pre- and postvictimization) | Client's need to tell trauma and life narratives; trauma narrative gaps; disrupted life narrative |
| *Meaning-creation* work for meaning protest | Cherished beliefs about self, others, or world challenged by trauma |
| *Clearing a space experiential Focusing* for an absent/unclear felt sense | Client is overwhelmed or distanced from experience; client has unverbalized troubling or painful experiences |
| *Systematic evocative unfolding* for self-understanding problems | Puzzling "flashbacks" of trauma; fear episodes; nightmares |
| *Active expression tasks* | |
| *Two-chair dialogue* for self-conflict splits | Self-criticism for victimization; approach versus avoid trauma-related experiences; self-induced "anxiety splits" with weak/bad self |
| *Two-chair enactments* for self-interruptions | Blocked trauma-related fear, anger |
| *Empty chair work* for unfinished emotional business | Lingering bad feelings (especially anger) toward unhelpful others or perpetrators |
| *Interpersonal contact tasks* | |
| *Empathic affirmation* with vulnerability (painful self-related experience) | Sense of personal fragility, foreshortened future |
| *Relationship dialogue* for alliance difficulties | Distrust, anger at therapist as real or potential unhelpful other |

*Experiential search tasks* involve some form of problematic experience which requires the client to pay attention to unclear, puzzling or problematic aspects of inner experience. These tasks reflect the client-centered heritage of Process-experiential therapy. In our experience, these are the most common tasks in Process-experiential therapy with PTSD. Five different experiential search tasks will be described, roughly in the order in which they might occur in a treatment:

1. *Empathic exploration* of trauma-related experiences is the "baseline task" because the therapist begins each session with it, because the markers for other tasks typically emerge from empathic exploration, and because client

and therapist return to this task when they pause or complete their work on one of the other tasks. Empathic exploration differs from the next task to be presented, facilitating retelling, in that exploration addresses key unclear or undifferentiated aspects of the victimization in a nonlinear, branching fashion, while retelling involves the linear unfolding of victimization-related narratives.

In a sense, any experience that captures the client's attention in the session is an *exploration marker* and can be empathically explored or differentiated, especially when it is incomplete, fuzzy, undifferentiated, or global, and even when it is expressed only in external terms. For example, one client stated: "I mean *it* [my fear] controls my life, every, step of my life, every action and every thing." This client's "it" provided the marker for an extensive, branching exploration of her experience of her trauma-related fear as a "thing." The therapist offered the client a variety of different "processing proposals" (see Sachse, 1992) to help her explore different aspects of her experience of her "fear as a thing," including "What kind of thing is it?"; "Can you locate it in your body?"; "As we talk has it changed or is it the same?"; and "What would you like to do with it?" The therapist balanced these process-directive exploratory questions with evocative reflections. (See Greenberg et al., 1993, for a description of the *experiential response modes* used by process-experiential therapists to carry out treatment principles and tasks.) These evocative reflections included, among others, "So the fear is like a *thing* that comes upon you," and "Oh, I see. It's the blob of stuff that comes from your being victimized."

Empathic exploration events can be said to be partially resolved if they lead to a marker for another therapeutic task (e.g., unfinished business); a greater degree of resolution occurs if the client is able to achieve a substantial differentiation of his or her experience. A complete resolution of this task requires some form of experienced shift in the targeted experience.

2. *Facilitating retelling* of the trauma and related stories is also very common in process-experiential therapy for PTSD. While telling the trauma narrative is usually painful, people who have been victimized typically have a strong need to describe the sequence of events in their victimization. The marker for facilitating retelling is a trauma-related *narrative marker*, that is, a reference by the client to some aspect of the trauma about which a story could be told (e.g., "When I was robbed, there was nothing I could do to stop them"). In addition to the victimization narrative markers, there are also previctimization narrative markers ("Before I was robbed, I was always careful") and postvictimization narrative markers ("Ever since I was robbed, I can't even go near that part of town"). A final type of trauma-related story is the victimization nightmare, involving the victimization or a variation of it.

In the first session of therapy, the therapist typically listens for victimization narrative markers and, if necessary, suggests a facilitating retelling task by encouraging the client to "Tell me the story of your victimization in as much detail as you feel comfortable giving." This provides a useful way to begin the therapy and signals the therapist's willingness to "hear the client through his/her pain" (Egendorf, 1995). Similarly, the therapist listens for pre- and postvictimization narratives in the first couple of sessions, and, if necessary, encourages the client to enter into the facilitating retelling task for these as well:

> "I wonder if you would be willing to tell me what your life was like up to the point when you were raped, you know, what you had been working toward in your life over time."

> "It might be useful for us to go over how your life has gone since the rape, what you've been through and how you've dealt with it over time."

As the client tells one of these stories, he or she often reexperiences it to some degree. Important features of it become clear, including the aspects of the story that continue to puzzle or trouble the client. It is generally useful for the client to retell the different trauma-related stories more than once in the course of therapy. This is because the story is expected to change over time, as the client comes to trust the therapist more, as he or she accesses additional memories, and as the meanings of the events in the story evolve and become clearer over time.

What does resolution look like in the facilitating retelling task? A resolved retelling is a relatively complete narrative experienced by the client as "making sense" or "fitting together," with a clear "point" or overall meaning for the client (Wigren, 1994). Resolved retellings may also be marked by an indication from the client that he or she has developed a greater awareness or understanding of something in the story. For example, as one client retold her postvictimization story near the end of her treatment, she began to see her debilitating fear as not only due to her victimization but also the result of her having since set aside her own needs in order to please her boyfriend, which blocked her life projects and led to lowered self-esteem, which then led to a return of her sense of vulnerability. This finally helped her to make sense out of the puzzling downward spiral of increasing fear that had brought her into therapy.

3. *Meaning creation* work occurs when a client seeks to understand the meaning of an emotional experience or crisis (Clarke, 1989, 1991). This task involves the symbolization of emotional experience in the presence of high emotional arousal. Clarke (1989) described the marker for this event as the expression of strong emotion arising from a discrepancy between a life event and a cherished belief. We refer to this as a "meaning protest" marker. Meaning protests often involve loss, disappointment, or other life crises, and so meaning creation work is very appropriate with PTSD. Therapist interventions that facilitate this task attempt to clarify and symbolize the client's cherished beliefs, the client's discrepant experience (i.e., the victimization), and the discrepancy between belief and experience. The client and therapist

work together to accomplish this, often using metaphors to capture aspects of the meaning protest in words and images.

Typically, resolution of a meaning protest passes through three phases: First, there is an initial phase in which emotional arousal increases and the elements of the meaning protest (event, cherished belief, reaction) are specified. Second, the client and therapist explore the cherished belief, including its basis and continued tenability. Finally, the client modifies some aspect of the cherished belief, symbolizes this change, and considers new behavior. For example, the depressed, physically abused client described in Labott, Elliott, and Eason (1992) wept intensely as she expressed her disappointment and anger with her alcoholic father for hitting her as a child; in exploring her reaction, she discovered that his behavior had violated her cherished belief that "If you love someone, you don't hurt them". Through examining this belief and her experience, she decided that her father hadn't really loved her and that his behavior was not really her fault. Finally, she realized that she needed to work on issues of trust in her marital relationship.

4. The next task, *experiential focusing* for an absent or unclear felt sense, has been described by Gendlin (1981, 1996) and is relevant to work with clients' immediate, in-session experiential processing difficulties. Focusing is really two different subtasks, *clearing a space* and *focusing on an unclear felt sense*, both of which are important in PTSD.

First, the client may feel overwhelmed by an immediate state of emotional hyperarousal or may become overwhelmed whenever he or she begins to explore painful feelings or memories ("overwhelmed" marker). In this case, it is very useful for the therapist to propose a variant of the "clearing a space" subtask (Gendlin, 1996) by suggesting that the client first imagine a favorite "place" or an internal mental "space"; the client is then asked to mentally list and imagine setting aside each of his or her problems, one at a time, until the imagined internal space is fully "cleared" and feels "safe." The client is encouraged to experience this cleared, safe space fully, and to use it when he/she begins to feel overwhelmed again. Resolution of this subtask involves the attainment and full appreciation of the imagined "safe space."

Second, focusing proper is also useful, especially at a "distanced" marker, which occurs when the client is experiencing emotional distancing within the session. Most commonly, the client will be speaking in an unemotional, externalizing manner, sometimes talking around in circles without getting to what is important to him or her or dwelling on details whose significance is not clear, in spite of the therapist's use of empathic and exploratory reflections. When this occurs, the therapist can suggest the use of experiential focusing, in which the therapist gently interrupts the client, as follows:

T1: I wonder, as you are talking, what are you experiencing?

C1: I'm not sure, I'm just going on [talking].

T2: Could you try something here? (*Client nods.*) Can you take a minute, maybe slow down, look inside yourself, where you feel things, and ask yourself, "What's going on with me right now?" And see what comes to you.

In focusing, resolution is indicated by the emergence of a clear and accurately labeled sense, accompanied by an experienced sense of easing or relief. Often, the clarified felt sense is a marker for another task.

5. *Systematic evocative unfolding* for self-understanding problems (see Greenberg et al., 1993) is the final experiential search task, used for posttrauma "flashbacks," in which the client suddenly and vividly reexperiences the victimization; and fear episodes ("anxiety attacks"), in which the client experiences strong, trauma-related fear. These episodes often trouble clients to such an extent that they bring them into the session to work on, providing the *problematic reaction point* marker, which indicates the client's readiness for the task.

The therapist then suggests the task to the client, asking the client to take him or her through the episode in which the reaction occurred, including what led up to it and exactly what it was that the client reacted to. The therapist helps the client alternately explore both what he or she noticed about the situation and his or her inner emotional reaction in the situation. Sometimes, with flashbacks, it can be useful to have the client enact the flashback situation in order to access subtle bodily cues. As with the other tasks, resolution is a matter of degree; at a minimum, resolution involves reaching an understanding of the reason for the flashback or fear episode. Unfolding tasks resemble retelling tasks in that both involve narratives, but unfoldings are driven by a need to understand how a specific recent puzzling reaction came about (they are like a personal mystery story), whereas retellings are driven by the need to share distress or to construct a general story that holds together and makes sense (they are like a history).

*Active expression tasks*, the next set of trauma-related process-experiential tasks, reflect the Gestalt and psychodrama heritage of process-experiential therapy. The client is asked to enact aspects of self or others in order to evoke and access underlying emotion schemes. Such tasks are particularly useful for helping the client to access disowned or externally attributed aspects of self, especially anger and sadness. The major active expression tasks have been extensively described elsewhere by Greenberg and colleagues (1993), so only adaptations for work with PTSD will be described here. Note that these active, evocative tasks generally require a stronger therapeutic alliance and thus are rarely attempted before session 3.

6. *Two-chair dialogues* for internal conflict splits are an important aspect of Process-experiential trauma work. Two kinds of conflict split occur often in PTSD: First, self-blame for one's victimization is a form of self-evaluation split (Greenberg et al., 1993) and is readily worked with as a conflict split between a blaming, critical aspect of self and a guilty or shame-

ridden aspect. Second, "anxiety splits" involve a vulnerable self facing a "coaching" or "catastrophizing" aspect of the self that dwells on fear-inducing situations. Anxiety split markers typically take the form of a description of some situation that "makes" the client afraid of revictimization, accompanied by some indication that the client recognizes his or her reaction as exaggerated or not wholly warranted. The coaching/catastrophizing aspect of self typically sees itself as trying to prevent future revictimization by continually scaring the other aspect of the self; unfortunately, the unintended consequence is making the self feel more weak and vulnerable.

The therapist initiates this task by suggesting that the client "be" the scary situation (e.g., the freeway) or the catastrophizing part of the self and "show how you scare _____ [client]." This gives the client the opportunity to identify with and reown the powerful, "frightener" part of the self; this reowning would constitute a partial resolution, while a full resolution would require some kind of mutual understanding and accommodation between the fearful and fear-inducing aspects of self.

7. *Two-chair enactments* for self-interruptions are relevant for addressing immediate within-session episodes of emotional avoidance or distancing. The underlying emotional processing split described earlier between reexperiencing and distancing aspects of self sometimes expresses itself in the form of a *self-interruption* marker, in which the client is experiencing or expressing painful experiences related to the victimization (e.g., anger, fear, terror, or disgust) but then suddenly becomes emotionally blocked, numb, or distanced.

Resolution of this task is facilitated by asking the client to enact the process of self-interruption. In a two-chair enactment, the therapist directs the client's attention to the blocked state, then suggests the experiment by asking him or her to "show how you stop _____ [client] from feeling [looking at] _____ [the victimization]." The intervention aims to help the client to bring the automatic avoiding aspect of self into awareness and under deliberate control; this in turn helps the client become aware of the previously interrupted emotion so that it can be expressed in an appropriate, adaptive manner. Minimal resolution involves expression of the interrupted emotion, with more complete resolution requiring expression of underlying needs and self-empowerment.

8. *Empty-chair work* for unfinished emotional business has been used extensively by therapists working with adults who were sexually abused as children (e.g., Briere, 1989). As noted earlier, a key element in almost all traumas is the perceived role of unhelpful and malevolent other(s) during and after the victimization incident. In interpersonal victimizations, there is a malevolent other who actively perpetrated violence or abuse against the person. There is some controversy about the therapeutic value of "putting the perpetrator in the empty chair" (Briere, 1989), and in any case the method appears to us to be less useful in single victimizations by strangers. On the

other hand, the victimization experience almost always involves significant others who are perceived by the person as having failed to provide adequate protection during and after the trauma.

The *unfinished business* marker has been described by Greenberg et al. (1993) and, briefly, consists of currently experienced, lingering bad feelings toward a developmentally significant other (e.g., a neglectful parent). In the presence of a strong therapeutic alliance, the therapist suggests that the client imagine the other in the empty chair and express any previously unexpressed feelings toward him or her. The therapist may also suggest that the client take the role of the other and speak to the self. Resolution consists, at a minimum, of expression of unmet needs to the other, with fuller resolutions requiring shifts toward more positive views of self and other.

We have two specific suggestions for using empty-chair work to work on traumatic experiences: First, it is generally best to begin empty-chair work with unhelpful or neglectful others, such as the nonabusing parent who ignored or allowed the abuse; direct work with a malevolent other or abuser may come later, but some clients never reach the point of being willing to do so (Rohn & Greenberg, 1994). Second, empty-chair work is highly evocative and emotionally arousing; if the client is already in a strong emotional state, he or she is likely to feel overwhelmed by even the suggestion to try speaking to the other in the empty chair. We agree with Clarke (1993) that when emotional arousal is high, it is generally better to use meaning creation, an experiential search task that helps the client to symbolize and contain painful emotion.

As may be apparent from our discussion about emotional arousal in empty-chair work, the therapist needs to be actively empathically attuned to the amount of emotional arousal that the client is experiencing at any given moment. We believe that experience can be optimally processed by the client if he or she has enough emotional arousal to be in contact with the experience but not so much as to be overwhelmed by it. This is referred to as "working distance" (Gendlin, 1981). Too much emotional distance and a person cannot make contact with his/her experience; too little distance and a person is overwhelmed by it.

*Interpersonal contact tasks* constitute the final set of process-experiential tasks we will discuss. These tasks return to the relational strands of the client-centered and Gestalt therapy traditions and include two kinds of genuine person-to-person contact between client and therapist, empathy and dialogue. Thus, a key aspect of resolution in these tasks is the establishment of the therapist as a helpful other; change emerges directly from the genuinely empathic and prizing therapeutic relationship.

9. *Empathic affirmation* with vulnerability is one of the most common tasks in working with traumatized clients, who struggle with powerful feelings of personal shame, unworthiness, vulnerability, despair, or hopelessness. In the course of facilitating other tasks, the therapist should be alert for the

emergence of any of these *vulnerability* markers, which are typically marked by the client's reluctant confession of a pervasive painful feeling of being "at the end of the road" (Greenberg et al., 1993).

In this situation, the client's need is to confront and admit to another person some intense, feared aspect of self that had been previously kept hidden. The therapist's task is to offer a nonintrusive empathic presence, accepting and prizing whatever the client is experiencing, and allowing the client to descend into his or her pain, despair, or humiliation as far as he or she cares to go. The therapist does not push for inner exploration and, indeed, does not try to "do" anything with the client's experience except understand and accept it. When the therapist follows and affirms the client's experience in this way, the client will express the vulnerability until he or she "hits bottom" and will then begin spontaneously to turn back toward hope. It is very important, but also very difficult, for the therapist to maintain the faith that the client's innate growth tendencies will enable him or her to come back up after "hitting bottom." Resolution consists of enhanced client self-acceptance and wholeness, together with decreased sense of isolation and increased self-direction.

10. *Relationship dialogue* for alliance difficulties and interpersonal problems between the client and therapist is relatively rare in brief process-experiential treatments for PTSD but is particularly important in longer-term work with clients who have extensive or severe histories of abuse or other forms of victimization. Such persons routinely perceive the therapist as just another unhelpful other. Furthermore, therapeutic errors, empathic failures, and mismatches between client expectations and treatment are inevitable in process-experiential therapy (as in all therapies!).

The *alliance difficulty* marker occurs when the client expresses some form of complaint or difficulty with the treatment, for example:

"I feel stuck, like I'm not progressing anymore, or maybe even going backwards."

"There you go, exaggerating again."

"I know you're not supposed to give advice, but I really think I need someone to tell me what to do about these fear attacks I keep having."

It is very important that therapists listen carefully for and respond to such alliance difficulty markers. The therapist begins by offering a solid empathic reflection of the potential difficulty, trying to capture it as accurately and directly as possible. The therapist suggests to the client that it is important to discuss the difficulty in order to understand what is going on, including what the therapist may be doing to bring about the problem. The difficulty is presented as a shared responsibility for the client and therapist to work on together. The therapist models and fosters this process by genuinely considering and disclosing his/her own possible role. In this way, the client is encouraged to examine his/her own part in the difficulty as well, and the client and therapist explore what is at stake for the client in the difficulty, as well as how it might be resolved between them. Resolution consists, at minimum, of the client and therapist together arriving at an understanding of the sources of the problem; full resolution entails genuine client satisfaction with the outcome of the dialogue, along with renewed enthusiasm for the therapy.

## RESEARCH IN PROGRESS ON PROCESS-EXPERIENTIAL THERAPY FOR PTSD

There is to date little or no research focusing specifically on the use of an experiential therapy with PTSD. Paivio and Greenberg (1995) reported on a study of the effects of a process-experiential therapy on unfinished business difficulties (emphasizing empty-chair work); a number of the clients involved had suffered physical, emotional, or sexual abuse, and some would be formally diagnosable with PTSD (Paivio, 1995). Paivio and Greenberg reported that clients in the process-experiential therapy obtained clinically significant pre–post change with substantial effect sizes. In addition, the process-experiential therapy was superior to a psychoeducational treatment condition.

Recently, with our colleagues at the University of Toledo, we carried out a pilot study comparing the process and outcome of process-experiential and cognitive-behavior therapy in short-term (16-session) treatment of crime-related PTSD (Elliott et al., 1996). Six clients (five female, one male) in the process-experiential condition completed treatment. Their results for the five main outcome measures are summarized in Table 11.3.

Because the sample is so small, no significance tests have as yet been conducted; however pre–post effect size values are given as estimates of how much the clients changed on average. Overall, these clients showed relatively minimal change at midtreatment: about a third of a standard deviation, when averaged across change measures. The amount of change increased, on average, to a little less than a standard deviation (.90) by posttreatment, which is a bit less than the mean pre–post value of 1.24 reported in the Greenberg, Elliott, and Lietaer (1994) meta-analysis of experiential therapy outcome research. It is also substantially smaller than the posttreatment value of 1.52 reported in the previous study of process-experiential therapy of depression in the same research program (Elliott et al., 1990). Larger amounts of change at posttreatment were obtained on the Keane PTSD Scale (effect size, *ES* = 1.28), the MCMI-A (*ES* = 1.09), and the SCL90-R GSI (*ES* = 1.04). Clients showed less change on the Impact of Events Scale (*ES* = .67) and on the Toronto Alexithymia Scale (.71), a theory-relevant measure that was used to evaluate changes in clients' ability to attend to and put their inner experi-

**TABLE 11.3. Early Outcome Data for Process-Experiential Therapy for PTSD**

| Measure | | Pretreatment | Midtreatment | Posttreatment | 6-Month follow-up |
|---|---|---|---|---|---|
| Impact of Event Scale | Mean | 26.7 | 23.4 | 16.8 | 14.8 |
| | (SD) | (14.7) | (14.7) | (10.5) | (10.5) |
| | Pre–post ES[a] | — | .22 | .67 | .81 |
| | n | 6 | 5 | 6 | 4 |
| Keane PTSD Scale | | 31.2 | 27.0 | 24.3 | 19.0 |
| | | (5.4) | (5.3) | (12.8) | (15.2) |
| | | — | .78 | 1.28 | 2.26 |
| | | 5 | 5 | 6 | 4 |
| MCMI-A | | 85.6 | 80.4 | 63.2 | 45.8 |
| | | (20.5) | (26.7) | (23.3) | (38.5) |
| | | — | .25 | 1.09 | 1.94 |
| | | 5 | 5 | 6 | 4 |
| SCL-90-R GSI | | 1.8 | 1.3 | 1.0 | 1.0 |
| | | (1.09) | (1.11) | (1.04) | (.97) |
| | | — | .46 | .73 | .73 |
| | | 6 | 5 | 6 | 4 |
| Toronto Alexithymia Scale total | | 2.81 | 2.77 | 2.31 | 2.52 |
| | | (.70) | (.71) | (.45) | (.42) |
| | | — | .06 | .71 | .41 |
| | | 4 | 5 | 5 | 4 |
| Mean change effect size | | — | .35 | .90 | 1.23 |

*Note.* MCMI-A, Millon Clinical Multiaxial Inventory, Anxiety Disorder Scale; SCL-90-R GSI, Symptom Checklist 90—Revised, Global Symptom Index.

[a]Pre–post ES (effect size) = $(M_{later} - M_{pre})/SD_{pre}$.

ence into words. It is worth noting that these effect sizes were obtained in spite of large variances on some of the measures (especially the Impact of Event Scale, MCMI-A, and SCL-90-R GSI), variances that were larger than those reported in previous studies or normative samples. It is possible that traumatized clients' responses to process-experiential treatment show greater variability than has been found in previous research. While we see these very tentative results as encouraging, more research and a larger sample are clearly needed.

## CONCLUSIONS

We have presented a process-experiential theory of PTSD, together with a complex, integrated therapy to address these difficulties. In particular, we focused on the relevance and particular application of a set of 10 therapeutic tasks in helping clients deal with their trauma-related difficulties. For more information, interested readers are encouraged to seek the sources referred to for each of the tasks, especially the more complete coverage of many of the tasks in Greenberg et al. (1993).

Consistent with our view of PTSD, process-experiential treatment of these difficulties emphasizes restoration of a helpful other in the form of the therapist, as the client seeks to regain a sense of self with adequate power to act in a "safe-enough" world.

On a closing note: In this chapter, we have tried to address differences between the difficulties that stem from single or "simple" traumas and those that derive from multiple or "complex" traumas. For these clients, recent traumas that bring the client to therapy are layered on top of earlier multiple or extensive traumas such as prolonged childhood sexual or physical abuse. Thus, the sense of self preceding the recent trauma was also fragile. Therapy with these clients is likely to be substantially longer than the 4–16 sessions typically needed for "simpler" traumas, and the new, empowered sense of self that begins to emerge from such work is likely to be an improvement over the older fragile or damaged self. Many clients with longstanding unresolved issues find themselves working directly for the first time on their traumatic experiences. As they do so, they begin to gain access to their internal experiences, clarity about self, empowerment, and self-direction. Moreover, they experience this not as a return to their former self, but rather as a novel and surprising development. We see the articulation and evaluation of therapeutic approaches for this population as an important next step for process-experiential therapy.

## ACKNOWLEDGMENTS

The research reported here was supported by grants from the University of Toledo Graduate School. We acknowledge the contributions of Leslie S. Greenberg and

Laura N. Rice, the main developers of the process-experiential approach; Frederick Wertz and Constance Fischer, for their analysis of the phenomenology of criminal victimization; the other members of the University of Toledo PTSD Project, including David Ensing, Julie Germann, Elisabeth James, Janie Manford, Chris McCullen, Laili Radpour-Markert, Robin Siegel-Hinson, Julie Reeker, Patsy Suter, Nicole Taylor, Missy Urman, and Sharon Young; and the clients involved.

## REFERENCES

American Psychiatric Association. (1994). *Diagnostic and statistical manual of mental disorders* (4th ed.). Washington, DC: Author.

Blake, D. D., Abueg, F. R., & Woodward, S. H. (1993). Treatment efficacy in post-traumatic stress disorder. In T. R. Giles (Ed.), *Handbook of effective psychotherapy* (pp. 195–226). New York: Plenum.

Briere, J. (1989). *Therapy for adults molested as children: Beyond survival.* New York: Springer-Verlag.

Clarke, K. M. (1989). Creation of meaning: An emotional processing task in psychotherapy. *Psychotherapy, 26,* 139–148.

Clarke, K. M. (1991). A performance model of the creation of meaning event. *Psychotherapy, 28,* 395–401.

Clarke, K. M. (1993). Creation of meaning in incest survivors. *Journal of Cognitive Psychotherapy, 7,* 195–203.

Egendorf, A. (1995). Hearing people through their pain. *Journal of Traumatic Stress, 8,* 5–28.

Elliott, R., Clark, C., Wexler, M., Kemeny, V., Brinkerhoff, J., & Mack, C. (1990). The impact of experiential therapy of depression: Initial results. In G. Lietaer, J. Rombauts, & R. Van Balen (Eds.), *Client-centered and experiential psychotherapy in the nineties* (pp. 549–577). Leuven, Belgium: Leuven University Press.

Elliott, R., Suter, P., Manford, J., Radpour-Markert, L., Siegel-Hinson, R., Layman, C., & Davis, K. (1996). A process-experiential approach to post–traumatic stress disorder. In R. Hutterer, G. Pawlowsky, P. F. Schmid, & R. Stipsits (Eds.), *Client-centered and experiential psychotherapy: A paradigm in motion* (pp. 235–254). Frankfurt am Main: Lang.

Fischer, C. T., & Wertz, F. J. (1979). Empirical phenomenological analyses of being criminally victimized. In A. Giorgi, R. Knowles, & D. L. Smith (Eds.), *Duquesne studies in phenomenological psychology* (Vol. 3, pp. 135–158). Pittsburgh: Duquesne University Press.

Gendlin, E. T. (1981). *Focusing* (2nd ed.). New York: Bantam.

Gendlin, G. T. (1996). *Focusing-oriented psychotherapy: A manual of the experiential method.* New York: Guilford Press.

Greenberg, L. S., Elliott, R., & Lietaer, G. (1994). Research on humanistic and experiential psychotherapies. In A. E. Bergin & S. L. Garfield (Eds.), *Handbook of psychotherapy and behavior change* (4th ed., pp. 509–539). New York: Wiley.

Greenberg, L. S., Rice, L. N., & Elliott, R. (1993). *Facilitating emotional change: The moment-by-moment process.* New York: Guilford Press.

Herman, J. L. (1992). Complex PTSD: A syndrome in survivors of prolonged and repeated trauma. *Journal of Traumatic Stress, 5,* 377–391.

Horowitz, M. J. (1986). *Stress response syndromes*. Northvale, NJ: Aronson.

Janoff-Bulman, R. (1992). *Shattered assumptions*. New York: Free Press.

Labott, S., Elliott, R., & Eason, P. (1992). "If you love someone, you don't hurt them": A comprehensive process analysis of a weeping event in psychotherapy. *Psychiatry*, *55*, 49–62.

Maslow, A. H. (1968). *Toward a psychology of being* (2nd ed.) New York: Van Nostrand Reinhold, 1968.

Paivio, S. C. (1995, December). *Difficulties in process-experiential therapy with sexually abused clients*. Presentation to Second Process-Experiential Therapy Workshop, York University, Toronto, Ontario, Canada.

Paivio, S. C., & Greenberg, L. S. (1995). Resolving "unfinished business": Efficacy of experiential therapy using empty chair dialogue. *Journal of Consulting and Clinical Psychology*, *63*, 419–425.

Rohn, R., & Greenberg, L. S. (1994, February). *Clients' perceptions of change in the resolution of unfinished business*. Paper presented at the annual meeting of the North American Society for Psychotherapy Research, Santa Fe, NM.

Sachse, R. (1992). Differential effects of processing proposals and content references on the explication process of clients with different starting conditions. *Psychotherapy Research*, *2*, 235–251.

Wertz, F. J. (1985). Methods and findings in the study of a complex life event: Being criminally victimized. In A. Giorgi (Ed.), *Phenomenology and psychological research*. Pittsburgh: Duquesne University Press.

Wigren, J. (1994). Narrative completion in the treatment of trauma. *Psychotherapy*, *31*, 415–423.

Yalom, I. D. (1980). *Existential psychotherapy*. New York: Basic Books.

Zajonc, R. B. (1980). Feeling and thinking: Preferences need no inferences. *American Psychologist*, *35*, 151–175.

Zlotnick, C., Zakriski, A. L., Shea, M. T., Costello, E., Bergin, A., Pearlstein, T., & Simpson, E. (1996). The long-term sequelae of sexual abuse: Support for a complex posttraumatic stress disorder. *Journal of Traumatic Stress*, *9*, 195–205.

# 12

\*\*\*\*\*

# Experiential Psychotherapy of the Anxiety Disorders

Barry E. Wolfe
Patti Sigl

*This chapter focuses* specifically on the anxiety disorders, a class of disorders that seem particularly likely to yield to the ministrations of an experiential psychotherapy. As we shall demonstrate, the anxiety disorders are characterized by a number of emotional processing difficulties that typically have been the focus of experiential psychotherapies. Moreover, we will also show that the cognitive-behavioral therapies that have shown such promising results with the various symptoms of specific anxiety disorders are also in fact ameliorating specific blockages in an individual's experiencing process.

The 13 specific anxiety disorders separately listed in the fourth edition of the *Diagnostic and Statistical Manual of Mental Disorders* (DSM-IV; American Psychiatric Association, 1994) are far too many to be adequately covered in the scope of this chapter. We will therefore limit our attention to four: panic disorder with agoraphobia, specific phobias, social phobias, and generalized anxiety disorder. The rationale for this selection is simply that the first author has had the most experience and success with experientially oriented therapies applied to these four anxiety disorders.

Our chapter begins with a consideration of the concept of experiencing and moves quickly to the more specific concept of "self-experiencing." We consider healthy and productive self-experiencing as a baseline for defining dysfunctional patterns of self-experiencing. We then will describe the specific forms of dysfunctional self-experiencing as they are expressed in the particular forms of anxiety disorders under consideration here. We will contrast this approach to defining an anxiety disorder with the descriptive, symptom-based approach that one finds in DSM-IV (American Psychiatric Association, 1994). Next, we illustrate how specific forms of dysfunctional self-experiencing may lead to a specific form of self-pathology. Case illustrations of patients suffering from panic disorder with agoraphobia, social phobia, and generalized anxiety disorder are presented. An experiential treatment model follows, one that addresses both the symptoms of a specific anxiety disorder as well as the specific forms of self-pathology and dysfunctional self-experiencing that underlie the anxiety disorder. Finally, the treatment model is be illustrated in the three aforementioned cases.

## THE CONCEPT OF EXPERIENCING

Increasingly, various authors have suggested that the process of experiencing and the facilitation of new experiences are common factors in all forms of psychotherapy (Arkowitz & Hanna, 1989; Bohart, 1993; Gendlin, 1979; Goldfried, 1980). This conclusion has been generally accepted even though definitions of experiencing have varied. Bohart (1993), for example, defines experiencing as a process of apprehending, one that is immediate, bodily, holistic, and contextual. Experiencing for Bohart is contrasted with cognition, which he views as an emotion-free process of information manipulation. By contrast, Greenberg, Rice, and Elliott (1993) define experiential processing as "an active, dialectically constructive process of creating emotional meaning" (p. 4). Experiencing and the creation of meaning involve a dialectic between reflexive or acquired conceptions and explanations of how things are or ought to be, on the one hand, and one's immediate experience of how things actually are, on the other. Both conceptualizing and immediate experiencing are included in their broader concept of experiencing.

Our view is closer to that of Greenberg et al. (1993). We view experiencing in the broader sense, which includes immediate felt experience and our reflexive awareness of our experience. Thus we conceive of a process that may involve immediate, felt experience, symbolization of that experience, and a reflexive awareness of our concepts of already symbolized experience. It is important to note, however, that what we experience is a function of where we focus our attention. We may focus our attention on the external environment, on our immediate felt experience, or, reflexively, on our awareness of our awareness, as it were. Again, we mostly agree with Greenberg et al. (1993) that the goal of such experiencing is the construction (or discovery) of personal, emotionally significant meanings. We maintain that different kinds of information are obtained depending upon where our attention is focused. Thus conscious experience results from the synthesizing of information from various sources, including (1) the perception of events in the external environment; (2) thoughts, images, and beliefs from memory; and (3) our immediate felt experience.

## THE EXPERIENCE OF SELF

Much of what we experience pertains to our "self." Therefore it is necessary to introduce the concept of self-experiencing. Self-experiencing refers to the continuous perception, evaluation, assimilation, or rejection of internally generated or externally imposed felt meanings relating to one's self. The experience of self (just like experiencing in general) is based on information from two different sources (i.e., two different ways of paying attention to the self), our immediate experience and our conceptualizations of self. These two different but interrelated forms of self-experiencing have been postulated by many writers since William James (1890). It was James who highlighted a dilemma in our efforts to understand the concept of the self. This difficulty is rooted in the fact that the self is both subject and object, both the knower and the known. These different ways in which one experiences the self involves, on the one hand, the experience of various senses of self, and, on the other, the experience of various beliefs that one holds about the self, that is, one's self-concept. As Stern (1985) has suggested, we experience directly many senses of self, including a sense of a single distinct integrated body, the agent of actions, experiencer of feelings, maker of intentions, designer of plans, translator of experience into language, and communicator and sharer of personal knowledge. At the same time, we have internalized many beliefs and images about the self, which, in the aggregate, make up our self-concept.

Rather than viewing the phenomenon of self as representing two different forms, our view is that the self as subject versus the self as object actually represent two different ways of paying attention to the self. The kind of information obtained about the self, whether it be one of the senses —or concepts—of self depends upon the way in which we focus our attention. Attention may be focused *sentiently* on the immediate, in-the-moment experience of our self acting and interacting in the physical and social world. When someone insults us we may immediately feel the pain of having our self presented in such a diminished light. Attention on the self may also be focused *reflexively*, which allows us to access the various beliefs that we hold about the self. For example, one may be attempting to teach a class but find oneself focused on the belief that one is a less than competent teacher.

While reflexive and sentient experiencing represent the two foci of self-attention, there is a third way in which attention can be focused. Human beings spend much of their time focused on the external world, that is, in *exterior* awareness. Experience obtained from exterior awareness ultimately, of course, has implications for the self, but such experience per se is virtually "selfless." Doing our taxes, engaging in a hobby, listening to a lecture, or collecting data for an experiment are all instances in which our attention is likely focused in exterior awareness.

# THE DYNAMICS OF SELF-EXPERIENCE

Self-knowledge is obtained through the dynamic interaction of the two ways of knowing the self—reflexively and through sentient experience. In the relatively undisturbed individual, there is an active oscillation between both sources of information about the self. Reflexive awareness allows us to consult the conceptualizations of our experiencing, whereas sentient awareness provides us with the "raw gold" of life experience that serves to either confirm or disconfirm our conceptualizations of self or lead to the development of new self-conceptions.

Other theorists have conceptualized the dynamics of self-experience in terms of a dialectical interaction between the acting and experiencing "I" and the observing and evaluating "me." Guidano (1991), for example, has argued that the "I" is always one step ahead of the current appraisal of the situation and the evaluating "me" becomes a continuous process of reordering and reconstructing one's conscious sense of self. Greenberg et al. (1993) postulate a similar dynamic between one's immediate experience of self and one's acquired conceptions of self: "Consciousness is thus the arena for the dialectical synthesis of the different sources of information about the self as the person encounters and resolves felt contradictions between aspects of the self, and between self and the world" (p. 60). It is clear that direct experience potentially can, but does not necessarily, impact on one's preexisting self-beliefs and that preexisting self-beliefs influence, constrain, and often distort the sentient experience of self.

# SELF-PATHOLOGY

In the most general sense, our theory suggests that self-pathology begins with an imbalance between the dual attentional foci of self-experiencing. Emotional difficulties arise whenever immediate self-experience is ignored or interrupted and one responds only to preconceived notions about the self. An example of this is the student who consistently earns "A's" in her/his courses but continues to think of her-/himself as not very bright. Emotional difficulties also arise, however, when one has no clear conceptualization(s) of the self. Patients suffering from borderline personality disorder often have no clear sense of self and therefore have difficulty creating meaning out of their experiences (American Psychiatric Association, 1994).

Most of the self-pathology associated with the anxiety disorders involves primarily only one of these extremes, namely, the interruption of immediate self-experience designed to protect a cherished self-belief from painful disconfirmation—that is, when the pathway from immediate self-experience to self representation is blocked or severed. There are three major sites of interruption: (1) preventing awareness of emerging thoughts, feelings, and motives; (2) inhibiting expressive action; and (3) interfering with awareness of the impact of one's actions on others and vice versa (Wolfe, 1992a). The principle underlying the defensive interruption of self-experience is that people try to regulate the experience of negative affect by reducing self-awareness. However, the price of these defensive interruptions is a shrinking of one's subjective perspective. Attention to internal or external events is often interrupted in order to avoid experiences of self-diminishment or, in the extreme case, trauma to one's self.

In addition to there being different *sites* of interruption, there are also different *ways* in which people interrupt their direct self-experience. In the course of attempting to cope with painful internal and external realities, individuals learn or develop a variety of ways of interrupting or deflecting their attentional focus. The entire catalogue of psychological defenses described by the psychoanalytic and Gestalt therapy traditions represent implicit and explicit strategies for interrupting one's subjective self-awareness. Thus, the psychoanalytic defenses such as repression, projection, denial, disavowal, and somatization (Horowitz, 1988), as well as defenses identified in the Gestalt therapy tradition such as clouding or dulling one's awareness and retroflected action and interaction (Smith, 1985), all have the same function: to help the individual avoid or deflect painful meanings and their accompanying feelings.

Such defensive processes automatically shift one's attention from sentient to reflexive self-experiencing. As we shall see, a cardinal characteristic of all anxiety disorders is the individual's inability to shift his/her attention out of reflexive awareness. These two processes, the defensive interruption of immediate self-experience and the relentless reflexive focus of attention, lead to the development—or maintenance—of specific forms of self-pathology. These include the following (see Wolfe, 1995, for details regarding the specific forms of self pathology):

- Dysfunctional content of specific self-beliefs
- Dysfunctional organization of information in the self-structure (which is construed here as the organization of self-relevant experience)
- Lack of ownership of self-experience
- Discrepancies between self-beliefs and self-standards
- Discrepancies between self-beliefs and immediate self-experience
- Attempts to escape a hated or disapproved-of self

## THE ANXIETY DISORDERS

Before presenting our model of the etiology of the anxiety disorders under consideration, we will present the criteria for classifying the anxiety disorders found in DSM-IV. These criteria, which are descriptive and symptom-based rather than etiologically based, are considered to be the standard for mental health professionals. This classification system is in clear contrast to the way in which anxiety disorders are diagnosed according to our perspective, not so much in terms of the symptoms that define the disorder, but rather in terms of what processes seem to be generating the symptoms in the first place.

## Panic Disorder with Agoraphobia

The essential feature of panic disorder is the presence of recurrent, unexpected panic attacks followed by at least 1 month of persistent concern about having another panic attack, or worry about the possible implications or consequences of the panic attacks. To identify panic attacks using DSM-IV diagnostic criteria, the individual suddenly develops a severe fear or discomfort that peaks within 10 minutes and is accompanied by 4 or more of 13 cognitive or somatic symptoms. These include the following: chest pain or other chest discomfort; chills or hot flashes; choking sensation; derealization or depersonalization; dizzy, lightheaded, faint, or unsteady feelings; fear of dying; fears of loss of control or becoming insane; heart pounding, racing, or skipping beats; nausea or other abdominal discomfort; numbness or tingling; sweating; shortness of breath or smothering sensation; and trembling.

## Social Phobia

The essential feature of social phobia is a persistent fear of situations in which the individual is exposed to the scrutiny of others, where he or she fears behaving in a way that will be embarrassing, shameful, or humiliating. For example, individuals with social phobia may fear that others will notice their hands or voice trembling when they are speaking or writing in public. Individuals with social phobia may be caught up in a vicious cycle of anticipatory anxiety of the feared social situation that leads to fearful cognition and anxiety symptoms when confronted with the situation. This becomes a self-fulfilling prophecy as it produces an actual or perceived poor performance in the feared situation, followed by embarrassment, and then generates increased anticipatory anxiety about the feared situation.

## Generalized Anxiety Disorder

Generalized anxiety disorder is characterized by anxious mood or worried preoccupations present on most days for at least 6 months. The anxiety tends to be low key and chronic, and the symptoms are relatively unfocused. The symptoms fall into three clusters: muscle tension (restlessness, shakiness, trembling, twitching, fidgeting, muscle aches, and easily fatigued); autonomic hyperactivity (rapid pulse, sweating, cold clammy hands, dry mouth, dizziness, digestive disturbances, frequent urination, hot or cold flashes, or a sensation of a lump in the throat); and vigilance and scanning (exaggerated startle response, difficulty concentrating, insomnia, irritability, and feeling on edge).

Some individuals are aware of and can state what makes them nervous, whereas others individuals cannot. The degree of impairment is usually not severe, and many individuals can experience these symptoms for years prior to seeing a therapist.

## Specific Phobias

Specific phobias involve intense anxiety when one is exposed to a specific phobic stimulus. The most common are phobias of animals, blood and injections, heights, travel by airplane, being closed in, and thunderstorms. Exposure to a phobic stimulus can produce generalized anxiety or a panic attack. This anxiety produces a persistent fear of the phobic stimulus, which is either avoided or tolerated only with intense anxiety. Generally, the closer an individual is to the feared stimulus and the more difficult it is to escape, the more anxious and panicky the person will feel. The focus of the fear may be anticipated harm from the feared object or situation, losing control, and panicking. People with a phobia involving blood or injections may fear fainting. They often experience a vasovagal response, which is characterized by an initial brief acceleration of the heart rate followed by a deceleration in the heart rate, and a drop in blood pressure resulting in the person actually fainting.

## SELF-PATHOLOGY AND THE ANXIETY DISORDERS

While we accept for the moment the DSM-IV classification of symptoms for the anxiety disorders, we feel that it is insufficient for us to understand where to intervene if we are in search of a comprehensive and durable treatment approach. Useful symptom-focused treatments have been developed based on the DSM-IV classification system, but the results of such treatments are insufficiently comprehensive and rarely durable even in the case of the symptoms. The underlying assumption of this perspective is that anxiety disorders have most to do with painful and dangerous self-experience, which in turn depends upon the underlying form(s) of self-pathology. There is observable in each of the anxiety disorders a chronic sense of self-endangerment. While different anxiety disorders reflect variations in the *contents* of threatening self-experience, they more importantly represent variations in the experiential *processes* employed to stave off the danger.

A common sequence can be described for the development of an anxiety disorder that reflects the importance of self-experiencing and its vicissitudes. This sequence typically begins with the impact of early traumatic experiences on the individual's capacity for *sentient* self-experiencing. Most of these early traumas occur in an interpersonal context and in each instance leave the individual feeling helpless, trapped, and unable to forestall what is perceived to be certain doom to one's experience of a subjective self (i.e., self-endangerment). Self-endangerment experiences appear to be confined to the psychological realm, to fears associated with separation, rejection, loss of a primary caretaker or loved one, intensely humiliating experiences, disillusioning experiences at the hands of primary caretakers or loved ones, and the experience of "self-loss" (i.e., the wholly subjective sense of the disappearance of self-experience entirely). Self-endangerment experiences can range from a painful self-awareness to extreme trauma. Trauma, however, is a relative term, referring to the amount of pain one experiences relative to one's ability to bear it. The same events may be processed quite differently by people with very different abilities to cope with or bear them.

The most fundamental impact, however, of self-endangerment experiences on sentient self-experiencing is that *dangerous self-experiences make sentient self-experiencing dangerous*. In other words, trauma makes it difficult for an individual to have in-the-moment experience of self. Therefore, anytime an individual finds him-/herself in a situation that resembles the context of a self-endangerment experience, he/she will experience anxiety. Anxiety serves as an alarm or signal that further sentient self-experiencing would be dangerous. But the individual interprets the anxiety to mean that a potentially catastrophic event is about to take place. This catastrophic interpretation, while incorrect, has a number of other important implications. The feared object, situation, or sensations relate to earlier traumas. Also, catastrophic interpretations indicate that the individual's attention has been shifted from direct experience of self and/or world to the reflexive experience of one's self being fearful.

Thus, a second phase of the anxiety disorder sequence involves the shift of the individual's attention from either sentient or exterior awareness to reflexive awareness. In reflexive awareness, the anxiety patient will inevitably experience dysphoric emotions and negative evaluations of their first-order anxiety. The result is a rapidly intensifying experience of anxiety.

A third phase in the anxiety disorder sequence is avoidance behavior. Very often, anxiety patients will associate the various contexts in which they experience anxiety or panic with the recurrence of anxiety and panic. Consequently, in an effort to control the anxiety, the individual will begin to avoid the contexts of prior self-endangerment experiences. Avoidance then increases the difficulty of reentering the feared situations. Thus the common anxiety disorder sequence can be summarized as follows: Self-endangerment experiences leads to compulsive, reflexive self·experiencing that increases the anxiety, which in turn leads to avoidance behavior in particular contexts as an attempt to control the recurrence or intensifying of anxiety.

## Reflexive Awareness in the Anxiety Disorders

Reflexive awareness is a frequently observed characteristic of any patient suffering from an anxiety disorder (Barlow, 1988; Borkovec, Metzger, & Pruzinsky, 1987; Ingram, 1990). This automatic shift of attention from sentient or exterior awareness to reflexive awareness can be observed across many different types of anxiety disorders. Ingram (1990) and Barlow (1988), among others, have referred to the phenomenon of "self-focused attention" as a cardinal characteristic of anxiety disorder patients, which is essentially identical to our concept of reflexive awareness. The anticipatory anxiety of a public speaking phobic, the worrying of a generalized anxiety disorder patient, and the painful public self-consciousness of a socially phobic individual are all examples of compulsive reflexive self-experiencing, as are the following fears associated with panic disorder:

- Fear of fear
- Fear of losing control
- Fear of being trapped
- Catastrophic interpretation of frightening bodily sensations

As the above examples illustrate, one of the characteristics that separates different anxiety disorders is the different ways in which individuals focus their attention reflexively.

From this theoretical vantage point, the bodily sensations that terrify a panic disorder patient are somatic traces of feelings associated with a past traumatic event. But these feelings cannot be articulated or reexperienced. Thus sentient self-experience is bypassed, and the patient reflexively focuses on him-/herself in danger. If the panic patient can stay focused on the sentient experience of these sensations, the tacit feelings will begin to emerge. In my own version of interoceptive exposure, attention is retrained to focus on the sentient experience of these frightening bodily sensations. This process seems to restart the emotional processing of painful or threatening feelings associated with either a past catastrophic experience or a particular form of self-pathology.

The various forms that reflexive self-experiencing take in the several anxiety disorders are easily observed and rich in their implications. The observation of reflexive experiencing and its close association with self-endangerment suggests that this process may be a key psychological marker of an anxiety disorder. The ubiquity of reflexive self-awareness in the anxiety disorders suggest the difficulties that anxiety patients have in directly experiencing their lives when they feel endangered. Moreover, it suggests the constraints that early trauma may place on the way in which an individual focuses his or her attention, and on the development and smooth functioning of the emotional processing cycle. Finally, it suggests that the restoration of sentient self-experiencing in the patient's feared situations may be a key treatment target for the resolution of an anxiety disorder.

## THE TREATMENT MODEL

The goals of the following experiential therapy model include the treatment of both the symptoms of specific anxiety disorders and the underlying issues of self-pathology. With respect to these underlying issues, the following goals are included:

- Altering specific self-representations and self-beliefs
- Enhancing self-efficacy or sense of agency
- Resolving discrepancies between self-beliefs and self-standards
- Increasing tolerance for—and ownership of—negative affects and perhaps affective experience in general
- Identifying and modifying defensive interruptions to organismic experience
- Increasing willingness to engage in authentic relationships (i.e., in which one allows oneself to be known and allows oneself to know the other)

In order to effectively treat both the symptoms of an anxiety disorder and the underlying issues of self-pathology, a four-stage treatment sequence has been delineated: (1) establishing the therapeutic alliance; (2) ameliorating the anxiety symptoms; (3) uncovering the deficiencies in self-experiencing; and (4) repairing the underlying forms of self-pathology (see Wolfe, 1989, 1992a, 1992b, 1995).

## Establishing the Therapeutic Alliance

One of the issues that tends to be deemphasized in the literature on the treatment of anxiety disorders is the importance of the therapy relationship for enabling and catalyzing all of the other specific treatments one might employ. Although the therapeutic alliance is critical to the success of treatment, it is often not all that easy to establish with patients suffering from an anxiety disorder. The reason for this is that anxiety disorder patients very often are quite distrustful of people in general and therapists in particular. This distrust highlights another deficiency of the anxiety disorder literature, and that is the close connection between anxiety symptoms and interpersonal problems.

The personal and interpersonal dynamics of "trusting" have their source in the close relationship between how one is treated and how one sees oneself (Guidano, 1991). If the actions and communications of others toward us suggest that we are not trustworthy, then the task of coming to trust ourselves is made all the more difficult. Repairing the patient's ability to trust another, therefore, contributes to their ability to trust themselves and vice versa. The source of distrust in both instances is often childhood interpersonal traumas inflicted by caretakers. The evolution of trust, therefore, is a difficult process for anxiety disorder patients and is usually the first issue negotiated in therapy, either as an explicit or implicit issue.

The first therapeutic task, then, is for therapists to establish their trustworthiness *and for patients to acknowledge to themselves this trustworthi-*

*ness.* To the extent that the therapist is being trustworthy, he or she is providing the patient with important information to be assimilated. But because of past disillusionments and resultant fears of disappointment, the patient may find it difficult to acknowledge the therapist's care and concern. Part of the alliance-building phase of therapy will include identifying the various ways in which the patient *defensively interrupts* his/her sentient experiencing of the therapist's trustworthiness. As these defenses are identified and found to be inapplicable in the *present* context, the patient may begin to experience sentiently the therapist's trustworthiness. The resurrection of sentient experiencing will begin to lead to a corrective emotional experience regarding the dependability of a significant other.

The sentient experiencing of the therapist's trustworthiness indirectly contributes to the rebuilding of the patient's sense of self-efficacy. With the therapist as an ally, the patient feels more confident of his/her ability to face the anxiety-inducing situations and to endure the automatically occurring anxiety.

## The Experiential Treatment of Anxiety Symptoms

Patients suffering from anxiety disorders require a sense of control over their symptoms before they can profit from any intensive therapeutic work repairing the deficiencies in their self-experiencing. Therefore, one must treat symptoms before self-pathology. A number of closely related exposure-based treatments have been developed from the cognitive-behavioral perspective that have been quite useful in the reduction and elimination of anxiety symptoms. In the case of panic disorder with agoraphobia, for example, a "panic-control treatment" has been developed by Barlow, Craske, Cerny, and Klosko (1989) that combines breathing retraining with interoceptive exposure and cognitive restructuring. A similar treatment has been developed for panic disorder at several centers around the world (Beck et al., 1992; Clark et al., 1990; Ost, 1991). This treatment has been reported to eliminate panic attacks in 80–90% patients completing treatment.

From an experiential point of view, the various components of panic control treatment have the effect of increasing a patient's ability to "allow" his/her direct, in-the-moment experience of the feared body sensations. Similarly, exposure therapy for specific phobias enhances the patient's ability to "allow" his/her sentient experience of the phobic object or situation. In fact, taken together, the various components of panic-control treatment seem to work synergistically in "interrupting" the various ways in which a panic patient defensively interrupts their sentient experience of the feared sensations and situations. With the clear goal in mind of restoring the sentient experience of the feared object, sensation, and situation, we employ a variety of exposure-based treatments to help a patient achieve a sense of control over the anxiety symptoms. For example, a driving phobic was treated by means of graduated exposure, which involved gradually increasing the distances he could drive a car. He soon learned that he could cope with the ensuing anxiety and later learned that the act of driving does not lead to catastrophic consequences.

## Uncovering the Deficiencies in Self-Experiencing and the Specific Forms of Self-Pathology

This phase of treatment usually begins with imaginal exposure to the feared object, situation, or sensations. In the case of phobias, the imaginal exposure is applied to the feared object or situation. In the case of panic patients, it involves a strict attentional focus (i.e., interoceptive exposure) on the bodily sites of fearful sensations. In both instances, the procedure begins the same way, with a breathing-induction exercise. This induction procedure helps the patient tune out competing stimuli from the external environment, allowing him/her to focus attention inwardly.

The patient is then invited to be receptive to his/her internal productions, that is, to any thoughts, feelings, images, or ideas that arise automatically. In the case of phobias, the patient is asked to imagine the feared object or situation and, while intensively focusing attention on the phobic scene, to notice any automatically arising feeling or thought. In the case of panic disorder, the patient is asked to identify the most prominent body sites of anxiety or fearful body sensations and to maintain a strict attentional focus on these sites. Typically, within one or two sessions, this procedure results in the appearance of several thematically related and emotionally laden images. The images are imbued with themes of conflict and catastrophe that the patient is helpless to prevent or terminate. The goals of this version of imaginal exposure depart somewhat from those of the more behavioral version. The experience of anxiety is not only for the purpose of learning that the feared disaster will not take place or that the anxiety will habituate but also for the patient to uncover the felt catastrophe and to experience the associated feelings.

## Ameliorating Specific Forms of Self-Pathology

For some patients, a symptom-focused treatment will be sufficient or all that they wish to undertake. For others, however, there is often a strong motivation to explore and resolve the underlying issues associated with an anxiety disorder. The final stage of this experiential treatment then is to identify and ameliorate the specific forms of self-pathology that underlie the patient's anxiety disorder. Imaginal focusing is typically employed to uncover the specific forms of self-pathology, and then a variety of experiential therapy techniques are employed to remedy the specific self-pathology. The empty-chair technique is, for example, quite useful in helping a patient express the heretofore inexpressible feelings to a loved one. The two-chair technique is useful in resolving splits between two different aspects of the self, as for example between one's actual self-experience and one's self-standards. Guided imagery techniques allow rapid contact with powerful emotions associated with tacit catastrophic themes. These are particularly useful with anxiety disorders for uncovering issues underlying the patient's fears. This technique is also useful in helping a patient to experience and reappraise disowned emotions. The experience of disowned emotions often has a profound effect on the patient's negative self-beliefs. For example, the experience of disavowed rage often can chip away at a patient's belief that he/she has no right to express a grievance toward a loved one. *All of these techniques are designed to restore sentient experiencing, but at the level of processing implicit or disavowed emotions.* To bring the treatment model more clearly into focus, let us consider three case illustrations: (1) panic disorder with agoraphobia; (2) social phobia, public speaking subtype; and (3) generalized anxiety disorder.

## CASE ILLUSTRATIONS

### Panic Disorder with Agoraphobia: The Case of Joan

Joan is a 30-year-old housewife with two young children. She developed the symptoms of panic disorder with agoraphobia 3 years before coming to see me. Joan had an unexpected panic attack while driving her children to an after-school activity and became so frightened that she had to pull the car off the road. Her husband had to come pick them up. As a result of this panic attack, Joan was unable to drive her car. Several interconnected fears inhibited her ability to get back into the car: fear of having another panic attack, fear of losing control and wrecking the car, and fear of seriously injuring herself or the children. She began to be very fearful of having additional panic attacks and clearly began to restrict her activities in an effort to control the venues in which she might have a panic attack. After some time, it became difficult for her to go into public restaurants that were too great a distance from home.

Joan had been married for almost 10 years to an attorney who was just beginning to become very successful. They had recently moved into their present affluent neighborhood from another suburb in the same metropolitan area. In her old neighborhood, she had made many friends and was very active in a variety of community services and volunteer activities. In her new neighborhood, she was having difficulty making friends and had not as yet become very active. The move represented a tangible sign of her husband's success, as the new house was much larger and much more expensive than their previous one. For her, the rise in socioeconomic level represented by the move meant a change in the kind of people that she would now encounter, people with whom she felt much less comfortable and, as the therapist posited, to whom she felt inferior. Joan clearly met DSM-IV criteria for panic disorder with agoraphobia, but there are many pieces of evidence that suggest that she also possessed some of the symptoms of social phobia. Traditionally, this diagnostic distinction has been difficult to make.

## Forms of Self-Pathology

Joan was weighted down by a number of negative self-beliefs that revolved around her diminished sense of self-efficacy and sense of inferiority. In addition, she was frightened by her emotional experiences, often not allowing herself to experience or "own" painful or rage-based emotions. Moreover, her behavior patterns frequently revealed a split between the "self" that she wished to present to the world and her actual self-beliefs. Often this involved wanting to present herself to the world as a nice, sweet person who harbors no angry or spiteful thoughts. She interrupted her immediate self-experience at all three junctures: (1) not allowing herself to experience pain or rage-based emotions; (2) allowing herself to experience these emotions but not to express them; and (3) sometimes expressing them but not allowing herself to take any action based on these emotions.

## Treatment

Joan began therapy quite reticently and was not eager to share any information that might lead me (BEW) to reject her or think her inferior. In fact, it took the first two sessions of therapy, characterized primarily by little else than empathic attunement responses from me, before she was ready to begin any kind of structured, symptom-focused program of anxiety management. However, I learned a great deal about the processes and content of her self-experiencing:

- She was in a constant state of self-monitoring and self-evaluation, what I have referred to as reflexive self-experiencing. She was very much trying to manage the impression that I should have of her.
- She appeared to have a number of grievances against her husband but would not allow herself to experience or express her apparent rage at him. She would refer often to how she saw herself as a nice person, and the few times she did get angry she would immediately say to herself that she "was not herself." In other words, there was a clear split between her "ought self" and her "actual self" (Strauman, 1994).
- She also referred several times to how she thought she was basically OK but was afraid that she would not be good enough for the people in her new neighborhood.

*An Experientially Based Treatment for the Symptoms of Panic Disorder.*  By session 3 Joan was ready to undertake the symptom-focused treatment. The rationale for beginning with the symptom-focused treatment involves two considerations: (1) she came into therapy in order to be freed of the panic attacks and her fear of them, so to begin here is to be responsive to what the patient wants; and (2) before she could undertake some of the other treatments designed to address her self-pathology, she would need a sense of control over the symptoms.

We began with diaphragmatic breathing, which apart from being an all-purpose anxiety reducer enables the individual to focus more easily on her/his sentient experience. Associated with the slow, deep, diaphragmatic breathing is the technique of awareness tracking that teaches an attentional focus on different locations on the body. A key element of this treatment is the acceptance of whatever the individual experiences, first at the level of bodily sensations and then at the level of affective experience. These techniques instruct the patient on how to remain with the experience of anxiety rather than automatically shifting to the reflexive mode of self-experiencing (e.g., fear of the fearful bodily sensations). The awareness tracking itself is a modification of the "interoceptive exposure" therapy employed by cognitive-behavioral therapists, which involves exposure to the frightening bodily sensations. In addition, "cognitive restructuring" is used in order to alter the patient's catastrophic thoughts regarding the frightening bodily sensations. This may include verbal prompts that the anxiety is not life threatening, that they have experienced these sensations before and have survived, and that they should recall a previous experience of these frightening sensations that they have successfully mastered.

*Diagnostic Interoceptive Exposure.* These techniques have proven to be quite useful for the reduction of panic and anxiety symptoms as well as giving the patient a sense of control. At this point, the patient will be invited to explore the underlying roots of his/her anxiety. If he/she chooses to undertake this exploration, we would begin with a strict attentional focus on the body locations of anxiety. In Joan's case, the chief location of her anxiety was a feeling of light-headedness that she found to be extremely frightening. Joan was instructed to maintain a rigid attentional focus on her head and just to notice what thoughts and feelings automatically arise. After a short period of time, the experience of light-headedness changed into an experience of intense rage directed at her husband. She was enraged by his decision to move the family without consulting her or obtaining her consent, and for his neglect of the family due to his professional ambition. The experience of rage, as mentioned before, was particularly frightening because it threatened her sense of herself as a "nice person." It became clear to her that the meaning of her initial, unexpected panic attack was that self-endangering rage was coming to the surface. What was particularly endangered was her self-concept of being a nice person, because it was axiomatic for her that "nice people" do not get angry.

*Resolving Specific Forms of Self-Pathology.* When it became clear to her that her panic attacks were rooted in the fear of rage, we spent an extensive period of time just having her experience and explore the rage to help her accept the fact that this was the way she really felt (i.e., the ownership of self-experience). We also had to work on her incorporating the experience of rage into her self-image as a "nice person" (i.e., expanding her self-concept to include the experience of rage). The next step was to employ the empty-chair technique so that she could express her rage to her husband. This would begin to complete the unfinished business that she experienced with respect to the move and to his neglect of the family. This also legitimated her ownership of the rage.

As she carried out the empty-chair work, she began to experience a "split" between viewing herself as a nice person and as a "rage-filled bitch who is never satisfied." To deal with this split, she began to carry out two-chair work between the actual self and the ought self (Strauman, 1994), that is, between the "nice woman" and the "angry bitch." Again, this dialogue helped her to transform her understanding of her own rage, to see it as based in legitimate grievances rather than as an expression of an unacceptable persona (i.e., an angry bitch).

In order to enhance her sense of self-efficacy, we carried out some guided imagery exercises that involved her focusing on a problem, making a decision about it, and carrying out the appropriate action to solve the problem without running to her husband for a solution. Finally, Joan did some empty-chair work, an imaginal encounter with three specific new neighbors in whose company she felt the most inferior. By expressing her feelings about how they had responded to her, she began a process of reducing the "felt gap" between her and these neighbors. At a subsequent real meeting with several of her neighbors, she noticed that she felt less inferior to even those neighbors who figured in her empty-chair work. By means of these experiential techniques, we were able to make significant progress in enhancing both her self-concept and her in-the-moment sense of self.

## Social Phobia: The Case of Glen

Glen is a 35-year-old college professor who presents with a moderately severe case of social phobia, which primarily involves speaking before large groups. Glen is afraid of revealing any signs of anxiety, including panicking. He construes the symptoms of anxiety in this context as incontrovertible proof of his incompetence. He is fearful of his voice cracking or tremors in his extremities. But he is most fearful of panicking. To panic in such a situation is extremely humiliating and feels to him like an annihilation of self. His major problem is anticipatory anxiety. If he can get into his talk, within a few minutes the anxiety subsides and he is able to perform. But there have been times when the anticipatory anxiety had been so great that he could not give his talk.

### Forms of Self-Pathology

I eventually learned that Glen has substantial doubts about his intellectual capacities, despite the fact that he has published often and that his work is valued by his colleagues. He often feels like an impostor whenever he is invited to give a talk. He believes he is intellectually inferior to all of his colleagues and that he has no right to speak at all, because his thoughts are so unintelligent or commonplace. Moreover, his fear of being found out as weak and incompetent is tied up with his views regarding his masculinity, so that deficiencies in his work possesses implications for his experience of gender identity (dysfunctional beliefs).

In addition, he is terrified that others may come to the same view of him, so he employs a number of different stratagems for presenting himself as intellectually superior. Thus his continual need to perform perfectly conflicts with his self-belief that he is far from perfect, and this conflict produces a wide gap between self-belief and self-presentation (actual self–ideal self split).

It was also noted that as his talk approaches, his attention automatically switches to reflexive self-experiencing during which he is so concerned about how he is seen by others that he cannot focus on the task at hand, which is to communicate the substance of his talk.

## Treatment

*Establishing the Therapeutic Alliance.* Because Glen was keenly aware that I (BEW) was an academic like him, he initially was very concerned about appearing intellectually inferior to me. Thus when I attempted to obtain information about his difficulties during our first session, he communicated in a very guarded fashion. His speech was loaded with polysyllabic words more often found in formal writing than in intimate conversation. When he saw that I was not going to engage in any form of intellectual competition with him, and when I disclosed the fact that I also had suffered from public speaking anxiety, our relationship began to gel. As he began to trust me, he began to talk in depth about his life-long struggle with the issue of intellectual inferiority. These feelings were exacerbated by his hypercritical father, who was also an academic,—indeed, one with an international reputation in his field. Glen always felt intimidated by his father's academic abilities and credentials.

*Experiential Therapy for the Symptoms of Public Speaking Phobia.* The symptom-focused treatment began in the same fashion as with Joan, with my teaching Glen diaphragmatic breathing. Secondly, using diaphragmatic breathing as an entrée, we did some awareness tracking and bodily focusing in order to heighten his awareness of bodily sensations. Thirdly, we did some attention retraining to help him move from reflexive self-awareness to direct self-experiencing. Attention retraining initially involves a mindfulness technique that trains an individual to notice but not honor reflexive thoughts and to maintain attention on the task at hand; the next step is behavioral rehearsal of the talk itself, first, as it normally happens and, then, with the individual—

in this case, Glen—keeping his attention on what it is he wants to communicate, that is, keeping his attention on the task at hand. These rehearsals allowed Glen to experience the contrast first hand between reflexive and sentient self-experiencing in the context of giving a talk. He was also enabled to use diaphragmatic breathing to reduce his anxiety.

*Exploring Issues of Self-Pathology.* As Glen began to achieve control over his anxiety symptoms, he expressed a desire to further explore the roots of the anxiety in the hope of resolving these issues. We began with imaginal probes of the felt meanings that automatically come up when he imagines himself giving a major address before a large audience. He began to allow himself to feel the humiliation that he has assiduously avoided as he imagines himself panicking during the address. This painful scene automatically shifted into memories of verbal abuse that Glen experienced at the hands of his father, when Glen's academic or intellectual performance was not up to his father's standards. Glen's father had no compunction about humiliating his son in front of his father's distinguished colleagues.

We segued into an empty-chair dialogue with his father regarding his verbal abuse of Glen. Glen eventually was able to express his rage at his father and began to question the perfectionistic intellectual demands that his father seemed to have placed on him. During another imagery probe, Glen was able to experience clearly the gap between his self-presentation and his self-belief. He typically presents himself as one of the foremost authorities in his field, simultaneously feeling like an impostor. To deal with this dichotomy, a two-chair dialogue was employed to help him experience both sides of the gap. After several of these dialogues, Glen was able to close the gap between self-presentation and immediate self-experience. He began to let go of the need to be the perfect academic, while allowing himself to experience whatever feelings came up in the moment as he gave a talk. He began to view himself as a competent academic but not necessarily the best in his field, whatever that means. The pressure to present himself as a superior intellect collapsed of its own weight—and with it the anxiety around public speaking.

## Generalized Anxiety Disorder: The Case of Don

Don is a 25-year-old single man who presents with more or less constant feelings of anxiety, restlessness, and muscular tension. He has insomnia periodically and lapses into irritability and depressed mood states from time to time. He has difficulty extricating himself from a state of constant worrying. Much of his worry is focused on relationships. He is obsessively concerned with what others think of him, and he experiences extreme pain if he learns that someone, anyone, dislikes him, or is critical of him. It is as if he has a constant monitor watching how he is coming across, lest he offend someone. If he receives any indication that he is being criticized, he criticizes himself harshly, resulting in extremely painful depressive affect. Yet, at the same time he becomes frightened if people try and get too close to him. He realizes that he is frightened of his feelings but becomes very angry with himself because of this characteristic. However, he finds it difficult to experience anger toward anyone else.

### Forms of Self-Pathology

- An exploration of his characteristic interpersonal behavior patterns indicates that he harbors a number of self-beliefs that suggest to him that he is inferior to others (*dysfunctional self-beliefs*).
- He finds it difficult to tune into his immediate self-experience, particularly feelings that deviate from the way he feels he either ought to be or wishes to be (*disallowing experience*).
- When he is able to tune into his direct experience, it often conflicts with the way he thinks he is supposed to feel (*actual self–ideal or ought self split*).
- Often, during our sessions, he would reveal indications that he was angry with me or others but would not "own" these feelings.

### Treatment

*Establish the Therapeutic Alliance.* The initial part of the therapy with Don was quite challenging because of his extreme need for approval and severe level of distrust. It was as if he were geared for rejection and consequently monitored himself very carefully lest he reveal some reaction that would lead to my (BEW) rejecting him. He seemed to desire unconditional positive regard but did not believe it even when I offered it. But a steady diet of empathic attunement allowed Don to begin to confide in me the extent of his difficulties. He began to share the history of several relationships, including those with his parents and with two girlfriends. A common theme emerged regarding his exquisite sensitivity to rejection. But before we became too deeply involved in these issues, we began the symptom-focused treatment.

*Treating the Symptoms of Generalized Anxiety Disorder.* We began by giving Don some control over his anxiety symptoms. I taught him diaphragmatic breathing and progressive relaxation. In addition, he learned awareness tracking and body focusing. These techniques not only gave him ways to cope with, reduce, or eliminate his anxiety symptoms, they also made it possible for him to increase his tolerance of affective experience in general.

*Resolving the Underlying Self-Pathology.* We began this portion of his therapy with imaginal probes designed to identify self-representations and self-with-other representations—in other words, his dysfunctional self-beliefs. We learned from these probes the extent of his feelings of inferiority, and the specific contexts in which these feelings and self-images arose. One of the interesting themes that emerged from this work was the absence of an attentional focus on his own reactions to other people. Instead, he focused only on others' reactions to him and his *anticipations* of others' reaction to him. Consequently, the next focus of treatment involved guided imagery exercises to help Don focus on his immediate self-experience of his reactions to the people with whom he interacted. This would involve his imagining specific relationship vignettes in which he would act out, first, as he habitually does and, secondly, with his attentional focus shifted significantly toward his own reactions to others rather than others' reactions to him. These vignettes would put him into contact frequently with feelings of rage and disappointment with people who were extremely important to him. In this way, he began to allow certain emotional experiences that he had forbidden to himself before. Moreover, this allowed him to tap into another source of information regarding his relationships, namely, his own reactions to others.

When he could allow such experiences, he became aware of the gap between how he thought he ought to be, feel, and act and the ways in which he really existed, felt, and acted. These discrepancies between self-beliefs and self-standards were addressed by means of a two-chair dialogue between his ought self and his actual self. For example, a two-chair dialogue was conducted between his "super nice" self and the self that was filled with anger, rage, and disappointment. Through this dialogue, Don was able to incorporate some of these "risky" affective experiences into his concept of self without his losing the belief that he was a decent and acceptable human being.

Another issue that became patently obvious in our work together was his belief in his powerlessness in relationships. In truth, his behavior had a tremendous impact on others, but indications from others that this was so were ignored by Don (i.e., defensively interrupted) and he continued to believe in his powerlessness. To address this issue, we did some reparative guided imagery in order to enhance his sense of self-efficacy in relationships. He would imagine interactions with particular individuals with whom he felt particularly powerless. He would focus first on his behavior, then on the individual's reactions, which clearly indicated the impact Don was having, and Don would attempt to absorb the felt meaning of his power in this relationship. This was quite difficult for Don to do because of his firm belief in his powerlessness. We did this exercise with several people who were important in his life. Don was able to make some progress in this area, but he has much work left to do on this issue.

Finally, we focused on the growing realization that he was often angry at me and unable to express it. I had him do this first in imagery and then directly. After several imaginal rehearsals, he was able to look at me directly and express at least some anger that he was feeling toward me. These experiences would echo the great fear he has always possessed regarding the expression of anger toward his parents, which inevitably would bring on feelings of guilt and fears of rejection.

## SPECIAL PROBLEMS IN THE APPLICATION
## OF EXPERIENTIAL THERAPY
## WITH ANXIETY DISORDER PATIENTS

As effective as experiential therapy can be for these anxiety disorders, it is not for everyone. Typically, the more interpersonal difficulties an anxiety disorder patient has, the less successful an experiential therapy of this nature is likely to be. As suggested before, the critical issue that will determine what a therapist can and cannot do is the level of trust the patient can develop. Some patients find it so difficult to trust anyone, but particularly a "doctor," that they cannot carry out the prescribed treatments or find ways to undermine them. One patient, for example, misinterpreted the difficulties associated with exposure therapy as a form of punishment and refused to comply. Another, when told that he needed to confront the phobic object, accused the therapist of not understanding that he was terrified of the phobic object. He thought the therapist was not listening to him. One patient rejected any emotion-based therapeutic approach by proclaiming, "I am not comfortable with the language of feelings." The more imaginative experiential techniques such as the empty-chair and two-chair techniques struck a number of patients as silly and embarrassing, and they refused to try them despite a number of entreaties by the therapist.

A second major difficulty involved in working with anxiety disorder patients is the intensity of their defenses against sentient experiencing. Some panic disorder patients, for example, have great difficulty in changing their catastrophic thinking, particularly with respect to frightening bodily sensations. The recurrence of a particular body sensation has been so frequently construed as a sign of a life-threatening illness that it becomes difficult to convince such a patient of its absence regardless of how favorable are the reports from frequent physical examinations. Such patients are so convinced that the occurrence of the frightening sensation signals the onset of a major illness that it is next to impossible to have them keep a strict attentional focus on the experience of this sensation. They require a much more graduated approach to contacting their sentient experience. This would entail initally brief periods of focusing work. Once they can tolerate this small amount of focusing on the frightening sensation, they are then instructed to increase the length of focusing time until they can contact the affective experiences that underlie the fearful body sensations.

## SUMMARY

We have presented a model of the development, maintenance, and amelioration of selected anxiety disorders that takes the patient's process of experiencing as the primary locus of disturbance and intervention. We have suggested that these disorders reflect difficulties in the patient's experiencing and processing of immediate, in-the-moment (i.e., sentient) self-relevant informa-tion. We have suggested further that these difficulties are rooted in a chronic sense of self-endangerment, which in turn reflect two dysfunctional processes of self-experiencing and a number of specific forms of self-pathology. We have also suggested that these specific forms of self-pathology are related to frequent or intense traumatic interpersonal experiences that occurred ear-lier in life and typically involved the patient's primary caretakers. But there are probably other sources of self-pathology as well.

We have also presented an experiential treatment model that attempts to remedy first the symptoms of an anxiety disorder and then, only later (and at the expressed wish of the patient), the underlying forms of self-pathology. The symptomatic treatment employs a number of techniques adapted from the cognitive-behavioral tradition that attempt to increase or enhance the patient's sentient experiencing of the situations and objects that co-occur with the patient's anxiety symptoms. Such techniques as diaphragmatic breath-ing, interoceptive exposure, and cognitive restructuring are designed to help a patient gain control over his/her symptoms through what is essentially a process of restoring sentient self-experiencing. In addition, several experien-tial techniques were employed to address specific forms of self-pathology. We illustrated by case examples that specific experiential techniques can address specific forms of self-pathology, which in turn were shown to be associated with specific anxiety disorders. While a standardized form of this treatment approach has not yet been tested empirically, it has shown prom-ise of resolving the underlying self-pathology as well as producing a durable elimination of the symptoms of anxiety disorders.

## REFERENCES

American Psychiatric Association. (1994). *Diagnostic and statistical manual of mental disorders* (4th ed.). Washington, DC: Author.

Arkowitz, H., & Hanna, M. T. (1989). Cognitive, behavioral, and psychodynamic therapies: Converging or diverging pathways to change? In A. Freeman, K. Simon, L. Beutler, & H. Arkowitz (Eds.), *Comprehensive handbook of cog-nitive therapy* (pp. 144–167). New York: Plenum.

Barlow, D. H. (1988). *Anxiety and its disorders.* New York: Guilford Press.

Barlow, D. H., Craske, M. G., Cerny, J., & Klosko, J. S. (1989). Behavioral treat-ment of panic disorder. *Behavior Therapy, 20,* 261–282.

Beck, A. T., Sokol, L., Clark, D. A., et al. (1992). Focused cognitive therapy of panic disorder: A crossover design and one year follow-up. *American Journal of Psychiatry, 147,* 778–783.

Bohart, A. C. (1993). Experiencing: The basis of psychotherapy. *Journal of Psy-chotherapy Integration, 3,* 51–67.

Borkovec, T. D., Metzger, R. L., & Pruzinsky, T. (1987). Anxiety, worry and the self. In L. M. Hartman & K. R. Blamkstein (Eds.). *Advances in the study of communication and effect: Vol. II. Perception of self in emotional disorder and psychotherapy* (pp. 219–260). New York: Plenum.

Clark, D. M., Gelder, M. G., & Salkovskis, P. M. (1990, May 15). *Cognitive therapy for panic: Comparative efficacy.* Paper presented at the annual meeting of the American Psychiatric Association, New York.

Foa, E. B. (1979). Failure in treating obsessive–compulsives. *Behaviour Research and Therapy, 17,* 169–176.

Gendlin, E. T. (1979). Experiential psychotherapy. In R. J. Corsini (Ed.), *Current psychotherapies* (2nd ed., pp. 340–373). Itasca, IL: Peacock.

Goldfried, M. R. (1980). Toward the delineation of therapeutic change principles. *American Psychologist, 35,* 991–999.

Greenberg, L. S., Rice, L. N., & Elliott, R. (1993). *Facilitating emotional change: The moment-by-moment process.* New York: Guilford Press.

Guidano, V. F. (1991). *The self in process.* New York: Guilford Press.

Horowitz, M. J. (1988). *Introduction to psychodynamics: A synthesis.* New York: Basic Books.

Ingram, R. E. (1990). Self-focused attention in clinical disorders: Review and a conceptual model. *Psychological Bulletin, 107,* 156–176.

James, W. (1890). *Principles of psychology.* New York: Holt.

Ost, L. G. (1991, September). *Cognitive therapy versus applied relaxation in the treatment of panic disorder.* Paper presented at the European Association of Behavior Therapy meeting, Oslo, Norway.

Smith, E. W. L. (1985). *The body in psychotherapy.* Jefferson, NC: McFarland.

Stern, D. N. (1985). *The interpersonal world of the infant.* New York: Basic Books.

Strauman, T. J. (1994). Self-representations and the nature of cognitive change in psychotherapy. *Journal of Psychotherapy Integration, 4,* 291–316.

Wolfe, B. E. (1989). Phobias, panic and psychotherapy integration. *Journal of Integrative and Eclectic Psychotherapy, 8,* 264–276.

Wolfe, B. E. (1992a). Self-experiencing and the integrative treatment of the anxiety disorders. *Journal of Psychotherapy Integration, 2,* 29–43.

Wolfe, B. E. (1992b). Integrative psychotherapy of the anxiety disorders. In J. C. Norcross & M. R. Goldfried (Eds.), *Handbook of psychotherapy integration* (pp. 373–401). New York: Basic Books.

Wolfe, B. E. (1995). Self-pathology and psychotherapy integration. *Journal of Psychotherapy Integration, 5,* 293–312.

# 13

\*\*\*\*\*

# Goal-Oriented Client-Centered Psychotherapy of Psychosomatic Disorders

## Rainer Sachse

*This chapter serves* to elucidate a specific client-centered psychotherapy (CCT) approach for those persons who suffer from so-called psychosomatic disorders. This therapy, called goal-oriented client-centered (psycho)therapy (GCCT), has proved to be very successful. It enables psychotherapy to be applied to clients who in the past were considered "very difficult" or hardly capable of being treated (Sachse, 1994b, 1995a, 1995b).

To clarify what this therapy is about, three aspects are dealt with in more detail after a brief introductory section: (1) the underlying theory of disturbances; (2) the specific form of GCCT applied; and (3) illustration of therapeutic principles by way of transcripts.

## DEVELOPMENT OF A DISTURBANCE THEORY

For a well-aimed formulation of therapeutic strategies and interventions it is necessary to develop a psychologically founded theory of disturbances that is capable of mediating between the disorder and the therapy. Such a disturbance theory must verify the therapeutic goals that are considered reasonable for a given disorder, must reveal the central therapeutic starting points, and must provide information about the type of therapeutic that is suitable to reach the desired goal.

When dealing with psychosomatic disorders—in our case with psychosomatic gastrointestinal tract disturbances (PGTD): ulcerative colitis, Crohn's disease (or regional ileitis), and duodenal ulcers—up to now there has been no disturbance theory that could be used to mediate between the disorder, on the one hand, and the CCT approach, on the other. For that reason, the prime intention of our current research efforts is to develop the essentials of a psychological disturbance theory as a basis for a CCT of psychosomatic disorders.

The starting points for developing the present disturbance theory stem from observations and examinations of the therapy process itself:

1. Observations and examinations have confirmed that clients diagnosed as being afflicted with psychosomatic ailments showed a very low degree of self-exploration in the therapy process (not only in CCT but in psychoanalytic therapy as well). They almost exclusively describe external facts and do not pay attention to self-aspects or even their own feelings, and a search for new associations in themselves does not take place (Atrops & Sachse, 1994; Ahrens & Mergenthaler, 1982; Tress, 1979). Such clients also show a very low degree of readiness to struggle with their internal problems (Sachse, 1994a, 1995a; Sachse & Atrops, 1991; Sachse & Rudolph, 1992a, 1992b). Psychosomatic clients often avoid any clarification—or explication—as to what extent they themselves contribute to their problems. These clients show almost no response to relevant interventions made by therapists (Sachse, 1990).

2. A second starting point was research work on the so-called alexithymia concept, which assumes that psychosomatic clients show or experience little emotion. They do not engage in introspection and seem to systematically avoid grappling with their feelings (see Ahrens, 1983, 1985).

3. Linguistic investigations of psychotherapy transcripts from psychosomatic clients show that these persons furnish a lot of redundant information. They give situational descriptions in a stereotyped manner and hardly deal with themselves at all.

These findings obtained by different methods (ratings, text analyses, questionnaires) in a variety of settings can be summarized as follows: *Clients suffering from psychosomatic disturbances systematically avoid coping and being confronted with negative self-aspects* (Sachse, 1995a).

We have systematically looked into this aspect of the condition and have asked ourselves what this finding would mean if it is understood as being not a peripheral but a central aspect of the disorder; if it is viewed not as a "symptom" of the disorder but as a central processing aspect; and if it is assumed that this not only takes place in therapies but is a consistent processing feature. If this is so, the following questions may be posed: How does this tendency to avoid dealing with self-aspects emerge? What are the consequences of such a tendency? To be able to answer these questions we evaluated several psychological theories that were likely to produce relevant information to this effect. Based on these theories a psychological function model of psychosomatic disturbances was formulated, as considered in the next section.

## A PSYCHOLOGICAL FUNCTION MODEL
## OF PSYCHOSOMATIC DISTURBANCES: THE THEORY
## OF THE DISTURBANCE OF SELF-REGULATION

### The Avoidance of Reflection

The first essential question is the following: What causes a systematic tendency to avoid grappling with relevant problematic self-aspects to develop? A theoretical answer to this can be derived from the theory of objective self-awareness (Duval & Wicklund, 1972; Buss, 1980; Carver & Scheier, 1981, 1985a, 1985b, 1987; Frey, Wicklund, & Scheier, 1984; also see Sachse, 1995a). According to theory such a systematic avoidance may emerge if the following prerequisites are fulfilled:

- There is a distinct discrepancy between what is desired and what is actually achieved in certain domains. For example, someone may have high professional ambitions but in fact may be far from reaching these specific goals.
- A person assesses his/her competence negatively. He/she has doubts as to whether he/she is capable of eliminating the above discrepancy, whether he/she can reach his/her objectives with reasonable efforts.
- A person is constantly confronted with these targets, the discrepancy, lack of competence, etc.
- The desired goals are of vital importance to this person. This may be the case, for instance, if "identity targets" are involved (Gollwitzer, 1986, 1987a, 1987b; Gollwitzer & Wicklund, 1985), that is, targets serving to define a person's identity.

In this case the person will be unable to give up or even to seriously question his/her objectives.

For such a situation the theory of objective self-awareness predicts a constant attitude of avoidance (Carver, 1979; Carver, Blaney, & Scheier, 1979): The person will uphold his/her goals and objectives as well as the pursuance of these goals, but avoids systematically any reflection upon objectives, the desire/fact discrepancy, or insufficient competence. Such reflection would be highly aversive and is therefore circumvented. However, as the person is again and again confronted with these relevant aspects (as he/she is still attempting to pursue his/her goals!) the avoidance process must constantly be reinitiated: He/she is unable to fundamentally solve the problem, cannot really evade it, but only succeeds in "escaping" from acute internal conflicts so that finally reflection processes are systematically avoided (see Merz, 1984).

The avoidance of reflection primarily causes one's own attentiveness to be "withdrawn" from problematic or potentially problematic self-aspects. This can be accomplished quite effectively by changing over from an internal to an external perspective: The person no longer regards his/her own feelings, thoughts, actions, etc., but instead focuses on external situations, the behavior of other people, and the like. The avoidance of reflection thus leads to the *observation perspective becoming externalized.*

Assuming an internal perspective is, however, essential for reflection and representation of relevant self-aspects (Sachse, 1992a, 1992b). Therefore, a restriction of private self-awareness leads to an inadequate representation of one's motives, goals, and the like (Kuhl, 1994a, 1994b; Kuhl & Beckmann, 1994; Kuhl & Eisenbeisser, 1986). An insufficient internal perspective, furthermore, impedes the *current* accessibility of the motive system. The person avoids updating, focalizing, and representing his/her relevant goals, motives, values, etc. because any self-awareness of such personally problematic schemata would almost *force* him/her to deal with his/her imperfections.

## Accessibility of the Motive System and Alienation

Thus, a direct consequence of reflection avoidance is alienation (Kuhl, 1994a; Kuhl & Beckmann, 1994), a state of estrangement from one's own motive system. The person is uncertain as to what he/she actually wants, what is important to him/her. He/she regards "borrowed" goals as his/her own motives and is no longer capable of verifying the appropriateness of goals (Kuhl, 1994a, 1994b; Kuhl & Beckmann, 1994). Affective processing is reduced, since evaluation processes as well as the activation of affective schemata are impaired due to an inadequate access to motives (Sachse, 1992a, 1992b, 1995a). These effects will then bring up the typical "alexithymic" behavioral patterns (Sachse, 1991, 1993).

Such a motivational "alienation effect" has a strong influence on decision making and verifying whether certain alternatives are compatible with one's own motive system. If there is no current access to one's own motive system and no reasonable representation, it can no longer be determined whether one's *own* intentions have initiated a given action. One's decision-making basis (i.e., the motivational foundation on which the selection of an action has been based) can thus neither be retrieved from memory (since there is no "entry" for this) nor is it possible to actually reconstruct the decision making basis ("Why did I choose X?") via one's own motive system (Kuhl, 1983a, 1983b). Even the selection of a given action may, to some extent, be governed by chance; that is, even when this selection is made, inadequate consideration is given to one's own motive system. In this case *there is no difference* at all, post hoc, between self-initiated and externally initiated actions. Action control is impeded.

# Reflection Avoidance Impairs the Establishment of One's Own Identity

Insufficient access to one's own goals and insufficient representation also impair one's *personal identity*: If I do not know what I want, what is important to me, I do not know anything about myself that defines me. I also start to doubt my own competences and capabilities. These reduce my self-definition, lead to self-insecurity (who am I, what governs me?), erode my self-confidence, and in this manner impede my self-worth and self-acceptance.

A significant feature of a self-concept or self-schema (see Markus, 1977) is the organized representation of self-aspects. Experience gained "from oneself," what one does, what one is capable of doing, etc., is compressed into a schema representing one's own person, the "self." If a person resorts to a systematic avoidance of reflections, as outlined above, he/she in fact systematically does *not* deal with certain self-aspects: All self-aspects that are (or may be) problematic are included in the avoidance process, are faded out of attentiveness and thus also excluded from representation. As a result of this, an incomplete, fragmentary self-concept develops a deficient representation of one's self.

## Reflection Avoidance Impairs the Sense of Self-Worth

The access to one's motive system also impacts the functioning of a *self-reinforcement system*. Self-reinforcement, the feeling of pride if something important has been accomplished, the feeling of competence, are indispensable for the development of self-worth (see Heckhausen, 1969, 1977, 1980; Meyer, 1972, 1973). However, these effects are only achievable if one has access to one's goals and motives. The feeling of pride, the experiencing of competence, the feeling of having accomplished an objective completely on one's own resources necessitates that one's own actions be adapted to one's own motive system.

*Building a well-functioning self-assertion system and thus developing self-worth depend on the degree to which a person has accessibility to his/her own motive system.* It thus follows that persons who have little access to their own motive system will not be able to develop a satisfactory self-reinforcement system.

## Lack of Self-Worth Strengthens Avoidance

Insufficient self-worth and a low degree of self-acceptance will lead a person to view his/her competence as being inadequate and maintain it at this low level. This will contribute to upholding the system itself because a low competence assessment promotes the tendency toward reflection avoidance and the like. In this case the system shows a *significant self-devaluation loop: It stabilizes itself.*

## Social Uncertainty and Anxiety

The factors hitherto described often entails uncertainty about how to act. The pursuance of one's goals even *against* the will of other people, the fighting out of social conflicts, etc. initially requires knowledge of what one wishes to do. To be able to pursue and defend one's own interests, one must first determine what one's interests are. For this purpose one must have access to one's own motive system, which also needs to be represented. Without access and representation the pursuit of goals and the development of social competence is hardly feasible. *Reflection avoidance* in conjunction with insufficient *representation* should therefore promote anxiety and uncertainty about how to act.

## External Orientation

Insufficient representation of one's motives as well as lack of access to one's motive system promote a norm orientation (Snyder, 1974, 1979; Kuhl, 1983b): People who cannot rely on their own norms of behavior, who cannot by themselves determine what they want to do, must necessarily be guided by external norms, by the expectations of others, or by social standards. In this way, these people become highly *externally oriented*. They are no longer guided by their own intentions (their "organismic valuing tendency" in the sense of Rogers, 1959) but focus on and adapt themselves to the demands of others.

This external orientation is strongly backed by feelings of social uncertainty and anxiety, as mentioned above. So one's inclination increases to direct one's attention to issues of whether one "is doing things right," "does not give offense to anybody," "is liked by people," and so on. This leads to the loss of social control; since one is unable to strive for things one needs against the opposition of others for fear of losing their approbation and is unable to resolve conflicts or fight for one's goals (which ones are right?), one feels controlled and at the mercy of others. The result is the feeling of being a "pawn"—a pawn on a chessboard being pushed around by others and having almost no control of one's life.

## Inability to Say No: Stresses from Social Demands That Cannot Be Curbed

Everybody is confronted at times with the need to respond to certain demands. A person must react to various situations, adapt to social settings, and the like.

A demand in itself need not be stressful. A person may decide to accept it or not. People are thus in a position to examine demands to determine whether they should be accepted and obligations taken on or whether they should be rejected.

Examining obligations can act as a method of stress regulation: If a person is already under great stress, one step toward stress regulation might certainly be to *reject* taking on further stressful commitments.

Self-obligation may, however, become even stronger due to a number of variables described in the model. If a person is highly *externally oriented*, that is, tends to abide by the expectation of others, conform to norms, etc. and attaches great significance to external recognition, he/she may find it hard to reject demands. A person anxious about being rejected for "nonconformist" behavior will often be unable to turn down a demand (see Froming & Carver, 1981; Carver & Scheier, 1981; Froming, Walker, & Lopyan, 1982; Cheek & Briggs, 1982). A high degree of external orientation impairs flexible self-regulation in the event of stresses.

Furthermore, a person's ability to access his/her own motive system is of great importance. When I am confronted with a request to perform a task, it is mandatory for me to examine this request with regard to not only whether it may involve a social commitment but also whether it is compatible with my own motive system: Is this what I really want? Does it fit with my own objectives? Should it turn out that it does not, this must be duly considered when I decide whether this self-obligation should nonetheless be assumed.

Persons subject to a high degree of reflection avoidance are generally unable in such a situation to "mediate" between and balance their own goals and external demands. They are prone to primarily abide by external demands and allow their own goals to pale into insignificance. In doing so they abandon the self-regulation processes that control their actions in conformity with their *own* goals, values, etc. and surrender to "external regulation."

## Unfavorable Strategies for Stress Control: Avoidance Instead of Confrontation

A distinction can be made between functional and dysfunctional stress control strategies (cf. Obrist, 1976; Obrist et al., 1978). Functional stress control strategies are those that bring about an actual change of the stress load: A modification of the stress source proper, experiencing the pressure as a positive challenge (i.e., as something from which positive feedback or support can be obtained). Dysfunctional stress control strategies are those that impede any active coping with stress sources and stress reactions. Although they may have a stress-reducing effect for a brief period, they are entirely unsuited to change the constellation of stress factors in the long run (Florin, Gerhards, Knispel, & Koch, 1985).

If one does not closely examine the sources or one's own reactions to stresses but instead avoids such a confrontation by assuming an attitude of evasion or running away, this will have a negative effect on the perception and processing of stresses. The person neither sufficiently perceives (potential or actual) strenuous effects caused by external demands nor adequately responds to the consequent internal demands. This leads to long-lasting stress effects that cannot be reduced.

Various stress theories (Selye, 1946, 1981; Henry & Stephens, 1977; Martin & Pihl, 1985, 1986) assume that a stress condition of "system over-exertion" occurs if there are long-lasting and/or highly burdensome factors of external or internal nature that are not modified (or cannot be modified) by the person and whose oppressive effects can neither be compensated nor "cushioned" by coping measures. Such a system overexertion results in various physiological processes (depending on the type of process) leading to organic symptoms. Stringent demands in conjunction with a high loss of control will massively influence the immune system and in this way assist the development of chronic inflammatory bowel diseases.

In everyday life stress is normally self-regulated, based to some extent on conscious control mechanisms and on automatic processing and action schemata. The latter will take effect in a stress-alleviating manner without conscious control or initiation of actions. For example, one may briefly stop reading, lean back, and look out of the window without even being aware of it.

It is further assumed that a form of cognitive avoidance, termed reflection avoidance, can contribute to a dysfunctional processing of stress, as it implies that discrepant aspects are *not* reflected on, or grappled with, and are *not* examined, discussed, or analyzed.

## The Disturbance of Self-Regulation

As has already been pointed out, psychosomatic diseases of the gastrointestinal tract may theoretically be said, on a psychological level, to be a severe disorder of self-regulation:

- Avoidance of reflection, caused by a chronic desire–fact discrepancy, leads to effects that strengthen the avoidance tendency and prevent a thorough reflection on dysfunctional goals. The system "preserves" its disorder.
- Reflection avoidance has as a consequence self-alienation, a loss of self-worth, identity, social autonomy, and social control. The person will experience an extreme loss in quality of life.
- The inability to say no, external orientation, and social uncertainty will cause stresses to increase.
- Dysfunctional processing of stress will prevent constructive coping with stress factors.

The person is "stuck" in a very unfavorable processing system that he/she is unable to abandon; effective self-regulation is no longer possible.

# A SPECIFIC CLIENT-CENTERED APPROACH:
## THERAPEUTIC WORK ON THE PROCESSING LEVEL

### Therapy Must be Adapted to the Client: A Client-Centered Method for Dealing with "Difficult" Clients

As can be seen from the foregoing discussion of the theory of the disturbance of self-regulation, the concept of reflection avoidance plays a vital role in the "functioning" of the disturbance. This has two major consequences for the formulation of an approach to therapy:

1. If reflection avoidance is linked with such massive dysfunctional effects that cause and maintain a disturbance of self-regulation, then such avoidance constitutes a central therapeutic point of approach. Reducing or eliminating reflection avoidance should result in largely constructive effects in the processing system and restore the functionality of the self-regulation system. So there is obviously an indication for a therapy aimed at promoting self-reflection, in particular, affective, emotional, and motivational self-reflection. This is what CCT is about (see Rogers, 1942, 1951; Gendlin, 1978; Finke, 1994; Sachse, 1992a, 1996).
2. On the other hand, a high degree of reflection avoidance, insufficient access to the motive system, and the like often lead to behavioral patterns of clients in therapy that make these clients "difficult," as noted earlier.

Therefore, female and male clients suffering from psychosomatic disorders have been considered "difficult" for a long time, especially for clarification-oriented forms of psychotherapy such as psychoanalysis or client-centered psychotherapy. These clients usually have not the prerequisite characteristics considered essential for these therapy forms, that is, a capability for introspection, self-exploration, etc., and for that reason are viewed as "unsuited" for these types of therapy. Therefore, by prior selection, these clients have been deemed no longer within the "reach" of these therapies. Such an attitude was strongly advocated by supporters of the so-called alexithymia concept, who suggested that, due to alexithymic characteristics, psychosomatic clients did not meet the prerequisites for effective therapy (see Kirmeyer, 1987; Shands, 1977; Franke, 1980).

If one were to follow this view, it would obviously be better for clients not to have these characteristics and preferably adapt to the rules prescribed by the therapy because then, and only then, could they expect help.

This problem—that a therapy form is basically indicated but clients do not meet certain prerequisites for its application—can logically be resolved only by means of a strategy of *adaptive indication* (Bastine, 1981): If there is a basic indication of a therapy form for group of clients and if this therapy form prescribes something that the clients cannot fulfill, this therapy must be modified such that it "agrees" with the starting conditions of the clients. It must meet the clients where they are situated, must make a "suitable" adjustment. (There are no "unsuited clients" but only ill-fitting forms of therapy!)

From a client-centered viewpoint the client need not adapt her-/himself to the particular therapy, but the therapist must adjust his/her approach to the client's needs. The therapist must tailor his/her efforts in such a way that the client is met where she or he is. In such a case, "alexithymic" features will no longer be seen as a interfering with the therapy or of the therapist but as *aspects of the disorder* that are of significance and must be taken into account in theory and practice. In other words, instead of being irritated by the client's behavior, one should attempt to understand it and utilize this understanding therapeutically (see Martin & Pihl, 1985, 1986).

## The Central Aspect of the Therapeutic Approach: Work on the Processing Level

Such an adjustment has been provided for in GCCT (Sachse, 1995a). It has been derived from the three-level model proposed by Sachse and Maus (1991) and Sachse (1992a). According to this model three levels of perception or analysis can be distinguished with respect to the psychotherapeutic process, as follows:

- The *content level*, encompassing questions such as "What are the client's problems and difficulties?" and "What are the central topics in the therapy?"
- The *processing level*, encompassing questions such as "How does the client cope with these problems?" and "Does she/he refrain from scrutinizing her/his problems?" On the processing level questions do not aim at the contents itself but are intended to find out how the client deals with content aspects.
- The *relationship level*, encompassing questions such as "How does the client arrange his relationship with the therapist?" and "Does the client enter into a trusting relationship with the therapist?"

A therapist may view the therapy process primarily on the content level. However, he/she may also attempt to ascertain how a client deals with her/his problems or how a client sets up the relationship with the therapist (see Grawe, 1988, 1992; Grawe & Caspar, 1984; Grawe, Donati, & Bernauer (1994); Caspar, 1989, 1996). These levels may not exclusively be regarded merely as levels of perception but also as levels of action. A therapist may make interventions chiefly directed toward the content level (e.g., to promote explication processes); but he/she may also make interventions aimed at the processing level (e.g., by making transparent how the client deals with her/his problems); the same applies to the relationship level (see Sachse, 1995a).

A therapist may lay emphasis on the processing level. In this case he/she intends to find out whether and in which way the client dysfunctionally deals with her/his problems. If the therapist finds the client uses a dysfunctional way of processing, he/she may propose more constructive processing modes, may draw the client's attention to the dysfunctional way of processing, work on the reasons for avoidance, and so on.

Such therapeutic "work on the processing level" is needed if a client effectively avoids reflection because content work in this case is not the main objective of the therapy; rather, the focus is on avoidance processes that significantly impair any effective content work. This means that if clients avoid reflection to a considerable extent, there is a therapeutic indication for a well-aimed "processing of the processing work."

## What Does Therapeutic Work on the Processing Level Mean?

If a therapist focuses attention on the processing level, he/she handles information that differs from that encountered on the content level and processes this information in a different way. The therapist does not so much take notice of what the client says and what it means in regard to its contents but rather attributes importance to how the client deals with, follows, and views a given content aspect. A therapist who works on the processing level addresses other types of questions and in doing so keeps track of other issues than those that concern a therapist who is working on the content level. Working on the processing level a therapist may, for example, address questions of the following nature:

- Is the client's representation concrete, conceivable, and conclusive?
- If not, is any inconcreteness linked with certain subjects or contents aspects?
- Does the client block the processing of certain subjects?
- Does the client systematically exclude her/his own share of the problem?

The interventions a therapist makes on the processing level serve therapeutic purposes:

- The therapist wishes to impart other, more constructive processing modes to the client; the client is meant to learn how to cope with problem aspects in a different manner so as to enable problems to be clarified.
- The therapist wants the client to produce a representation of her/his dysfunctional way of processing. The client is expected to gain knowl-

edge about how to handle problems and how these strategies prevent
her-/himself from clarifying and resolving her/his problems.
- The therapist wants the client to recognize the reasons why certain
processing strategies should be adopted. The client is expected to
understand that she/he evades certain self-aspects and should also
understand why she/he evades them.

These three therapeutic goals constitute the "processing of processing work":
The way in which the client processes her/his problem itself becomes the
subject matter of the therapy.

## A Central Aspect of Processing the Processing Work: The Therapeutic Approach to Avoidance Strategies

As explained earlier, the therapy process with psychosomatic clients is marked
by the phenomenon that the clients avoid being confronted with self-aspects
and refuse the reflection, clarification, and thus processing of relevant schemata, which is at least the case in the initial phase of the therapy.

In their avoidance efforts clients very frequently use a "standard form";
that is, they follow simple strategies that can be easily described. Nevertheless, therapists who are not familiar with these strategies and their functions
may well have some difficulty in handling them. Therapists are often "check-
mated" by these client actions and do not know how to react constructively.
Therefore, some of the most frequently employed strategies and ways to take
therapeutic action that straightforwardly illustrate what in fact is meant by
"processing the processing work" are described in the following subsections.

### Normalization

*Description of the Client Action.* The client names a problem. She/he
may even see her/his own determinants of the problem. However, she/he
speaks of this problem and/or the relevant determinants as if they were normal. The problem is said not to deviate from (mostly social) norms; it is an
*average* problem.

Such an effort at normalization may in fact take place in various ways.
A psychosomatic client may say, for example, "Well, isn't it the accepted
thing to have gastric ulcers? In our company you are expected to." A client
suffering from alcoholism says, "I don't drink more than what's normal. If
you think me to be an alcoholic, 60 million people in Germany must also
be." The message to the therapist is clear: "Either there is no problem at all
[because it is unimportant] or it is a problem that most people have. If there
is no problem, there is no need to deal with it. If it is a problem that most
people have, then it is *not specifically* mine. If this is so, there no need for me
to look at it. On the contrary, looking at it would mean for me to take on a
responsibility others should accept. Of course, I'm not willing to do so."

In this case the client creates a pattern of argumentation either explicitly or implicitly insinuating that (1) there is no reason for her/him to clarify her/his problematic aspects, and (2) such a course of action would be an outright impertinence or intrusion. The client thus insulates her-/himself against interventions offered by the therapist. All approaches aimed at internalizing the perspective and inducing the client to process her/his internal aspects are thus defined as impermissible.

*Possible Therapeutic Interventions.* A strategy such as normalization serves to eliminate one's own share of the problem. If something is deemed "normal" or considered to be "general" it has nothing to do with me specifically. The message sent to the therapist thus is as follows:

I have a problem $X$.
This is a normal/widespread problem.
It must therefore be due to general factors (my company, society).
Obviously, I have nothing to do with it.
Since this is so, there is no need for me to look at it.
So let's stop talking about it.

With this chain of conclusions the client (explicitly or implicitly) has terminated therapeutic work and said goodbye. Were this accepted by the therapist, a clarifying psychotherapy would practically come to an end (checkmate in six moves). Therapists often sense such a development but allow themselves to be bluffed by the argumentation pattern since they are not familiar with it.

Basically, the therapeutic counterstrategy is quite simple. It is based on the "basic postulate of explicating psychotherapy" (Sachse, 1992b). The chain of reasoning the therapist follows in this case is straightforward:

The client has a problem $X$.
Problem $X$ is that the client reacts to situation $Y$ by response $Z$.
This response is not mandatory.
Even if many people react to $Y$ by $Z$, there may be others who react completely differently.
If there are people who react in a different way, then $Z$ is not an inevitable reaction.
But if the client's reaction is not inevitable, $Z$ must have something to do with the client.
If $Z$ has something to do with the client, the specific idiosyncratic internal determinants of the client have to be scrutinized.
Therefore, the focus of the therapy must be on the client.

The argumentation presented by the therapist thus produces quite a different result. While the client concludes that her/his person should not be examined any further, the therapist draws the conclusion that precisely this has to be done. The decisive difference between the two lines of argumentation is that in the second the reaction is *not* thought of as being inevitable: Even if 8 million people react similarly this need not necessarily be due to an external incentive. These people may have similar goals and schemata according to which they react in this and in no other way. Now if this involves the people, it is the people who must be examined more closely because this is where the underlying cause will be found.

For that reason, the therapist should never permit himself to be bluffed by normalization or generalization arguments. If, for example, the client says, "Gastric ulcers are normal in our company," the therapist might reply, "I believe that work in the company is quite stressful. But we still know that people react differently to stress. And what we don't know is how *you* react to stress. Until we have found that out, we are unable to help you. So we must take a closer look at it now." Here, the therapist strictly avoids any argumentation with the client. He/she accepts the client's assumption that the company causes stress but draws different conclusions from it and points out to the client that this course of action is mandatory if she/he wants to bring about a change.

The therapist should follow these rules: (1) whether the problem is normal, widespread, esoteric, or whatever does not make any difference at all; (2) what is important is how the client reacts, what the client does, what the client's processing is; (3) if the client does not make any mention of these aspects, the therapist directs the focus on them.

## Downplaying

*Description of the Client Action.* Another way of impeding the processing of a problem and preventing explicating work is by playing it down. The client describes a problem, certain symptoms of it, and so on. The therapist then asks relevant questions (e.g., "What makes this problem so serious to you?"). It would now be appropriate for the client to start explicating work. But to avoid this she/he may underplay the issue, stating that the problem was not that acute, need not be dealt with, and in fact was not worth looking into any more. If the therapist accepts this, the problem has vanished; it is out of focus and thus has escaped processing.

If a client uses this downplaying strategy excessively, it may well develop that problems are no longer visible at all. This was the case with one of our female psychosomatic clients at the beginning of therapy. She had her bodily ailments, but beyond that all problems immediately ran through the therapist's fingers like water; allegedly, there was really nothing so important or burdensome that it needed to be discussed.

*Possible Therapeutic Interventions.* Downplaying is a strategy enabling the client to block the processing of a content aspect: If there is not anything really that bad happening, it is hardly worthwhile talking about it in detail.

I think a therapist should not let him-/herself be impressed by this. Especially at the beginning of therapy (when this strategy is most frequently encountered) the processing of vital problem aspects is not so decisive. Rather, it is essential for the client to learn how to work in the course of the therapy. However, this cannot be taught by the therapist giving lectures; instead the client will learn from appropriate interventions that the therapist offers with a view to elucidating important issues. Moreover, from a therapeutic angle it is not important where a client starts. *A stringently working therapist will arrive at central content aspects with clients who show cooperation no matter where the client starts in therapy.*

For that reason, the client's statement that something is "not so bad," "not so important," and the like is to be regarded as highly irrelevant. There is absolutely no reason not to start with therapeutic work at that point. In fact, the main thing at the beginning of therapy and at the beginning of every new therapeutic subject is *just to start.* Therefore, the therapist replies, "You say it's not that bad. But it's bad enough. What's so bad about it?" or "You say it's not bad, just a little bit unpleasant. I'm not quite sure what "unpleasant" means to you. Can you be a bit more specific?"

## "I Don't Know"

*Description of the Client Action.* A particularly favored blockage of processing is at the same time a very simple one: If clients are asked to look into an aspect a bit more closely, or if they are asked what in fact they want, they often answer, "I don't know." This reaction has an absolutely paralyzing effect on inexperienced therapists as a rule. They are perplexed and do not know how to proceed.

The reply "I don't know" is mostly resorted to when therapists direct clients' perspective inwardly and request them to deal with their own relevant motives, values, or convictions with respect to certain problems. It is a standard reply to questions such as the following:

What of X is important to you?
What crosses your mind in this situation?
What do you want to achieve by it?
What makes this situation so hard for you?

Now it is important to understand that the reply "I don't know" may mean that either the client does not have a "good" answer or the client wants to block the process. Let us consider each of these possibilities in turn.

*The Client Does Not Have a Good Answer.* Sometimes clients answer a deepening (or concretizing) question by "I don't know" because they think the therapist wants a "good" and detailed answer that they do not have. In such a case the reply actually means, "I'm not so sure about it, and I don't dare to express what I know." Here, the client does not intend to block the process but rather cannot go on as the result of unfavorable circumstances.

*The Client Wants to Block the Process.* However, quite a different intention may be linked with the answer "I don't know": By that reply, clients may be refusing to follow a certain aspect. Processing a specific content may be an unpleasant experience, too "hot" to handle. In this case they may say that they don't know what they feel or what has crossed their minds. In this way, they succeed in hiding information from the therapist that is needed to address further unpleasant issues. Thus the process is halted at this point, and such clients are in a position to prevent any aversive aspects from being looked into.

So an "I don't know" is often more than just an indication of the client's difficulties; it may be an *active blockage of the process.*

*Possible Therapeutic Actions.* How the client's "I don't know" reply ought to be responded to depends on whether the therapist is under the impression that the client wishes to continue the process but does not know how to do this or is blocked by her/his own excessively high expectations, on the one hand, or whether the therapist feels that the client wants to prevent any further processing of the subject, on the other.

In the first case, if the therapist thinks the client's "I don't know" reply is due to the client's inability to provide a "good" and elaborate answer, the therapist should put the client at ease. The therapist may say, for example, "I know you don't have a perfect answer yet. After all, these are aspects that are still indistinct and, obviously, that's why we are working on them. So I don't want a perfect answer from you. All we need now is a hint, some traces on which we can base our further work. Therefore, I would like you to stay on this point [or this situation] and take a closer look: What's crossing your mind? What do you feel?" Here, the client is expected to learn that therapy is in fact meant to deal with aspects that are *still* unclear. Consequently, any piece of information furnished must be taken seriously and any traces, vague though they may be, must be followed.

Clients impeding themselves in the process in the above manner usually make every effort to achieve clarification. They *endeavor* to answer the questions the therapist poses, but in doing so they experience difficulties. On the other hand, clients that actively block processing do not *attempt at all* to answer the therapist's questions. Rather than even trying to do what the therapist has proposed, without having looked into a situation and their own feelings in that particular situation, they simply reply, "I don't know." For a valid assessment of whether a client is circumventing contents, some other aspects need to be taken into account, however: lack of explication, missing "work order," and the like.

If a therapist comes to the conclusion that the client is using "I don't know" in an effort to actively block processing work, the therapist must adhere to the "contrary" principle. In this case, the client's message to the therapist is "I don't want to look into this content aspect any further (or more closely) and prefer to leave it right away." However, the therapist's intervention signifies to the client that "On the contrary, let us take a very close look at these content aspects." The mere fact that the client prefers to circumvent an aspect is evidence that it not only has relevance to the client but has not yet been clarified and integrated. This again is indicative of the fact that it *needs to be processed.*

Accordingly, the therapist might say, "I know it is hard for you to stay here and take a closer look. That's quite understandable. If you could tell me about it, everything would soon be cleared up and nothing would be left to look into. Therefore, I would ask you to continue with this point and tell me exactly what you are feeling or what is crossing your mind. . . . " In this way, the therapist at first exerts considerable "pressure." But if the client maintains her/his "I don't know" attitude, the therapist then *increases* the pressure: "I know it's difficult for you, but please continue with it. There is always something at the back of one's mind: You always feel or think about something, no matter how diffuse it is." In this way, the therapist establishes a "counternorm"; that is, he/she assumes that from a psychological perspective a person must have data of some nature available, which undoubtedly is true. By this course of action the client's obligation to continue with the particular issue at hand becomes stronger and being evasive has been made more difficult.

If the client insists that she/he has no idea the therapist will change over to the meta-processing level and make the client's behavior itself the subject matter: "I would like to talk with you about why it is so difficult for you to stay with it and take a closer look." On the other hand, the therapist may also resort to confrontation, saying for instance, "When I ask you a question you immediately say, 'I don't know.' You don't even take time to look and see if there is something else happening. Why not try to further clarify the subject at this point?" Here, the therapist offers a *processing the processing work* approach: The avoidance attitude itself becomes the subject matter of the therapy.

If a therapist carries out interventions in this manner it will be of decisive significance that these are integrated into a durable therapeutic relationship. The therapist must point out to the client that it is the sole aim of the approach to direct the client's attention to her/his own processes so that she/he will finally be in a position to recognize them and reflect upon them. There should be no doubt whatsoever that the aim is not to criticize the client or "forbid" anything. The basic idea that the therapist should impart to the client is that a client can only tackle a problem if she/he is aware of it; and if the problem is situated on the processing level, the client must recognize her/his way of problem processing and its dysfunctional consequences. Only then can she/he restore her/his capability to act and decide.

## Answering Questions That Are Not Asked

*Description of the Client Action.* Another especially elusive strategy, one often difficult for the therapist to recognize, seeks to change the subject and bring something new into focus by answering questions that have not been asked. The therapist asks a question to which the client replies at some length. If one now attempts to conclude from the answer just what the question to this answer might have been, it turns out that the question so reconstructed has very little to do with the original question. In the course of answering, the client has implicitly modified the question in such a way that she/he in fact has replied to quite another question. But the answer, and this is of significance, still has a slight association with the contents of the original question. Therefore, the strategy can be viewed as a pseudocommunicative approach. Apparently and seen cursorily, the client has continued the communication process, but what she/he has actually done is to "stifle the contents."

And this is what bothers the therapist: He/she is under the impression that the client has responded "somehow," yet knows there is something wrong with that answer without being immediately able to pinpoint the mistake. To find out what is wrong he/she is particularly attentive to what the client says—and so he/she follows the newly laid track.

*Possible Therapeutic Actions.* When coming across this avoidance strategy in therapy, the therapist acts according to the principle: "OK, let's start over."

If the therapist notices that the client does not answer a relevant (e.g., concretizing or deepening) question, he/she poses the question again. In doing so, he/she may take the responsibility for the problem by saying, for example, "I think I've not made myself clear enough. My question was . . . " The therapist may also attempt to formulate a clearer, shorter, more concrete question than before to rule out any misunderstanding. If the client still fails to answer the question, the therapist may elect to put the question again, saying, "There is still an aspect I'm not sure about . . ." So, the therapist does not allow him-/herself to be deceived but instead always focuses the client's attention on central aspects.

Should the client again proffer an evasive reply, the therapist may change over to a meta-level of processing by pointing out to the client that the question in fact *has not been answered*, in which case the therapist makes this the subject of the therapy; for example, "I would like you to note what you are actually doing in the therapy. I've asked you twice about X, but you twice have answered Y. So, please, let us discuss why it is so difficult for you to answer this question." If the therapist has already drawn the client's attention to such aspects several times, confrontation may even become more direct; for instance, "I've frequently noted that you evaded my questions by giving answers that did not fit—and I've often told you about it. I would urgently prefer to talk about what makes it so difficult for you to address my questions."

When dealing with this (and also other) avoidance strategies it is essential that a therapist takes a stringent approach. In the process, he/she must remind the client of these aspects again and again. This is vital, because a single intervention of the therapist will not be sufficient to enable a client to recognize her/his own strategies and their underlying intentions and motives.

## ILLUSTRATION OF THERAPEUTIC PRINCIPLES BY MEANS OF TRANSCRIPTS WITH COMMENTS

### Objective

Excerpts from two transcripts of therapies are given below to illustrate some of the relevant therapeutic principles. Obviously, since only short transcripts can be analyzed here, the number of principles illustrated is quite limited; nevertheless, transcripts are better suited than mere descriptions to elaborate the underlying principles.

Both transcripts are from the beginning of the third therapy session. They present some typical processing difficulties experienced by psychosomatic clients and indicate ways to handle these difficulties in therapy. To improve legibility and understanding the transcripts were slightly modified from spoken to written language but without any substantive changes having been made in the transcripts' contents.

### Client S: "Clarifying Feelings Does Not Make Any Sense"

Mr. S came to the therapy project because of ulcerative colitis. From the start he appeared to be very stressed and under pressure but told the therapist everything was not that bad really and "nothing could be done about it anyway"; it would be best if the disturbing feelings could be eliminated by the therapy. It took Mr. S 16 sessions of "processing the way of processing" before any noteworthy clarification work could start. The therapist had to tackle processing difficulties again and again and avoid getting too involved in the client's arguments. The therapy turned out to be a success, and Mr. S was very satisfied with what had been achieved.

*Transcript*

T1: (1) What do you want to talk about today?

C1: (1) Don't know.

T2: (1) Isn't there anything that bothers you at the moment? (2) Do you have a subject you want to discuss?

C2: (1) It's always the same. (2) Every day looks the same. (3) So what shall I tell you?

T3: (1) That sounds as if you were bored to death.

C3: (1) Bored? (2) No. (3) Only, nothing happens.

T4: (1) Do you find it difficult in this setting, with me, to name a subject you can or want to talk about?

C4: (1) There is not anything to tell, really. (2) It's always the same.

T5: (1) Last session you named three subjects. (2) Three fields that irritate you occasionally: your work, the relationship with your wife, and the way you manage your financial affairs. (3) Do you want to talk about one of these topics now?

C5: (1) I have already commented on all of these. (2) Mind you, I'm not feeling irritated all the time. (3) Such is everyday life, you know.

T6: (1) Yes, that's how your everyday life is. (2) But I'm not yet sure what in particular is eating you. (3) And, likewise, I don't know exactly what's happening with you when you feel irritated. (4) For example, if you are annoyed about your foreman, what do you feel?

C6: (1) I feel upset about him all the time. (2) Everybody does. (3) Actually, he is absolutely crazy. (4) Everybody in the workshop thinks he is.

T7: (1) OK, everybody knows the foreman is a difficult guy. (2) But I still don't know what upsets *you*. (3) May I ask you to think it over again and tell me what about the foreman annoys *you*?

C7: (1) Yesterday again there was such an incident. (2) I was told to paint a door. (3) He expects that we work overtime to do the job. (4) But you won't be paid for this. (5) If you say no, you are possibly bullied into doing it.

T8: (1) What exactly irritates you about this?

C8: (1) You certainly feel annoyed. (2) Well, of course, you can't help it. [Client stays completely cool and at ease; his anger is not noticeable at all.]

T9: (1) When you are talking about it now, do you still feel angry?

C9: (1) No. (2) There is no point in being angry. (3) It's useless. (4) It wouldn't change the foreman, would it?

T10: (1) You prefer not to feel angry. (2) What you are saying is—Feelings are useless. (3) It would be better to have no feelings at all.

C10: (1) Yes, that's right.

T11: (1) But you feel annoyed day after day. (2) Being angry shows you there is something wrong. (3) Your anger is like a lit oil pilot lamp. (4) But what you do, in fact, is disregard it.

C11: (1) But what shall I do? (2) I can't go and kill the foreman, can I? (*laughs*)

T12: (1) (*laughing*) You'd better not. (2) But I would like to understand what you are doing with yourself. (3) You say to yourself: I can't change anything. (4) And being unable to make changes, I would rather leave my feelings alone. (5) Is that correct?

C12: (1) Of course it is. (2) No point in being angry. (3) Won't help me in any way.

T13: (1) Yes, you are right. (2) The way you have handled your anger in the past won't help you at all.

C13: (1) What do you mean?

T14: (1) Well, I think the anger does exist. (2) It is real. (3) You feel irritated frequently, day after day. (4) But you say you can't do anything about it. (5) So there is no need for you to look at your anger more closely. (6) So you are not doing anything. (7) And that is why nothing changes.

C14: (1) And what am I supposed to do?

T15: (1) What can I say? (2) I'm convinced it would be very good if you come to a clear understanding—with my help—of what the anger tells you. (4) We will then understand what's going on. (5) We will then, and only then, understand what the problem is. (6) And understanding the problem is mandatory to arrive at a solution.

C15: (1) But I've tried everything.

T16: (1) Is that so? (2) Have you ever tried before to analyze your anger with me?

C16: (1) No, I haven't, of course. (2) But what's the point in doing so?

T17: (1) An analysis is meant to clarify what exactly happens inside you. (2) What do you think, shall we give it a try? (3) Is there anything against the two of us trying this out together?

C17: (1) No, not at all.

## Comments

In the case of this client the main processing problem involved normalizing, relativization, and downplaying combined with resignation, which however did not lead to depression but rather to externally oriented brooding, as is customary with psychosomatic clients.

The client thinks it useless to take his feelings seriously and accept them as a basis for analyzing the problem because "You can't do anything about it anyway" and therefore there is no point in having feelings. Of course, this doesn't prevent his feelings from causing constant trouble and a consistent state of stress accompanied by permanent feelings of discontent.

This attitude is evident from statement C2: It doesn't pay to work in therapy since nothing can be done. When the client said this he by no means made a depressive impression but appeared to be very tense and "under pressure."

In C3 it is quite clear that the client has assumed a highly external perspective and is experiencing extreme difficulties in directing his attention inward. Therefore, this sets a significant process target for the therapist: Internalize the perspective!

In T5 the therapist makes an effort to "process the processing work." He wishes to induce the client to direct his focus on own aspects, address questions, activate affective schemata. Therefore, the therapist deliberately *refrains* from dealing with the content aspects in C4; the therapist also views the therapeutic alliance between himself and the client as intact and for that reason does *not* refer to the relationship level. Rather, his process target is to familiarize the client with another way of dealing with problems.

In C5 the client responds to this by relativizing and normalizing: Everything is quite all right and, thinking about it, completely normal.

In T6 the therapist does not question the normality (1) but proceeds by asking a clarifying question: What happens to *you* (2–4)? As a pretext the therapist claims his *own lack* of understanding as being the reason, the "motive," for this question: He, the therapist, would like to have more clarity! This should help the client to accept this approach.

But in C6 the client again responds in a normalizing and generalizing way. He does not see the problem as being specific to him; everybody has this kind of problem. This, again, is not contested by the therapist; rather, he uses the same processing approach, saying in T7, "I would like to know what annoys *you*."

C7 again shows that the client "normally" assumes an external perspective and not an internal one. He has no intention of finding out what is happening to him but he reports events and concludes by accepting the inevitable: That's the way it is.

T8 illustrates something of the greatest significance for our access to processing: The therapist does not allow himself to be led astray. He wants the client to take a close look at his feelings, to focalize and clarify them.

If the client does not follow this prompting the therapist tries again and again (T9), or he investigates with the client the reason why the client does not internalize and clarify the perspective (T10). In this way the therapist consistently pursues a "processing of the processing work" and does not let himself be diverted!

In T10 the therapist puts the client's assumption to the test that it is better not to have feelings. Again, it is the therapist's goal that the client should internalize, focalize, and clarify his feelings. If there are obstacles impeding this for the client, these obstacles must be processed in the course of the therapy process.

In T11 the therapist uses a metaphor that he thinks the client, who works in an automotive paint shop, will understand: the red oil pilot lamp that the client disregards.

Following this, in C11, the client himself gives some elucidation about his construction that "There isn't anything to be done" and for that reason there is no point in understanding the problem. The therapist in T12 makes this construction transparent and offers a proposal (T15, T16, T17) after he has pointed out to the client the consequences of such a construction (T13, T14). The therapist tells the client (in T13) very pointedly that he considers the client's previous strategies as dysfunctional and is not at all surprised at the client's inability to solve his problem in this way. Such clear-cut remarks are often necessary to attack a client's attitude that may be plausible to him though hardly helpful. They are also necessary to restart the clarification process.

## The Perfect Millionaire

Mr. T came to the therapy project because he had suffered from severe recurrent and chronic gastric and duodenal ulcers for 16 years. Medical measures that included treatment to attack *Helicobacter* bacteria did not result in recovery. Therefore, Mr. T was completely frustrated and strongly opposed to further medical treatment. To attend a therapy session he had to travel 120 kilometers and so must be viewed as having been highly motivated.

Mr. T was co-owner of a large construction company and very affluent. Nevertheless, he was under the impression that he could not do anything enjoyable with his money because he was either working or experiencing severe pain or both.

In comparison with other psychosomatic clients, Mr. T was found to perform a comparably high degree of intrapersonal exploration that resulted in beneficial clarification work starting after only 8 hours of "processing the processing work." The therapy was altogether extremely successful. Mr. T was highly satisfied with the therapy and as of this writing, some 1½ years later, has not suffered any relapse. (In 35 sessions psychotherapy alone had achieved what medical treatment could not do in 16 years.)

Although Mr. T was a "good" client, he showed typical processing difficulties. However, the therapist was able to counteract them effectively, as reported below.

*Transcript*

T1: (1) Last session we started to talk about your work, (2) especially about your impression that you must be very thorough all the time. (3) Where do you want to continue, today?

C1: (1) I think I told you everything that is important here. (2) Come to think of it, I can't tell you any more about this. (3) At the moment, there is nothing I consider important.

T2: (1) It's difficult for you to start over at that point. (2) But I would still ask you to go back to the subject. (3) Perhaps, you should look again at aspects that make you angry, that strike you as remarkable. (4) Take your time, don't feel rushed.

C2: (1) You know, I keep forgetting everything we discussed here very quickly. (2) At the moment I'm not sure what else I can tell you about the whole affair.

T3: (1) I understand quite well that it's difficult for you to talk again about the subject of "work." (2) But last time I felt that you mentioned many things that gave you a great deal of trouble. (3) I know it's hard and maybe even unpleasant for you to get that out again. (4) But if we want to clarify what is putting a strain on you, this is a real must. (*pausing briefly*) (5) Now, if you look at the whole work situation again what is it that bothers you most?

C3: (1) Well, bothering is perhaps not the right expression. (2) Sometimes I just feel annoyed. (3) On the one hand, I'm very correct, very pedantic. (4) But as a self-employed person you have to be, don't you think? (5) But if I see how my partner is handling matters, too fast, not in the least less effective . . .

T4: (1) Then you would wish you could sometimes "stretch a point," make concessions now and then?

C4: (1) Yes, maybe that wouldn't be bad sometimes.

T5: (1) And what stops you? (2) What gives you trouble if you try to be more permissive?

C5: (1) I don't know. (2) Come to think of it, there isn't very much that could go wrong. (3) Operations in the company are checked over several times. (4) No need for me to do everything myself. (5) But still . . . (*pausing briefly*) (6) Of course, it would be a disaster if anything turned out badly because . . .

T6: [Interrupts the client] (1) Now, keep looking at yourself! (2) What keeps you, personally, from being more relaxed or permissive.

C6: (1) I don't know.

T7: (1) Please, do not turn away from this question—think about it. (2) Take your time.

C7: (1) I really don't know (*pausing*) (2) I'm a guy who must have every-thing functioning well. (*emphatically*) (3) That's simply the way it must be! (4) Of course, I know that it's not that serious to make a mistake now and then! (5) No doubt I've made quite a number of mistakes myself in the past!

T8: (1) You said you *know* that mistakes are not that bad. (2) But your *feelings* tell you something different. (3) Your feelings tell you that mistakes are in fact horrible!

C8: (1) Yes, that's true! (2) It just must not happen! (3) And, what is more, you are under an obligation to your customers to perform excellently.

T9: (1) The customers, OK. (2) But actually I think it is a horrible situation for you personally to make a mistake! (3) Can you tell me the reason for that?

## Comments

Although Mr. T was a comparatively willing exploratory client he also faced the difficulties characteristic of psychosomatic persons.

The problem starts with the client thinking that the problem list prepared by him and the therapist can be checked off in one session and that will be all that needs to be said about it: "In fact, everything is quite normal; in fact, I don't have any problems; and, in fact, there is little sense in getting involved in personal issues." This is a message quite frequently received from psychosomatic persons, and it is important for therapists not to allow themselves to be deterred by this.

The therapist accepts here that the client faces problems with processing his personal difficulties (T2/1), but nevertheless she induces the client to stick to his task (T2/2–4): Look for personally relevant subjects and focus your attention on these!

The same is repeated in C2 and T3 when the therapist explains why she asks the client not to turn away from this task (T3/4) and then tells him to cope with the task again.

Now the client attempts to provide something like the definition of a problem (C3/C4) actively supported by the therapist (T4), who then (maybe a little bit too early) asks a deepening question (T5).

From C5 it is evident that the client is not yet ready to access this level of processing, but he nevertheless sticks to the subject until he clearly "takes off" (in C6): Whereas he at first showed an internal perspective and directed his attention to *himself* and his norms, he now starts focusing again on external aspects and tells the therapist something about professional constraints. [Listening to the transcript we notice here that the client says sentence 6 faster than the previous sentences; we say the client "goes into higher gear" and thus again abandons the clarification process.]

The therapist, obviously noticing this change in processing mode, interrupts the client and explicitly requests that he should maintain the internal perspective and should stick to the question already addressed (T6). In this way she is very process-directive and induces the client not to disregard his clarification task.

Moreover, she does not allow herself to be irritated by an "I don't know" (C6) but again requests that he fulfill his task (T7). The client complies and resumes his internal perspective and again addresses the question, "What makes it so difficult for me to be permissive" (C7).

In T8 the therapist carries out an intervention we call "separating a cognition–emotion bond": The client "in fact knows" that he can react differently (cognitive constituent), but he still feels that way (emotional constituent). The client is now expected to explicitly disregard and remove from his focus the cognitive constituent accepted by the therapist and concentrate solely on the emotional aspect and the clarification *of this aspect*.

As C8 shows, the client experiences difficulties in reacting in this way (otherwise, there would probably not be a need for therapy). But the therapist proceeds by persistently requesting that the client try again (T9).

Having presented the theory, practice, and a case example of a GCCT approach to the treatment of psychosomatic disorders, a research study of this treatment is summarized below.


## A THERAPY STUDY

Based on the principles and approaches of a processing-oriented CCT as outlined here a therapy study was conducted involving 87 male and female clients suffering from psychosomatic gastrointestinal diseases.


### Phases of the Therapy

In the first phase of the therapy the therapists were instructed to lay emphasis on "processing of the processing work." The content aspects of the relevant client problem would be dealt with in later therapy phases.

The following phases of therapeutic work can be distinguished:


### Phase 1. Establishing Contact (1 to 2 sessions)

The clients furnish information about their somatic symptoms, their previous symptom history, etc. Together with each client the therapist prepares a *psychological problem list*. For this purpose clients report all the difficulties (as trifling as they may appear) they face in everyday life (during work, in relationships etc.)

The somatic symptoms are *not* included in the list of problems. The client is requested to address one of these psychological problems.

## Phase 2. Processing the Processing Work (10 to 15 sessions)

During this phase the therapist makes major efforts in a process-directive manner to draw the client's attention to dysfunctional types of problem processing and offers constructive problem-processing alternatives to the client.

At this time the focus is not yet on clarifying or changing the contents. Therefore, it is not essential that clients address central problems at this stage. Rather, it is important that clients, for example, assume an internal perspective, perceive their own feelings as an important source of information, respond to questions by the therapist, and notice and reduce avoidance strategies.

## Phase 3. Clarifying and Changing Content Aspects (10 to 20 sessions)

If the client's way of processing changes, the amount of clarification work increases and the transition is fluid.

During this phase clients endeavor to understand their experiencing and to understand and represent their motives, targets, and values. For example, clients may want to find out whether it is actually important to them to be always "functioning" individuals or whether they have other goals and motives they want to realize by actions. Clients may find that they do not want to be at the disposal of others all the time but instead have their own needs and wishes they would like to have by other people.

At this point clarification and change of (affective) schemata is desirable, contributing to a change of self-worth, increased access to clients' own motives, and diminished anxiety and fear.

## Phase 4. Transfer (5 to 8 sessions)

During this final phase the therapist can help clients to actively apply the knowledge they have gained about everyday life, which they may already have started to do on their own.

Together with the therapist clients draw up a plan as to what they actually want to change, for example, how to say no, or making a response where they can try out their self-awareness.

### Therapy Outcome

The empirical results show that, when compared to control groups, the clients achieved major significant improvements, some examples of which were the following:

- Self-acceptance increases.
- The conviction that one is controlled externally lessens.

- "State orientation" (Kuhl, 1994a) decreases, indicating a diminution of alienation.
- The ability to be successful and conduct oneself in society improves.
- Active coping with stresses improves and passive coping diminishes.
- Due to the resultant stress reduction and improved coping with stresses, the psychosomatic gastrointestinal symptom complex often significantly improves as well.

### GCCT: A Successful Psychotherapy for Psychosomatic Diseases

The results show that a specially adapted GCCT can effectively help clients suffering from psychosomatic gastrointestinal diseases (duodenal ulcers, ulcerative colitis, and Crohn's disease). It is not true that only a behavioral therapeutic approach is helpful for so-called alexithymic clients (Tönnies, 1986; Tönnies, Gades, & Pieper-Raether, 1987). The therapeutic improvements are numerous. They cover improvement of self-acceptance, the capability to act, improved social authority, adoption of active stress-coping strategies, as well as marked improvements of the physical symptoms. The duration of the therapy is rather short, and thus the effects can be achieved quite economically. Two things are evident from the results:

- CCT appears to be an indicated form of therapy for PGTD clients.
- To provide effective help CCT must, however, be adapted to the particular starting conditions and capabilities of each client.

Furthermore, the results show that it is essential for PGTD clients to systematically improve existing dysfunctional problem processing patterns. For that reason, it takes a considerable time in the therapy to "process the processing work." This type of therapeutic approach seems to be particularly expedient for clients suffering from psychosomatic disturbances, and it may even be specifically expedient for PGTD clients. On the other hand, the approach does not appear to be expedient for clients with "neurotic disorders" who have different prerequisites with respect to contents processing at the beginning of therapy. Moreover, it may not be expedient for clients with personality disorders (see Fiedler, 1994) who exhibit special interaction patterns when starting therapy; in this case, it is expedient to conduct therapeutic work on the relationship level.

### REFERENCES

Ahrens, S. (1983). Zur Affektverarbeitung von Ulcuspatienten: Ein Beitrag zur "Alexithymie-Diskussion." In H. H. Studt (Ed.), *Psychosomatik in Forschung und Praxis* (pp. 339–357). Munich: Urban & Schwarzenberg.

Ahrens, S. (1985). Alexithymia and affective verbal behavior of three groups of patients. *Social Science and Medicine, 20,* 691–694.

Ahrens, S., & Morgenthaler, B. (1982). Erfassung von Gefühlsprozessen bei Ulcuspatienten, somatisch Kranken und Neurotikern. *Medizinische Psychologie, 8,* 67–82.

Atrops, A., & Sachse, R. (1994). Vermeiden psychosomatische Klienten die Klärung eigener Motive? Eine empirische Untersuchung mit Hilfe des Focusing. In M. Behr, U. Esser, F. Petermann, R. Sachse, & R. Tausch (Eds.), *Jahrbuch für Personenzentrierte Psychologie und Psychotherapie* (vol. 3, pp. 41–59). Cologne: GwG-Verlag.

Bastine, R. (1981). Adaptive Indikation in der zielorientierten Psychotherapie. In U. Baumann (Ed.), *Indikation zur Psychotherapie* (pp. 158–168). Munich: Urban & Schwarzenberg.

Buss, A. H. (1980). *Self-consciousness and social anxiety.* San Francisco: Freeman.

Carver, C. S. (1979). A cybernetic model of self-attention processes. *Journal of Personality and Social Psychology, 37,* 1251–1281.

Carver, C. S., Blaney, P. H., & Scheier, M. F. (1979). Focus of attention, chronic expectancy, and responses to a feared stimulus. *Journal of Personality and Social Psychology, 37,* 1186–1195.

Carver, C. S., & Scheier, M. F. (1981). *Attention and self-regulation: A control theory approach to human behavior.* New York: Springer-Verlag.

Carver, C. S., & Scheier, M. F. (1985a). Aspects of self and the control of behavior. In B. R. Schlenker (Ed.), *The self and social life* (pp. 146–174). New York: McGraw-Hill.

Carver, C. S., & Scheier, M. F. (1985b). Self-consciousness, expectancies, and the coping process. In T. M. Field, P. M. McCabe, & N. Scheidermann (Eds.), *Stress and coping* (pp. 305–330). Hillsdale, NJ: Erlbaum.

Caspar, F. (1989). *Probleme und Beziehungen verstehen: Eine Einführung in die psychotherapeutische Plananalyse.* Bern: Huber.

Caspar, F. (1996). Die Anwendung standartisierter Methoden und das individuelle Neukonstruieren therapeutischen Handelns. In H. S. Reinecker & D. Schmelzer (Eds.), *Verhaltenstherapie, Selbstregulation, Selbstmanagement* (pp. 23–47). Göttingen: Hogrefe.

Cheek, M. S., & Briggs, S. R. (1982). Self-consciousness and aspects of identity. *Journal of Research and Personality, 16,* 401–408.

Duval, S., & Wicklund, R. A. (1972). *A theory of objective self-awareness.* New York: Academic Press.

Fiedler, P. (1994). *Persönlichkeitsstörungen.* Weinheim: PVU.

Finke, J. (1994). *Empathie und Interaktion: Methode und Praxis der Gesprächspsychotherapie.* Stuttgart: Thieme.

Florin, I., Gerhards, F., Knispel, M., & Koch, M. (1985). Objektive Belastung, subjektives Belastungserleben und Formen des Umgangs mit Belastung bei Migränepatienten und kopfschmerzfreien Personen. In D. Vaitl, T. W. Knapp, & N. Bierbaumer (Eds.), *Psychophysiologische Merkmale klinischer Symptome* (Vol. 1, pp. 244–257). Weinheim, Germany: Beltz.

Franke, A. (1980). Verhaltenstherapie und Gesprächspsychotherapie bei Patienten mit psychosomatischen Störungen. In M. Hautzinger & W. Schulz (Eds.), *Klinische Psychologie und Psychotherapie* (pp. 181–191). Berlin: DGVT & GwG-Verlag.

Frey, D., Wicklund, R. A., & Scheier, M. F. (1984). Die Theorie der objektiven Selbstaufmerksamkeit. In D. Frey & M. Irle (Eds.), *Theorien der Sozialpsychologie: Vol. 1. Kognitive Theorien* (pp. 192–216). Bern: Huber.

Froming, W. J., & Carver, C. S. (1981). Divergent influences of private and public self-consciousness in a compliance paradigm. *Journal of Research in Personality, 15,* 159–171.

Froming, W. J., Walker, G. R., & Lopyan, K. J. (1982). Public and private self-awareness: When personal attitudes conflict with societal expectations. *Journal of Experimental Social Psychology, 18,* 476–487.

Gendlin, E. T. (1978). *Focusing.* New York: Everest House.

Gollwitzer, P. M. (1986). Striving for specific identities: The social reality of self-symbolizing. In R. F. Baumeister (Ed.), *Public self and private self.* New York: Springer-Verlag.

Gollwitzer, P.M. (1987a). Suchen, Finden und Festigen der eigenen Identität: Unstillbare Zielintentionen. In H. Heckhausen, P. M. Gollwitzer, & F. E. Weinert (Eds.), *Jenseits des Rubikon: Der Wille in den Humanwissenschaften* (pp. 176–189). Berlin: Springer-Verlag.

Gollwitzer, P. M. (1987b). The implementation of identity intentions: A motivational–volitional perspective on symbolic self-completion. In F. Halisch & J. Kuhl (Eds.), *Motivation, intention, and volition* (pp. 349–369). Berlin: Springer-Verlag.

Gollwitzer, P. M., & Wicklund, R. A. (1985). The pursuit of self-defining goals. In J. Kuhl & J. Beckmann (Eds.), *Action control: From cognition to behavior* (pp. 61–85). Berlin: Springer-Verlag.

Grawe, K. (1988). Heuristische Psychotherapie: Eine schematheoretisch fundierte Konzeption des Psychotherapieprozesses. *Integrative Therapie, 4,* 309–324.

Grawe, K. (1992). Komplementäre Beziehungsgestaltung als Mittel zur Herstellung einer guten Therapiebeziehung. In J. Margraf & J. C. Brengekmann (Eds.), *Die Therapeut-Patient-Beziehung in der Verhaltenstherapie* (pp. 215–244). Munich: Röttger.

Grawe, K., & Caspar, F. M. (1984). Die Plananalyse als Konzept und Instrument für die Psychotherapieforschung. In U. Baumann (Ed.), *Psychotherapie: Makro-/Mikroperspektive* (pp. 177–197). Göttingen: Hogrefe.

Grawe, K., Donati, R., & Bernauer, F. (1994). *Psychotherapie im Wandel: Von der Konfession zur Profession.* Göttingen: Hogrefe.

Heckhausen, H. (1969). Förderung der Lernmotivierung und der intellektuellen Tüchtigkeiten. In H. Roth (Ed.), *Begabung und Lernen: Ergebnisse und Folgerungen neuer Forschungen* (pp. 193–228). Stuttgart: Klett.

Heckhausen, H. (1977). Motivation: Kognitionspsychologische Aufspaltung eines summarischen Konstrukts. *Psychologische Rundschau, 28,* 175–189.

Heckhausen, H. (1980). *Motivation und Handeln: Lehrbuch der Motivationspsychologie.* Berlin: Springer-Verlag.

Henry, J., & Stephens, P. (1977). *Stress, health and the social environment: A sociobiologic approach to medicine.* New York: Springer-Verlag.

Kirmayer, L. J. (1987). Languages of suffering and healing: Alexithymia as a social and cultural process. *Transcultural Psychiatric Research Review, 24*(2), 119–136.

Kuhl, J. (1983a). *Motivation, Konflikt und Handlungskontrolle.* Berlin: Springer-Verlag.

Kuhl, J. (1983b). Emotion, Kognition und Motivation: II. Die funktionale Bedeutung der Emotionen für das problemlösende Denken und für das konkrete Handeln. *Sprache und Kognition*, 2, 228–253.

Kuhl, J. (1987). Action control: The maintenance of motivational states. In F. Halisch & J. Kuhl (Eds.), *Motivation, intention, and volition* (pp. 279–291). Berlin: Springer-Verlag.

Kuhl, J. (1994a). A theory of action and state orientation. In J. Kuhl & J. Beckmann (Eds.), *Volition and personality* (pp. 9–46). Göttingen: Hogrefe.

Kuhl, J. (1994b). Handlungs- und Lageorientierung. In W. Sarges (Ed.), *Managementdiagnostik* (2nd ed.). Göttingen: Hogrefe.

Kuhl, J., & Beckmann, J. (1994). Alienation: Ignoring one's preferences. In J. Kuhl & J. Beckmann (Eds.), *Volition and personality* (pp. 375–390). Göttingen: Hogrefe.

Kuhl, J., & Eisenbeisser, T. (1986). Mediating versus nonmediating cognitions in human motivation: Action control, inertial motivation, and the alienation effect. In J. Kuhl & J. W. Atkinson (Eds.), *Motivation, thought, and action* (pp. 288–306). New York: Praeger.

Markus, H. (1977). Self-schemata and processing information about the self. *Journal of Personality and Social Psychology*, 35, 63–78.

Martin, J. B., & Pihl, R. O. (1985). The stress–alexithymia hypothesis: Theoretical and empirical considerations. *Psychotherapy and Psychosomatics*, 43, 169–176.

Martin, J. B., & Pihl, R. O. (1986). Influence of alexithymic characteristics on physiological and subjective stress responses in normal individuals. *Psychotherapy and Psychosomatics*, 45, 66–77.

Merz, J. (1984). Erfahrungen mit der Selbstaufmerksamkeitsskala von Fenigstein, Scheier und Buss (1975). *Psychologische Beiträge*, 26, 239–249.

Meyer, W. U. (1972). *Überlegungen zur Konstruktion eines Fragebogens zur Erfassung von Selbstkonzepten der Begabung.* Unpublished manuscript, Psychological Institute, University of the Ruhr, Bochum, Germany.

Meyer, W. U. (1973). *Leistungsmotiv und Ursachenerklärung von Erfolg und Misserfolg.* Stuttgart: Klett.

Obrist, P. A. (1976). The cardiovascular behavioral interaction as it appears today. *Psychophysiology*, 13, 85–107.

Obrist, P. A., Gaebelein, C. J., Shanks-Teller, E., Langer, A. W., Grignolo, A., Light, K. C., & McCubbin, J. A. (1978). The relationship between heart rate, carotid $dP/dt$, and blood pressure in humans as a function of the type of stress. *Psychophysiology*, 15, 102–115.

Rogers, C. R. (1942). *Counseling and psychotherapy.* Boston: Houghton Mifflin.

Rogers, C. R. (1951). *Client-centered therapy.* Boston: Houghton Mifflin.

Rogers, C. R. (1959). A theory of therapy, personality and interpersonal relationships as developed in the client-centered framework. In S. Koch (Ed.), *Psychology: A study of science* (Vol. 3, pp. 184–256). New York: McGraw-Hill.

Sachse, R. (1990). Schwierigkeiten im Explizierungsprozess psychosomatischer Klienten: Zur Bedeutung von Verstehen und Prozessdirektivität. *Zeitschrift für klinische Psychologie, Psychopathologie und Psychotherapie*, 38, 191–205.

Sachse, R. (1991). Probleme und Potentiale in der gesprächspsychotherapeutischen Behandlung psychosomatischer Klienten. In J. Finke & L. Teusch (Eds.), *Gesprächspsychotherapie bei Neurosen und psychosomatischen Erkrankungen* (pp. 197–215). Heidelberg: Asanger.

Sachse, R. (1992a). *Zielorientierte Gesprächspsychotherapie: Eine grundlegende Neukonzeption.* Göttingen: Hogrefe.

Sachse, R. (1992b). Zielorientiertes Handeln in der Gesprächspsychotherapie: Zum tatsächlichen und notwendigen Einfluss von Therapeuten auf die Explizierungsprozesse bei Klienten. *Zeitschrift für klinische Psychologie, 21,* 286–301.

Sachse, R. (1993). Gesprächspsychotherapie mit psychosomatischen Klienten: Die Explizierung der Krankheitslehre der GT auf der Ebene eines sprachpsychologischen Modells. In L. Teusch & J. Finke (Eds.), *Krankheitslehre der Gesprächspsychotherapie: Neue Beiträge zur theoretischen Fundierung* (pp. 173–193). Heidelberg: Asanger.

Sachse, R. (1994a). Herzschlagwahrnehmung bei psychosomatischen Patienten: Abwendung der Aufmerksamkeit von eigenen Körperprozessen. *Psychotherapie, Psychosomatik, medizinische Psychologie, 44,* 284–292.

Sachse, R. (1994b). Veränderungsprozesse im Verlauf Klientenzentrierter Behandlung psychosomatischer Patienten. In K. Pawlik (Ed.), *39. Kongress der Deutschen Gesellschaft für Psychologie* (pp. 601–602). Hamburg: Psychological Institute I, University of Hamburg.

Sachse, R. (1995a). Zielorientierte Gesprächspsychotherapie: Effektive psychotherapeutische Strategien bei Klienten und Klientinnen mit psychosomatischen Magen-Darm-Erkrankungen. In J. Eckert (Ed.), *Forschung zur Klientenzentrierten Psychotherapie: Aktuelle Ansätze und Ergebnisse* (pp. 27–49). Cologne: GwG.

Sachse, R. (1995b). *Der psychosomatische Klient in der Praxis.* Stuttgart: Kohlhammer.

Sachse, R. (1996). *Praxis der Zielorientierten Gesprächspsychotherapie.* Göttingen: Hogrefe.

Sachse, R., & Atrops, A. (1991). Schwierigkeiten psychosomatischer Klienten bei der Klärung eigener Emotionen und Motive: Mögliche Konsequenzen für die therapeutische Arbeit. *Psychotherapie, Psychosomatik, medizinische Psychologie, 41,* 155–198.

Sachse, R., Lietaer, G., & Stiles, W. B. (1992). *Neue Handlungskonzepte der Klientenzentrierten Psychotherapie.* Heidelberg: Asanger.

Sachse, R., & Maus, C. (1991). *Zielorientiertes Handeln in der Gesprächspsychotherapie.* Stuttgart: Kohlhammer.

Sachse, R., & Rudolph, R. (1992a). Selbstaufmerksamkeit bei psychosomatischen Patienten. *Zeitschrift für klinische Psychologie, Psychopathologie und Psychotherapie, 40,* 146–164.

Sachse, R., & Rudolph, R. (1992b). Gesprächspsychotherapie mit psychosomatischen Klienten?: Eine empirische Untersuchung auf der Basis der Theorie der Objektiven Selbstaufmerksamkeit. In M. Behr, U. Esser, F. Petermann, W. M. Pfeiffer, & R. Tausch (Eds.), *Jahrbuch für Personenzentrierte Psychologie und Psychotherapie* (Vol. 3, pp. 66–84). Cologne: GwG-Verlag.

Seleye, H. (1946). The general adaptation syndrome and the diseases of adaptation. *Journal of Clinical Endocrinology, 6,* 117–230.

Selye, H. (1981). Geschichte und Grundzüge des Stresskonzeptes. In J. R. Nitsch (Ed.), *Stress* (pp. 163–187). Vienna: Huber.

Shands, H. C. (1977). Suitability for psychotherapy: II. Unsuitability and psychosomatic disease. *Psychotherapy and Psychosomatics, 21,* 28–35.

Snyder, M. (1974). Self-monitoring of expressive behaviour. *Journal of Personality and Social Psychology*, 30, 526–537.

Snyder, M. (1979). Self-monitoring processes. In L. Berkowitz (Ed.), *Advances in experimental social psychology* (Vol. 12, pp. 86–131). New York: Academic Press.

Tönnies, S., (1986). Die Bedeutung der Alexithymie-Diagnose für die Verhaltenstherapie psychosomatisch Erkrankter. In A. Schnorr (Ed.), *Bericht über den 13. Kongress für angewandte Psychologie* (Vol 2, pp. 158–163). Bonn: Deutscher Psychologenverlag.

Tönnies, S., Gades, H., & Pieper-Raether, M. (1987). Die Effekte verhaltenstherapeutischer Gruppen mit psychosomatischen Patienten unter besonderer Berücksichtigung alexithymen Verhaltens. *Verhaltensmodifikation und Verhaltensmedizin*, 8, 193–211.

Tress, W. (1979). Die diagnostische Bedeutung der "Alexithymie": Eine vergleichende Untersuchung an vier Gruppen neurosenpsychologisch verschiedener Erkrankungstypen. *Medizinische Psychologie*, 5, 95–106.

Voigt, K. H., & Fehm, H. L. (1990). Psychoendokrinologie. In Th. von Uexküll (Ed.), *Psychosomatische Medizin* (pp. 153–167). Munich: Urban & Schwarzenberg.

# 14

\*\*\*\*\*

# Experiential Psychodrama with Sexual Trauma

## M. Katherine Hudgins

*The effects of childhood* sexual trauma (CST) present both conceptual and treatment challenges to the practicing clinician (Beutler & Hill, 1992; Briere, 1992; Green, 1993; Terr, 1991). The particular clinical configuration that has gained prominence—denial and/or flooding of body sensations, distorted perceptual processes, interruptions in information processing, dissociated intense affects, primitive defenses, and behavioral reenactments—points to the use of experiential psychotherapy as a treatment method of choice with patients with a history of severe trauma, specifically sexual abuse (Ellenson, 1986; Gelinas, 1983). Experiential psychotherapy targets interventions directly at the somatic, perceptual, cognitive, affective, adaptive, and behavioral processes that are of a critical nature in healing for these patients (Courtois, 1988; Ratican, 1992; Van der Kolk, 1996, 1997).

While classical psychodrama has the power to treat core trauma, many clinicians do not use experiential methods with survivors of sexual trauma because of the potential for uncontrolled regression or retraumatization. To avoid these pitfalls the therapist must always emphasize safety and utilize clinical judgment and modify classical psychodramatic methods as needed. While there has been little empirical research on psychodrama specifically with sexual trauma (Altman, 1993; Burge, 1996; Reynolds, 1996; Wilkins, 1997), the model presented in this chapter has been developed carefully over 15 years of clinical practice with survivors of sexual trauma and eating disorders, as well as in discussion with the clinicians who have participated on our treatment teams (Hudgins, 1989; Hudgins, in press; Widlake, 1997). Patient's self-reports, therapists' assessments, and videotapes of actual psychodrama sessions substantiate the effectiveness and safety of this approach.

A number of recent theoretical and empirical studies do validate many of the psychodramatic interventions and therapeutic constructs used in this model (Blatner & Blatner, 1988; Buchanan, 1984; Holmes, 1992; Hudgins & Kiesler, 1987; Kellerman, 1992; Kipper, 1989, 1992). Recent research also documents clearly that group psychotherapy is often the preferred method of treatment with sexual trauma (Mennen & Meadow, 1992; van der Kolk, McFarlane, & Weisaeth, 1996).

This chapter presents clinical goals, the use of an Action Trauma Team, types of reexperiencing dramas, and advanced action interventions (Hudgins, 1993b, Hudgins & Drucker, in press). A composite transcript of a psychodrama session also walks the reader through the steps of conscious reexperiencing developed to prevent uncontrolled regression and retraumatization (Hudgins, 1993a)

## THEORETICAL FRAMEWORK OF PSYCHODRAMA

Psychodramatic techniques seek to tangibly present all aspects of the client's internal experience, both verbal and nonverbal (Blatner, 1996; Dayton, 1997; Hare & Hare, 1996). Concretization and enactment are the main tools to produce new experience in psychodrama (Moreno, 1977; Moreno & Moreno, 1969). Concretization covers the use of expressive arts materials, visualization, projective objects, and personification of abstract qualities. Enactment includes role playing of parts of self, significant others, and various living beings such as dogs or cats.

Psychodrama changes experience in the here and now so that sensations, perceptions, images, feelings, and behaviors from the past can be accessed and modified at the core level (Blatner, 1997; Holmes, 1992). Developmental repair is a key ingredient of change. What did not happen in the past—a comforting mother, a protective father—can be created in psychodrama so that the new experience can be integrated into new meaning structures.

## STRUCTURE OF A PSYCHODRAMA SESSION

A psychodrama session consists of warm-up, action, and sharing (Remer, 1997). The warm-up focuses the group's attention on a certain theme or process and may include structured experiential tasks. For example, the therapist/director (in psychodrama, the therapist is called the director) might begin the group by asking group members to "draw their trauma" on a piece of paper and discuss how that felt in dyads. Action begins when a client chooses to be the protagonist for the session. The protagonist is the person who enacts a personal story using other group members to role play significant others and abstract qualities. Sharing of group members' experience ends the psychodrama.

In classical psychodrama the first scene is an assessment of the problem in the here and now (Goldman & Morrison, 1990). For example, a protagonist with a history of CST began by describing and enacting how emotion-laden, intrusive memory fragments interrupted a conversation with her boyfriend. The protagonist picked another group member to be her boyfriend and demonstrated how he responded to her when they were at a restaurant. Group members enacted internal roles for the protagonist, such as "the voice inside telling me I'll get hurt" and "the feeling of turning into a little child—I'm so scared."

Additional scenes are guided by clinical judgment of what aspect of the protagonist's reality needs to be experienced, explored, expressed, and processed. In this case, we followed the thread of primary affect and changed the enactment from the scene with her boyfriend to a scene with the teacher who sexually abused her at age eight. Exploring this earlier scene allowed the protagonist to adaptively release primary feelings that had been dissociated, allowing new meaning structures to emerge from the new experience in the psychodrama.

The final scene in a psychodrama is one of developmental repair and can let the protagonist experience a healing scene that did not happen in life. Here the protagonist watched as a group member played her mother confronting the teacher and reporting him to the principal. With these new experiences, the protagonist gained a sense of self-protection and being cared for by a "good enough mother" that changed her core sense of self as well as her cognitive and emotional schemes for the future.

Additionally, role training can be practiced for the future. This protagonist created the role of "calm self-supporter" and practiced saying, "This is the present. I am here with John, not that teacher. I can breathe and look at John and feel safe and calm today."

Sharing is the final stage in the structure of a psychodrama session. It is important that all group members verbally share what they experienced during the drama in order to cognitively anchor new awareness and/or adaptively release feelings. The man who played the protagonist's boyfriend shared that he is a survivor of CST and that this role helped him understand what his partner experiences with him. The group member who played the protective mom shared that she found out that her mother probably wanted to protect her from her uncle's abuse but that she didn't know how. Sharing helps integrate the protagonist back into the therapeutic community by connecting her story with others' experiences.

## CLINICAL THERAPEUTIC GOALS

### Goal 1: Establish Intrapsychic Roles of Safety and Build Interpersonal Connections among Group Members to Support Enactment

The protagonist must be safely anchored into the interpersonal support of the group as well as connected to an experiential sense of personal safety.

Even if the protagonist does not spontaneously produce roles of safety, the director prescribes them prior to further enactment. As director, I say to the protagonist who wants to enact a confrontation or uncover further memories, "Well, OK, but let's begin by building a safe place to do that. Pick someone to be the part of your self that is healthy, whole, and supportive. What roles/parts of self do we need here with you to be able to confront your uncle?" Positive roles need to be available to the director and protagonist when needed for containment (Hudgins & Drucker, in press).

Concretizing interpersonal roles also increases safety for the protagonist. Putting in a supportive friend or "good enough mother" gives the protagonist permission to explore unknown areas with less fear. If he or she has difficulty accessing personal roles of intrapsychic safety or interpersonal support, the director can also intervene with the suggestion that the protagonist bring his or her spirituality in for additional support. For many people in 12-step programs this is a known and valued role.

## Goal 2: Structure Enactment to Promote Regression in the Service of the Ego in Order to Access Dissociated Material while Preventing Retraumatization

In psychodrama scenes, the protagonist can return to the original traumatic moment when fixation in self-development occurred. Intense dissociated primary affect can be adaptively released, supported by the director's clinical judgment and the protagonist's informed consent, resulting in changes to meaning structures. Added spontaneity and creativity support this regression in the service of the ego by providing roles that were not available at the time of trauma.

An important issue requiring clinical assessment is the following: Does the protagonist have enough positive roles and adaptive capacity to stay conscious and able to observe the action while reexperiencing a core trauma scene? If so, the psychodrama progresses to the original trauma scene by following the *principles of conscious reexperiencing with developmental repair* (Hudgins, 1993a), discussed in a later section of this chapter. Unprocessed emotion-laden experiences become consciously experienced and are integrated into present reality step by step with the support of a trained clinical team to prevent retraumatization.

## Goal 3: Enact Original Core Trauma Scenes so That the Protagonist Can Consciously Reexperience Dissociated Material for the Purpose of Developmental Repair

The clinical question when one is conducting conscious reexperiencing of core trauma scenes is this: In which role does the protagonist need to experience developmental repair? Psychodrama scenes can focus on self-repair where one or more parts of the self or internal role relationships enact a dialogue and find a compromise solution for co-consciousness and/or integration. An auxiliary can create a healing experience of the "good enough father," "the friend who never leaves," or "the forgiving god." For others, a present-centered scene of interpersonal support from the group members themselves may be the moment of developmental repair.

There is a theoretical and clinical rationale for a protagonist to reexperience original trauma scenes from the role of the child who actually experienced the horror. Due to state-dependent learning, dissociated material must be accessed through the state in which it was learned. Primary emotions must be released and cognitive structures changed from the point of the original decision making. This level of conscious reexperiencing is always done with the support of a "containing double," the protagonist's positive roles, and full informed consent to prevent retraumatization.

The developmental repair scene must always be generated from the protagonist and be congruent with the individual set of internal object relations. This repair scene is never contrived or forced by the director. The protagonist's spontaneity creates what is needed for repair and healing.

## USE OF AN ACTION TRAUMA TEAM

As the clinical work I did with sexual trauma survivors became more experiential, I found these methods to be exceptionally healing and simultaneously found the need for structure imperative to prevent retraumatization. This level of depth required a team, so the Action Trauma Team was developed to guide the safe reexperiencing of core traumatic material with modified psychodramatic methods.

The Action Trauma Team includes a director, an assistant leader, and a minimum of two trained auxiliary egos. Each clinician is educated in traditional methods of healing—medicine, psychology, social work, counseling, education—with postgraduate training in psychodrama, sociometry, and group psychotherapy. All team members are board certified as Practitioners or Trainers of Psychodrama, Sociometry, and Group Psychotherapy or are working on these national graduate certification levels under clinical supervision. Team leaders are certified at the national level as Trainers in Psychodrama and Group Psychotherapy.

### Director/Team Leader

The therapist uses her/his clinician skills in the role of psychodrama director to provide safety and guide enactment for the protagonist, group, and team. The director assesses the protagonist's strengths and self-support and makes directing decisions based on clinical knowledge of diagnosis, adaptive functioning, treatment planning, timing, and goals of the session. She/he contracts with protagonist and group for the type of reexperiencing drama and establishes safety precautions needed for enactment and expression of intense emotion and dissociated material prior to action. The director then concretizes trauma scenes using the step-by-step principles of conscious reexperiencing with developmental repair (discussed later). She/he adeptly utilizes the Action Trauma Team to provide containment of experiencing and support affective expression as clinically indicated.

## Assistant Leader

The role of assistant leader (AL) was developed to provide extra clinical support to the director, protagonist, and other group members. It is a team effort to allow the protagonist to enact the chaos of the inner symbolic world while integrating group members who may become triggered into their own unconscious material. The AL is the gatekeeper between the spontaneous action of the audience and the enactment by the director and protagonist, and, like the director, utilizes clinical skills to prevent retraumatization.

The AL assesses group members' levels of personal safety, positive roles, and interpersonal support throughout the drama and intervenes for containment or expansion of intense affect and/or dissociation. She/he codirects the trained auxiliary egos to implement the director's interventions through use of the team. The AL integrates spontaneous auxiliary roles from group members and team members and makes therapeutic role assignments.

## Trained Auxiliary Egos

Trained auxiliary egos (TAEs) are a rich resource for the protagonist and group alike when they are reexperiencing past trauma scenes, promoting adaptive release of primary affect, and achieving developmental repair. TAEs provide structure for safety, expansion, and integration. For example, often while the protagonist is disclosing abuse, an audience member will start to shake and cry. In this case, a TAE will sit beside the group member and intervene with specific gentle instructions to reduce the intensity of the primary emotion that has been triggered.

Trained auxiliaries also support exploration and release of primary affect that has been stored in unconscious awareness. When directed to do so by the AL, a TAE stands beside the protagonist and gives encouragement in a role such as the "best friend" and says, "It's OK to express your feelings. You can handle it. You are not alone here." Intense primary emotion is then released with conscious support and is not only a purging of dissociated affect but integrated into future meanings.

A third function of the TAE is to promote cognitive integration of affect at the moment of emotional release. Emotional expression of dissociated affect can result in time distortion and uncontrolled regression, placing the trauma survivor at risk of retraumatization. To prevent this from happening, a TAE stands beside the protagonist and supports a level of conscious awareness with statements from the cognitive role of the self when directed to do so by the AL—for example, "I can feel my rage and also remember what it is about now as I express it. I can stay present and say what I mean." By making cognitive statements while the protagonist is in the process of intense affect, the TAE helps keep the dual awareness of emotion and thought alive and integrated into new meaning structures.

## TYPES OF REEXPERIENCING DRAMAS

The types of reexperiencing dramas are a further structure developed in this approach to prevent retraumatization (Hudgins, 1993b). Each type of drama has a contract, clinical session goals, and action descriptions to guide experiential methods of treatment.

### Renewal and Restoration

*Session goal:* To access the protagonist's active experience of a sense of personal and collective renewal and restoration.

*Action description:* In this first and most general type of drama, the protagonist contracts to focus on building and experiencing positive roles in order to build strength to (1) begin the work of uncovering, (2) get refueled during the process, and/or (3) celebrate termination and progress. This is an often overlooked though very necessary type of drama when one is working with trauma survivors, who need the positive role development to balance out the attentional focus on traumatic roles, intense primary affect, and problematic interpersonal relationships.

### Dreams and Metaphors

*Session goal:* To explore unconscious symbols of past trauma that are projected into dreams, metaphors, or myths as the vehicle for increased awareness and change in meaning structures.

*Action description:* When the protagonist contracts for a drama to enact a dream or metaphor, the director keeps the enactment at the level of symbolic projections. Relying on this contract for structure maintains a level of safety for the protagonist. Many survivors report becoming consciously aware of childhood trauma for the first time through recurring dream images that contain elements of trauma. Dissociated thoughts, feelings, defenses, and behaviors will, no doubt, intrude upon the symbolic projections concretized in dreams and metaphors, but the director must not be tempted to follow the strands of unconscious awareness to deeper levels of experiencing. A metaphor may also yield unconscious fragments of dissociated material in a safe and abstract manner.

## Initial Discovery and Accurate Labeling of Core Trauma

*Session goal:* To enact partially conscious memories, feelings, and behaviors, in order to connect them with accurate meaning arising from the client's own experiential awareness and processing.

*Action description:* The contract is not for emotional expression, but for the emergence of experiential meaning and new narrative labels. The protagonist enacts consciously remembered experiences—thoughts, images, feelings, behaviors, even ego states—for the purpose of exploration and clarification. The protagonist explores his/her internal reality and works with primitive images, defenses, and feelings, all of which promotes working through of perceptual distortions and inaccurate labeling of past experience. Doing it in a group setting both lifts shame and presents an immediate opportunity for feedback from others.

## Uncovering and Exploring of Core Trauma

*Session goal:* To access, consciously reexperience, express, and work through unconscious elements of the core trauma scene for the purpose of memory retrieval, emotional processing, and integration into information processing systems.

*Action description:* The protagonist contracts to find the unconscious affect and meaning behind repetitive trauma symptoms after sufficient spontaneity, positive roles, adaptive strategies, and interpersonal support are established. The director and protagonist begin with some conscious fragment of memory—demonstrated in the body, mind, emotions, defenses, and behaviors—and contract to move into active experiencing and expression of unconscious awareness. The use of an Action Trauma Team is necessary for clinical safety when uncovering and exploring dramas are conducted, as well as dramas where the contract is for conscious reexperiencing.

## Conscious Reexperiencing and Developmental Repair

*Session goal:* To support the protagonist to consciously reexperience all aspects of past trauma in order to retrieve, express, and process unconscious material to achieve developmental repair.

*Action description:* During the action of this type of drama, the protagonist contracts to reexperience core trauma scenes with the safety of positive and prescriptive roles available to prevent retraumatization. After the core trauma scene is experienced, primary affect is expressed, and new meanings made, the final scene is one of developmental repair.

This level of psychodramatic enactment should only be performed by an experienced protagonist who has the spontaneity, adaptive functioning, and group support needed for conscious reexperiencing of the full horror of trauma. When the protagonist and group are ready, it is very healing to honor the true intensity of the past and find new creative solutions in the present.

# ADVANCED ACTION INTERVENTIONS WITH TRAUMA

Several modifications of classical psychodramatic interventions are detailed below to increase safety and treatment effectiveness when one is working with survivors of sexual trauma. All of the presented interventions are woven into the clinical vignette that follows. A fuller description of the role structure and manualized interventions used to guide action with trauma survivors is found elsewhere (Hudgins, in press).

## The Containing Double

When working with trauma, a group member takes the role of the "containing double" (a modification of the classical double), an inner voice of the protagonist, and is instructed to only make affirming, supportive, and healing statements using "I" such as "I know that this is difficult, and I know that today I can take some small steps toward my healing" or "I know that today this is a safe group and I can tell a little bit of my story." The containing double supplies internal support and cognitive balance when needed by the protagonist. The technique is further defined and operationalized elsewhere (Hudgins, Drucker, & Metcalf, 1998).

## Concretizing the Observing Ego

The protagonist can be role reversed into an observing-ego role to prevent uncontrolled regression at any given moment. The director asks the protagonist to take the role of her/his observing ego while a trained auxiliary takes the role of protagonist who is slipping into the trauma scene from the past. The director asks, "What do you see happening now with yourself? How can we slow your feelings down?" And the protagonist in the observing role answers, "I see myself slipping into the past, but I know I can feel the support of my 'containing double' and stay present even though I'm terrified." The balance of experiencing and observing roles keeps primary affects from overwhelming cognitive functions and prevents retraumatization.

## Holder of Dissociation

A third intervention that helps prevent retraumatization is to have someone take the role of "holder of the dissociation" for the protagonist. There is a paradox in enacting the role of holding dissociation that decreases dissociation and creates consciousness. This group or team member is instructed to make statements such as "I can feel myself floating up to the ceiling, but I can stay here" to alert both the protagonist and director that dissociation is increasing. The protagonist can also be role reversed into this role for assessment and distance from the trauma if indicated.

### Role Reversal with the Victim and Perpetrator Roles

In this approach, trained auxiliaries (TAEs) are initially used for victim and perpetrator roles unless, through careful assessment of group members' strengths, the director determines that it is therapeutic that the protagonist and/or other group members take these roles.

### *Enacting the Role of Victim*

The victim/child role holds the primary emotions that were experienced but not expressed during the original trauma—terror, horror, rage, shame, despair. These primary emotions are usually well known to the protagonist, who may collapse into them early on in the drama. If this happens, a TAE is brought in to enact this role and free up the protagonist for other positive roles.

However, the child role may be enacted by the protagonist when there is sufficient strength, support, and positive roles to uncover and explore core trauma material that is unconscious. A TAE then supports the protagonist in this role so that she/he is not alone (as she/he was in the original trauma). Enactment of this role can allow memory retrieval to happen, intense affect to be released, and healing to occur.

It is in this child/victim role that the protagonist needs to be rescued and protected, which often occurs from the role of "observing ego" or one of the "positive strengths." The director does not allow the protagonist in any child role to fight or confront the perpetrator. That would be recapitulating the original trauma because of the powerlessness of that role, but as you can see there are clinical indications for when and how to enact the child role.

### *Enacting the Role of Perpetrator*

The perpetrator role is also concretized in psychodrama with trauma survivors, but initially the role is enacted by a TAE in this model. The enactment of the perpetrator role is structured in short experiences, so the warm-up to the role is broken into manageable experiential chunks. This structured role playing allows the protagonist the opportunity to master the role—without losing the observing ego to the experience of the perpetrator role.

The TAE develops the perpetrator role in response to the demonstrated strength of the protagonist so as not to overwhelm her/his adaptive capacities. This auxiliary enactment allows the protagonist to engage in interpersonal dialogue, confrontation, and healing as strength builds, affect is expressed, and new meanings emerge.

The protagonist can play perpetrator roles when there is enough containment to prevent uncontrolled regression. Clinical indications for enactment of the perpetrator role are (1) to gain accurate information about state dependent memories, (2) to work through idolization of the aggressor, and (3) to reintegrate personal power that the perpetrator role holds in the experiencing of self.

## PRINCIPLES OF CONSCIOUS REEXPERIENCING WITH DEVELOPMENTAL REPAIR

The principles of conscious reexperiencing with developmental repair were developed to guide the safe enactment of dramas dealing with unconscious trauma material (Hudgins, 1993a). Step by step the protagonist is guided to the core scene that ends with developmental repair. The steps are talk, observe, witness, reenact, reexperience, and repair and can be completed in a single protagonist's psychodrama or over a period of several dramas. The following subsections describe each step using one protagonist and details the director's clinical judgments.

### Talk

After a contract is negotiated for a "conscious reexperiencing" drama, the first step is for the protagonist to verbally describe the core scene to be enacted. Talking allows both the protagonist and the group to warm up to what they will see, hear, feel, and experience during the enactment, while the director and Action Trauma Team assess safety and plan ahead for interventions to control regression and dissociation.

In this example, the protagonist, Judy, states that she wants to reexperience a childhood scene where she was forced to have oral sex with the male neighbor next door when she was 5 years old in order to "make the pictures stop in my head."

DIRECTOR: Judy, Let's start by you telling us the scene you remember as if it is here in the present. What happens? How old are you?

JUDY: The man next door used to talk to us sometimes. One day he comes over and asks me if I want to see his new kittens? I say yes, and he takes my hand and leads me down the basement stairs. (*She stops and looks up at me with fear in her eyes.*)

DIRECTOR: Would you like a "containing double" to help? (*She picks Susan, who knows the role from previous group participation.*) OK, what happens next?

JUDY: Just as we get to the bottom of the stairs, he pushes me ahead into the wall. He grabs my ponytail and puts his hand over my mouth. I start to cry. I'm so scared. I want my mommy. (*She starts to become teary eyed in the session.*)

CONTAINING DOUBLE: It's OK, I can say what I remember. I'm scared, but I'm not alone now. It's not happening now, I'm only talking about it to the group.

JUDY: (*Takes a deep breath.*) Yes, I can talk about it now . . . (*pause*). He whispers that he will take his hand off my mouth if I stop crying. No noise, just do what he says and then I can go home. He says not to tell anyone what happens here or he'll kill my dog and tell mommy I am a bad girl and she won't love me anymore . . . (*pause*). I nod OK. He jerks me around and makes me sit down against the wall. (*Starts crying again.*)

CONTAINING DOUBLE: I'm OK, these are normal feelings. I was little and scared then, but I am an adult now . . .

JUDY: Yes, I am scared. He starts unzipping his pants and his thing comes out (*speaking rapidly*). It's big and red and he pushes it at me . . . against my head . . . in my face. Then he kneels down and grabs my cheeks and squeezes . . . really hard and says I better open up and do as he says or my dog is dead. (*Starts coughing and crying and a group member brings her a glass of water.*)

CONTAINING DOUBLE: I can breathe and take a drink of water. I'm OK. I'm here on the psychodrama stage and I'm OK. I can feel scared, and I still feel safe.

JUDY: (*Takes a deep breath and drinks a sip of water.*) Yeh, I'm OK. The water helps. Anyway . . . he is hurting my mouth so I have to open it up and . . . he pushes it in . . . just keeps doing it (*voice gets little girlish and goes up in pitch*) 'til . . . 'til . . . (*pause*) . . . 'til it's yucky all in my mouth (*speaking rapidly*). I want to throw up. I want to go home. He throws a dirty shirt at me and tells me to clean up, go home and never tell anyone or I know what will happen.

DIRECTOR: Then what happens? What do you do when you are so scared and so little?

JUDY: I go home and run and hide in the bushes. I just sit there in a little ball until my mommy lets Chris—our beagle—out, and he comes and licks my face and my mommy is calling me. I hug him and kiss him, and then I go inside for dinner. I don't tell her 'cause I love Chris and I don't want him to be hurt.

DIRECTOR: Take a breath. That's a lot to talk about. Let's walk around the stage (*to decrease affect and increase cognition*), and you tell me what you want to get out of the session today. What do you want when we go through this scene?

JUDY: This scene goes over and over in my head, especially at night when I'm trying to sleep and I want to stop it. Put a new ending on it. Can we do that?

DIRECTOR: Yes, we can. Step by step, we'll go back through what you just told us and you can stop the action whenever you want, change whatever you want. You are in control of what happens now. You'll have your containing double and other supports with you so you won't be alone.

## Observe

In the second step the protagonist sets up the scene with trained auxiliaries in the victim and perpetrator roles and group members in prescriptive roles of safety. We begin with the prescriptive roles to establish safety as part of the pretrauma scene and then move to the trauma scene itself. The goal is to have the scene set up on the stage and have the protagonist watch it for accuracy without affect added.

DIRECTOR: Before we concretize the scene you told us about, let's get some more help up here. Pick someone to be a support for you.

JUDY: Can I have my mommy up here?

DIRECTOR: You can have your mommy up here if that will help. The mother you have today, or the mommy from when you were little? Pick someone for the role you want.

JUDY: Evie, will you be my mommy? My mommy was a good mommy, and I know if I had told her what happened she would have protected me.

DIRECTOR: Evie, is that OK? Come up here and stand in the protagonist's space. Judy you role reverse and become your mommy when you were five. Be your mommy so Evie can see how she's supposed to be. What are you wearing? What are you like? Talk like mommy.

JUDY IN THE ROLE OF MOMMY: Judy, honey . . . I think there's something wrong. Do you want to tell me something? It's OK. I can hear you. Look, I have some Kleenex here in my apron.

DIRECTOR: Reverse roles and come back to your protagonist role. Evie, just remember those lines and stand there close to Judy 'til we see the scene she wants to tell you about. Do we need anyone else to help you?

JUDY: It's silly, but I want my dog, I want Chris here. He licked my face clean. He loved me no matter what.

DIRECTOR: Pick someone to be Chris.

JUDY: John, will you be Chris? (*She laughs.*) Chris used to howl . . . you know how beagles do? Ahh roo . . . with your nose up in the air.

DIRECTOR: (*Does not role reverse into this role as she has already increased the experience of safety with her laughter.*) Where do you want Chris to be? John, come up and let's hear you give a beagle howl!

JUDY: Laughing . . . good . . . that's good . . . you stay by your water bowl.

DIRECTOR: Now, let's pick someone to be your "observing ego." We want to make sure you have a part of you here that can observe at all times so you can make sense of this scene and not get overwhelmed with your feelings. Pick some one for that role.

JUDY: I'll pick Tim. Tim, you're always so serious. Can you be my observing ego?

DIRECTOR: Judy, reverse roles with Tim and enact your observing ego. Are you serious? Funny? What are you like as Judy's observing ego?

JUDY IN THE ROLE OF OBSERVING EGO: I can see whatever happens here. If it gets scary, I'll just move over to where Chris is, pet him, and we can watch together. I already know what happened anyway.

TIM AS OBSERVING EGO: (*Role reverses and starts off by Judy's side and slowly walks over to where Chris and the water bowl are.*) I can see whatever happens here. If there's a lot of feelings going on, I can pat Chris and we'll all be OK.

DIRECTOR: Now, let's move toward the scene itself. Where on the stage is the basement going to be? Where is the wall? Mark it off with some scarves, and put a scarf or a pillow for the wall (*this is for containment*).

DIRECTOR: (*Pretrauma scene is now complete, and the trauma scene is ready to be set up.*) Pick someone to be 5-year-old Judy and someone to be the neighbor next door. The trained auxiliaries can take these roles, or you can ask a group member.

JUDY: I'd like Ann (*a TAE who has a young, innocent face*) to be my little self. I had blond hair like that when I was five. And I want Stephen (*a TAE*) to be the guy next door. His name is Mr. M.

DIRECTOR: Now, Ann and Stephen, I want you to slowly walk through the scene just as Judy told it.

DIRECTOR: Judy . . . before little Judy and Mr. M come on stage, I want you to feel the support of your containing double, your mommy, Chris, and your observing ego. (*Judy gathers them all close to her; there's a brief pause.*) OK, Mr. M . . . go ahead. (*The scene is walked through slowly without any violence or sexual contact. When it is time for the push toward the wall, Stephen gently nudges Ann and she falls against the wall and sits down. When it is time for the oral sex scene, Stephen stands about a foot away from Ann, who is seated and moves his body slightly back and forth.*)

JUDY: (*As Mr. M says he'll kill her dog, she sits down and starts to pat Chris.*) I love you. I don't want anything to happen to you. That's why I didn't tell. I love you.

DIRECTOR: (*To decrease affect at this point.*) Reverse roles into your observing ego, and watch the rest of the scene from there.

## Witness

In the third step the protagonist witnesses the core trauma scene and moves into action. The director increases the spontaneity and affective expression in the scene by the TAEs, and the protagonist responds to the enactment of victimization from one of the positive roles on stage. Witnessing the past horror often results in the protagonist spontaneously rescuing the victim self. The protagonist must be able to demonstrate the ability to rescue the child self from the core trauma scene before the reexperiencing proceeds further in order to prevent retraumatization.

DIRECTOR: Judy, in this next part of consciously reexperiencing your trauma scene, you can witness it from any role you want for safety.

JUDY: I want to be in the role of my mommy. I wanted her there when it happened, and now she can be here today.

DIRECTOR: Judy, pick someone to be the adult you. (*She picks Cindy.*) Now, take the role of your mommy when you were five.

JUDY AS MOMMY: (*To adult Judy*) It's OK, I am here this time. I won't let you down. (*To little Judy*) It's OK, honey, I won't let him hurt you this time.

DIRECTOR: (*To TAEs*) Start the scene and play it with feeling this time. (*Affect is increased through movement, tempo, and voice tone.*)

JUDY AS MOMMY: (*Turns to adult Judy as Mr. M whispers that her mother won't love her.*) That's not true! If you had told me, I never would have stopped loving you. This is not right!

DIRECTOR: Mommy . . . tell that to Mr. M. Speak to him directly for little Judy.

JUDY AS MOMMY: (*Goes in and grabs Mr. M's arm and demonstrates ability to rescue self.*) Stop that . . . stop that . . . you leave my little girl alone. You are a dirty old man! I thought you were a friend of our family! Now I see what you were really like. You stop that! (*To little Judy*) Come here, honey . . . you're safe. Mommy won't let him hurt you.

DIRECTOR: (*To further expand the witnessing role and to check for introjection of the mother's caring.*) Judy, reverse roles back to your adult self. Evie, be mommy just like we saw, and Judy you respond from the adult role as mommy helps little Judy.

JUDY: (*Watches as Mommy goes in and brings little Judy out of the base-ment.*) Mommy, mommy, thank you. I knew you loved me. I knew you would help!

DIRECTOR: (*Assesses that she is in the child role and needs to develop the adult role a bit more.*) Judy . . . good, that is what the 5-year-old might say. What do you as the adult you are today say? Do you respond to your mother, to your little self, to Mr. M?

JUDY: (*Kneels down and embraces the TAE in the role of little Judy.*) It's OK. I've carried around that image of Mr. M hurting me for years and years, and now it's over. He can't hurt you again. Mommy took care of that. It's OK now. You don't have to keep going through that again and again.

## Reenact

This fourth step is the switch from the protagonist's experience of observing the scene to actively experiencing the roles of victim and perpetrator. This time Judy experiences the scene from the more vulnerable role of the child. Her containing double is always with Judy no matter what role, so retrauma-tization is prevented.

The director gives the protagonist a chance to "walk through" the en-actment from the wounded child/victim role before moving fully into reex-periencing. The director increases the level of active experiencing gradually so that there is a clear distinction between the processes of re-enactment and of reexperiencing with full informed consent.

DIRECTOR: Judy, this is good. You have rescued your child self from the role of good mommy and as your adult self. Often, as we step into reenact-ment and reexperiencing the protagonist or group may start "floating around the room," so I'd like you to pick someone to be the holder of dissociation for you (*prescriptive role*).

JUDY: I'll choose Gertrude. She's the most grounded person in the group, so maybe she can keep us all here.

DIRECTOR: Direct Gertrude in the role of "dissociation" to where you want her to be as we reenact the entire trauma scene. (*There is no role rever-sal here, as this is a preventive intervention and the protagonist is not showing dissociation.*)

JUDY: You can stand over by the wall there in the scene. When I see you, I can remember not to dissociate . . . that my goal is to stay present, feel what is here, make some meaning out of it all, so I can let it go.

DIRECTOR: Now, let's set up the scene. We are going to slowly walk through the entire scene as you originally described it, but you know there will not be any violence or sexual touching here. It is just a walk through, and you can stop at any time you want. OK?

## Reexperience

The fifth step deepens the protagonist's active experience of all roles in the drama—victim, perpetrator, self, mother—to reach a controlled regression, expression of primary affects, and changed perceptions.

After Judy walks through the core trauma scene from the role of the 5-year-old, she extends her active experiencing by going more fully into reexperiencing the vulnerability of being a child, but this time with support.

DIRECTOR: OK, Judy, you take the role of your 5-year-old self, and Ann, you stand beside her to support the role if she needs help.

LITTLE JUDY: (*Begins to dissociate almost immediately in the child role.*) I want my mommy . . . I'm scared . . . (*and then she is quiet and looks up to the ceiling*).

CONTAINING DOUBLE: I'm OK, I am in my psychodrama. I can see and feel what is happening to me as a little girl, and I can feel my hand on my double and I know Ann is here to support me. I'm scared and I'm determined to do this work and stop this memory.

HOLDER OF DISSOCIATION: I am holding the dissociation here. It's me that can't see and feel. You're OK, you can tolerate what you know . . . you have support.

LITTLE JUDY: Yes, I know where I am and that Ann is here. I can do this. I am OK. It's just really scary to be so little. (*Judy now goes back through the scene with her supports keeping her anchored in the dual awareness of past and present.*)

DIRECTOR: (*As the scenes ends and she runs up the stairs from the basement.*) Judy, little Judy, come here to your adult self and your mommy.

LITTLE JUDY: (*Rushes toward her mommy, embraces her, and starts crying.*) Mommy, mommy, he hurt me. He's a bad man. I love you. Do you love me?

MOMMY: Honey, of course I love you. I'm glad you're telling me about him, about what happened. Now we can keep you and Chris both safe.

DIRECTOR: Good, now come over here and take your adult role for a minute, and let's see what you have to say to little Judy.

JUDY: (*To Ann in the role of the 5-year-old*) See, he was wrong . . . mommy does love you, no matter what happened . . . and I love you too. It'll be OK from now on. No more images. No more bad guys.

In this psychodrama we did not have Judy take the role of the perpetrator, as the goal was to change the intrusive images, which was accomplished by expressing the dissociated primary affect and modifying the internal scheme of the original trauma.

## Repair

The final step in conscious reexperiencing is developmental repair. A healing scene emerges out of the action and must be congruent with the protagonist's models of self, others, and the world but is otherwise unlimited in creativity. In this example, the protagonist has already demonstrated the reparative scene of the mother rescuing the child self before the trauma occurs, so this is the scene that is set up.

DIRECTOR: Judy, we have one more step to complete. That is to go back into the scene one more time. But this time your mommy will come and rescue you as we have already seen . . .

JUDY IN CHILD ROLE: (*Goes along with Mr. M easily, but when she gets to the bottom of the stairs and falls against the wall she freezes.*) She says, I want my mommy.

MOMMY: (*Rushes into the scene.*) Get away from her. You can't hurt her. I love her. You are a dirty old man. I thought you were a friend of our family, but now I know better. (*Turns to little Judy.*) It's OK, honey, it's OK. I love you.

DIRECTOR: Little Judy, take all the time you need to feel your mommy taking care of you. (*When she indicates that she is complete by looking up toward the director, the director says to her.*) Now, role reverse into your adult self and let's finish this drama. How do you want to end? How do you want to rearrange all the parts of your self now that you have experienced your truth?

JUDY: Well, I am in the center (*adult role*). Chris is lying down at my feet. Little Judy is sitting down petting him, but also holding onto mommy's hand. Mommy is standing beside me, while she hold little Judy's hand. My observing ego and dissociation are linked together there off to the side still near the water bowl. And Mr. M is locked in the basement.

DIRECTOR: Take a moment to really look at this new self . . . Now we can have some sharing.

GROUP MEMBERS: (*Each group member now walks around the stage and deroles by saying his or her own name and then sitting in a circle to share the experience with the protagonist.*)

## DISCUSSION

One of the major strengths of this model is the emphasis on clinical safety. The structure provided by the types of reexperiencing dramas, principles of conscious reexperiencing with developmental repair, and modified psychodramatic techniques gives the clinician many new tools to contain and expand the experiential process. Using an Action Trauma Team allows both depth and containment to promote healing.

This psychodramatic approach provides an advantage over traditional verbal psychotherapy. What cannot be verbally expressed can be expressed in action, providing the perfect match for many of the symptoms of trauma survivors that cannot be expressed in words. As we have seen, perceptual, cognitive, affective, and behavioral processes can all be experienced, expressed, and processed into new meaning structures.

This psychodramatic model can be used in individual as well as group therapy settings. Individual sessions use one or two modified techniques directly targeted at a specific symptom. The model has been successfully adapted into small manageable chunks as well as expanded into an intensive workshop format.

Residential and inpatient settings allow full reexperiencing dramas to be completed with plenty of time for safety and the step-by-step process of controlled regression with conscious awareness. This model has also been expanded to working with other traumas—domestic violence, torture and trauma in political refugees, generational cultural trauma, eating disorders, and substance abuse.

While this modified psychodramatic model prevents retraumatization, there are many cautions to its use with severely traumatized individuals. First and foremost is the need for the clinician/director to be adequately trained in psychodramatic methods. Additionally, time and energy is always given to debriefing the Action Trauma Team so that they do not experience secondary posttraumatic stress disorder. When used by competent mental health professionals with advanced training in experiential methods, this psychotherapeutic approach provides a chance for profound healing in a brief period of time.

## REFERENCES

Altman, K. A. (1992). Psychodramatic treatment of multiple personality disorder and dissociative disorders. *Dissociation, 5*(2), 104–108.

Altman, K. A. (1993). Psychodrama in the treatment of post-abuse syndromes. *Treating Abuse Today, 2*(6), 27–31.

Beutler, L. E., & Hill, C. E. (1992). Process and outcome research in the treatment of adult victims of childhood sexual abuse: Methodological issues. *Journal of Consulting and Clinical Psychology, 60,* 204–212.

Blatner, A. D. (1996). *Acting-in: Practical applications of psychodramatic methods* (3rd ed.). New York: Springer.

Blatner, A. D. (1997). Psychodrama: State of the art. *The Arts in Psychotherapy, 24*(1), 23–30.

Blatner, H. A., & Blatner, A. (1988). *Foundations of psychodrama: History, theory, practice.* New York: Springer-Verlag.

Briere, J. (1992). *Child abuse trauma: Theory and treatment of the lasting effects.* Newbury Park, CA: Sage.

Buchanan, D. R. (1984). Psychodrama. In T. B. Karasau (Ed.), *The psychiatric therapies: Part II. The psychosocial therapies*. Washington, DC: American Psychiatric Association.

Burge, M. (1996). The Vietnam veteran and the family "both victims of post traumatic stress: A psychodramatic perspective." *The Journal of The Australian and New Zealand Psychodrama Association*, 5, 25–36.

Courtois, C. (1988). *Healing the incest wound: Adult survivors in therapy*. New York: Norton.

Dayton, T. (1997). *Heartwounds: Unresolved grief and trauma*. Deerfield Beach, FL: Health Communications, Inc.

Ellenson, G. S. (1986). Disturbances of perceptions in adult female incest survivors. *Social Casework*, 67, 147–159.

Gelinas, D. J. (1983). The persisting negative effects of incest. *Psychiatry*, 46, 312–332.

Goldman, E. E., & Morrison, D. S. (1984). *Psychodrama: Experience and process*. Dubuque, IA: Kendall/Hunt.

Green, A. H. (1993). Child sexual abuse: Immediate and long-term effects and intervention. *Journal of the American Academy of Child and Adolescent Psychiatry*, 32(5), 890–902.

Hare, P. A., & Hare, J. R. (1996). *J. L. Moreno*. London: Sage Publications.

Holmes, P. (1992). *The inner world outside: Object relations theory and psychodrama*. London: Tavistock/Routledge.

Hudgins, M. K. (1989). Experiencing the self through psychodrama and gestalt therapy in anorexia nervosa. In L. Hornyak & E. Baker (Eds.), *Experiential therapies with eating disorders*. New York: Guilford Press.

Hudgins, M. K. (1993a). Principles of conscious reexperiencing. In videotape: *Healing sexual trauma with action methods*. Madison, WI: Digital Recordings. (Monograph also available)

Hudgins, M. K. (1993b). Types of reexperiencing dramas. In videotape: *Healing sexual trauma with action methods*. Madison, WI: Digital Recordings. (Monograph also available)

Hudgins, M. K., Drucker, K., & Metcalf, K. (1998). *The Instructional Manual for the Containing Double Intervention Module*. Charlottesville, VA: The Center for Experiential Learning, Ltd.

Hudgins, M. K., & Kiesler, D. J. (1987). Individual experiential psychotherapy: An analogue validation of the intervention module of psychodramatic doubling. *Psychotherapy*, 24(2), 245–255.

Hudgins, M. K. (in press). *The therapeutic spiral model: An experiential practice approach to heal sexual trauma*. New York: Guilford Press.

Hudgins, M. K., & Drucker, K. (in press). The Therapeutic Spiral Model: Use of the containing double to prevent uncontrolled regression with trauma survivors. *The International Journal of Action Methods: Psychodrama, Skill Training and Role Playing. Special Edition on Trauma*.

Kellerman, P. F. (1992). *Focus on psychodrama: The therapeutic aspects of psychodrama*. London: Kingsley.

Kipper, D. A. (1989). Psychodrama research and the study of small groups. *International Journal of Small Group Research*, 5, 4–27.

Kipper, D. A. (1992). Psychodrama: Group psychotherapy through role playing. *International Journal of Group Psychotherapy*, 42(4), 495–521.

Mennen, F. E., & Meadow, D. (1992). Process to recovery: In support of long-term groups for sexual abuse survivors. *International Journal of Group Psychotherapy*, 42(4), 29–44.

Moreno, J. L. (1977). *Psychodrama* (Vol. 1). Beacon, NY: Beacon House.

Moreno, J. L., & Moreno, Z. T. (1969). *Psychodrama: Vol. 3. Action therapy and principles of practice*. Beacon, NY: Beacon House.

Ratican, K. (1992). Sexual abuse survivors: Identifying symptoms and special treatment considerations. *Journal of Counseling and Development*, 71, 33–38.

Remer, R. (1997). Chaos theory and the Hollander psychodrama curve: Trusting the process. *The International Journal of Action Methods: Psychodrama, Skill Training and Role Playing*, 50(2), 51–70.

Reynolds, T. (1996). Dissociative identity disorder and the psychodramatist. *The Journal of The Australian and New Zealand Psychodrama Association*, 5, 43–62.

Terr, L. C. (1991). Childhood traumas: An outline and overview. *American Journal of Psychiatry*, 148, 10–20.

van der Kolk, B. (1996). The body keeps score: Approaches to the psychobiology of posttraumatic stress disorder. In B. van der Kolk, A. McFarlane, & L. Weisaeth (Eds.), *Traumatic Stress: The effects of overwhelming experience on mind, body, and society*. New York: The Guilford Press.

van der Kolk, B. (1997). Keynote address. Presented at the annual conference of *The American Society of Group Psychotherapy and Psychodrama*, New York, NY.

van der Kolk, B. A., McFarlane, A. C., & Weisaeth, L. (Eds.). (1996). (Eds). *Traumatic stress: The effects of overwhelming experience on mind, body, and society*. New York: Guilford Press.

Widlake, B. (1997). Barbara's bubbles: The psychodrama of a young adult recovering from an eating disorder. *The British Journal of Psychodrama and Sociodrama*, 12(1–2), 23–43.

Wilkings, P. (1997). Psychodrama and research. *The British Journal of Psychodrama and Sociodrama*, 12(1–2), 44–61.

# 15

***

# The Treatment of Borderline Personality Disorder

## Jochen Eckert
## Eva-Maria Biermann-Ratjen

### THEORETICAL OUTLINE

Client-centered therapists assume that if a therapeutic process that leads to constructive changes in personality and behavior is to get under way, the therapist, as a representative of the real outside world, has to establish a certain kind of relationship with the client who is trying to understand or make sense of his/her own experiences. The therapist needs to empathize with the client and relate to him/her with unconditional positive regard; the therapist therefore needs to be congruent and not withhold any emotional reactions from consciousness.

Likewise according to client-centered thinking, patients taking part in group psychotherapy gain insight into how they relate to others. They discover that they too can empathize with other people and that others can empathize with them, and that their feelings and attitudes, the way they experience themselves and the outside world, may be respected by themselves.

The changes in personality and behavior that take place in psychotherapy are understood to be forms of self-development, that is, changes in the emotional value a person gives to experiences made in relationships. A successful psychotherapeutic process enables clients to relate to themselves in the way the therapist relates to them: to understand themselves and accept themselves with unconditional positive regard (see Biermann-Ratjen, Eckert, & Schwartz, 1995).

According to client-centered thinking, what applies to the process of self-development during psychotherapy equally applies to the process of self-development in early childhood. Developing a sense of self or identity depends on the baby gradually realizing that its significant others are showing empathy and unconditional positive regard for what it is experiencing, so that right from the beginning of life the child can come to believe or predict that any other experiences it may have will meet with similar support and approval (see Rogers, 1959, p. 199; Biermann-Ratjen, 1996).

So self-development begins with the anticipation of how another person will react to one's own experiencing. Client-centered therapists postulate that as soon as the self-concept has gained a first shape, there is a split in the meaning-making process. On the one hand, the organism as a whole continues to strive to make sense of what it is experiencing, integrating emotional experiences into the self-concept. On the other, the person tries to banish any experiences from consciousness that do not fit in with those integrated into the self-concept. Defending oneself against experiences that contradict the self-concept results in the state known as incongruence.

Over the past years it has become customary worldwide to diagnose patients as suffering from borderline personality disorder (BPD) if their experiencing meets the criteria outlined in Table 15.1.

In the psychoanalytic literature there are diverse theories on what brings about this syndrome. The most authoritative of these assume that it is the

---

**TABLE 15.1. DSM-IV Diagnostic Criteria for Borderline Personality Disorder**

A pervasive pattern of instability of interpersonal relationships, self-image, and affects, and marked impulsivity beginning by early adulthood and present in a variety of contexts, as indicated by five (or more) of the following:

(1) Frantic efforts to avoid real or imagined abandonment. **Note:** Do not include suicidal or self-mutilating behavior covered in Criterion 5.
(2) A pattern of unstable and intense interpersonal relationships characterized by alternating between extremes of idealization and devaluation.
(3) Identity disturbance: markedly and persistently unstable self-image or sense of self.
(4) Impulsivity in at least two areas that are potentially self-damaging (e.g., spending, sex, substance abuse, reckless driving, binge eating). **Note:** Do not include suicidal or self-mutilating behavior covered in Criterion 5.
(5) Recurrent suicidal behavior, gestures, or threats, or self-mutilating behavior.
(6) Affective instability due to a marked reactivity of mood (e.g., intense episodic dysphoria, irritability, or anxiety usually lasting a few hours and only rarely more than a few days).
(7) Chronic feelings of emptiness.
(8) Inappropriate, intense anger or difficulty controlling anger (e.g., frequent displays of temper, constant anger, recurrent physical fights).
(9) Transient, stress-related paranoid ideation or severe dissociative symptoms.

*Note.* From American Psychiatric Association (1994, p. 654). Copyright 1994 by the American Psychiatric Association. Reprinted by permission.

result of some fundamental disturbance in the relation between mother and child at a very early stage, more specifically during the phase when the child has developed the rudiments of a personal identity but is still highly dependent on the "mother's" emotional support.

Kernberg (1975) suggests that the borderline personality disorder sets in when very early, powerful, possibly even inborn, aggressive impulses have to be brought under control, as they seem to be a mortal threat to the person and his love objects. Mahler (1975) describes BPD as being fixed in the rapprochement phase, in which the child discovers that it is not omnipotent and is dependent on the help and affection of others. Searles (1958) sees the development of both schizophrenic and borderline symptoms as a sign not so much of rage stemming from disappointment or disillusionment but rather of the child's rejected love and admiration for its mother, which are vigorously warded off. In Wolberg's view (1973) BPD is the result of the child having to identify with a part of the parents that they themselves reject, thereby preventing the child from realizing this.

According to Rohde-Dachser (1995) the common factor in all these theories is that the pathological fixation comes about sometime during the second or third year:

> where the child already perceives the mother as a clearly separate object to itself and where its efforts to be autonomous in the anal phase have reached a climax. The child fails to achieve the autonomy it craves because one of the parents, usually the mother, misusing the child as a narcissistic extension of herself, actively refuses to permit this and because insults and disappointments which cannot be coped with at this stage prevent it developing further. . . . So there is a taboo on experiencing the whole realm of one's own impulses which include such elementary needs like the wish to give and receive love, the wish to be admired, to possess somebody, aggressive impulses and outgoing urges in general, including sexual desires. (p. 140)

In the client-centered context it is helpful to distinguish between three developmental phases in the course of which (e.g., according to Stern, 1985) the self develops into a structure that—

1. Can allow the felt sense of emotional experiences to develop and can symbolize or become aware of this, in conjunction with the physical relaxation which accompanies it
2. Enables the individual to realize that he/she is (a) the author of his/her experience (b) as a coherent being who (c) experiences his/her emotions as (d) one and the same being
3. Allows the individual to communicate his/her experiences as and if he/she wants to do so
4. Enables him/her to make sense of what he/she experiences by using words

During the first phase the process of integrating self-experiences into a rudimentary identity is entirely bound up with the baby's need for empathic and unconditional positive regard from significant others; if this need is satisfied, the child can then relax. Experiencing both this need and that it is satisfied are elements that become integrated into the core self. This in turn means that the self is the outcome of interpersonal relations.

During the second phase the feelings associated with evaluating each new experience—does it confirm or question the core self?—are also integrated, but only if the baby's experiences meet with empathy and unconditional positive regard.

Finally, in the third phase, the child's potential as an individual, experiencing the world for instance as a boy or a girl, can be added to create a distinct sense of self.

In our view BPD comes about because the empathic understanding the child required was not available during the second phase of development. If the feelings with which persons gauge their experience of themselves—surprise, fear or shame, and above all the desperate, frightening, and mortifying rage that wells up when the child cannot make itself understood or behave "acceptably" or cannot understand or accept itself—are not understood and accepted for what they are by significant others, the child will not be able to include them in its self-concept. As a consequence, whenever the same feelings are experienced later in life they will seem to challenge the person's idea of him-/herself and will be felt or symbolized as a personal threat. Bohart (1990) infers that borderline patients have grown up in "dangerous, chaotic or non-limit-setting environments" in which they have had no chance to develop "good differentiated and/or coherent 'maps' for functioning in certain important areas" (p. 615).

Patients suffering from BPD are likely to complain that they feel chronically bored or empty. When they are depressed, anxious, or irritable—and they feel these emotions very keenly—they have the impression that they are under assault from external enemies insinuating that they are worthless, wicked, or in mortal danger. The same applies to their so-called impulses to take care of themselves; these too seem like onslaughts from outside. Patients with BPD are chronically in a state of pent-up rage and deeply afraid of their own "impulses" to attack others or themselves, as these seem to threaten their whole personal identity.

Before looking more closely at our treatment of borderline patients it is important to stress that our psychotherapeutic approach is closely linked to the way we assume this disorder comes about. The American psychiatrist and psychoanalyst Otto F. Kernberg (1975) has argued that BPD is a disturbance in ego development. He has proposed that one of the central features of this disorder is a characteristic weakness in the defense functions that forces the patient to fall back on "primitive" forms of defense, in particular splitting and denial. This is accompanied by an internalized pattern of object relations in which both the self and the object are perceived exclusively in either/or terms of black or white; they are either "utterly good" or "utterly bad," without any shades of gray in between. As a result borderline patients oscillate between idealizing and denigrating themselves and others, and are victims of wild swings of mood. Above all they suffer from two feelings: deep anger and depression.

Kernberg dates the emergence of this ego disturbance in the second and third years of life, when an excessively high and, as he postulates, often in-born level of aggressiveness prevents the self and object introjects from losing their sharp division into good and bad and becoming integrated as a mixture of both. The split is strictly maintained to avoid at all costs contaminating the good self and object with the bad self and object. Borderline patients, according to Kernberg, find their own aggressive impulses so overwhelming and destructive that they assume they can only preserve their good, life-saving objects by protecting them from this rage. So the issues we are mostly confronted with when treating borderline patients are their intense, unstable relationships with other people, including the therapist, reflected in their efforts to avoid feeling angry by falling back on mechanisms such as splitting and denial.

As we have already mentioned, in the literature one finds several contrasting explanations for how this deep anger comes about. One position, which we would like to term the drive hypothesis, is, as already hinted, shared by Kernberg (1975). He sees the genetic roots of the borderline structure in a possibly inborn level of pregenital aggressiveness that is unusually high and cannot be dealt with properly during the appropriate phase. Under its influence there is an "premature oedipalization" (Kernberg, 1975; Rohde-Dachser, 1995, p. 32). According to this hypothesis the rage is fueled by unintegrated pregenital aggressive impulses; that is, the borderline patient's fury is the result of a developmental deficiency.

## A Client-Centered Perspective

The client-centered position has not been as widely discussed in the literature as has drive theory. A client-centered explanation of borderline functioning is arrived at by tracing Rogers's (1959) view of how humans gain a sense of self. They do so by accepting experience into the self-concept. Seen in this light, being exceedingly angry or having highly aggressive impulses is nothing but a natural reaction to a threat to the self (Biermann-Ratjen, 1989, 1990, 1993). Since only experience that has met with unconditional positive regard can be integrated into the self-concept, nobody can integrate "traumatic" experiences, and especially the feelings associated with them, without the assistance of an empathic other. In other words, everyone needs a sympathetic listener to cope with painful experiences.

Borderline patients find it impossible to reconcile their profound anger and aggressive feelings with their ideas of themselves; they cannot accept that these feelings really belong to them and are part of their experience. This leads us to infer that when they felt like this in childhood they and their feelings were not accepted by their caregivers. This is why the rage and hatred seem like adversaries threatening their very existence. Being very angry is in their eyes the same as being wicked, and this is wickedness understood in a truly archaic sense: if they are wicked, the patients imagine, then they have no right to exist, or, even more drastically, they are convinced that they deserve to be abandoned.

The two theories differ particularly on the meaning of the patients' rage and their defense against it. The drive hypothesis explains the defense as a deep fear of destroying the other, and the client-centered hypothesis explains it as a deep fear of being destroyed oneself. These contrasting positions naturally imply different therapeutic approaches, and the aims of therapy differ widely as far as treating the aggressive impulses is concerned. The drive hypothesis suggests it is helpful to reduce or channel the impulses we all have but these patients have in excess, so that the destructive feelings can be integrated into the patient's personality. The client-centered hypothesis, on the other hand, concentrates on other goals: first, that the patients gradually become aware of the existential fears concealed behind their rage; and, second, that the rage should in time become intelligible and acceptable as a (natural) reaction to the "traumatic" experiences they have undergone.

The drive hypothesis has led to borderline patients being offered an unnecessarily restricted type of therapy that seems to be regaining favor (see Aronson, 1989). The most common recommendation is "supportive" "face-to-face" psychotherapy 30 minutes a week during which the patient should above all be prevented from "regressing" too far. Just what might happen if there were a strong regressive transference reaction does indeed sound alarming; we are warned to beware of transference psychoses, micropsychotic episodes, suicide, murder, loss of employment, and hospitalization (Aronson, 1989, p. 514). Even though supportive elements play a more important role in the therapy of borderline patients than of neurotic ones, usually both the psychodynamically oriented psychotherapists taking up the line of thinking of Kernberg, Selzer, Koenigsberg, Carr, and Appelbaum (1989/1993) and client-centered therapists (e.g., Swildens, 1990) do not treat borderline patients in a merely supportive way. They assume that lasting changes in the patients' minds and feelings can only be achieved as usual by increasing their "insight" into the psychodynamics of their disorder or helping them to understand and accept their experiences better. This is a long-drawn-out process in borderline patients, as the duration of therapy shows; as a rule it lasts between 2 and 5 years.

## THERAPEUTIC GOALS

Despite the diverging explanations on how borderline disorders come about, there is common agreement on what therapy seeks to achieve. So as client-centered therapists we can go along with Kernberg et al. when they describe the general purpose as follows:

The therapy should increase the borderline patient's ability to experience himself and others as coherent [we would say, *congruent*], integrated and realistically perceived individuals. At the same time it should reduce the need to fall back on defense mechanisms [we would say, *a certain kind of incongruence*] which weaken the ego-structure [we would say, *indicate that the self-concept is unstable*] by restricting the number of ways of reacting available. So one can expect that the patient develops an enhanced ability to keep his impulses under control, to tolerate anxiety, regulate his affects, sublimate his drives—and while at the same time developing stable and satisfying interpersonal relationships—experience intimacy and love. (1989/1993, p. 17)

The routes taken by psychoanalysts and client-centered psychotherapists to reach these goals differ from one another. In what follows we intend to describe the course we have chosen. Our report is based on our work with patients in nine groups and a series of individual therapies, most of which took place after group therapy. The group therapies all had time limits: For inpatients they consisted of approximately 50 sessions within a 3-month period, and for outpatients about 100 group sessions within 1 year.

## SOME PRINCIPLES OF CLIENT-CENTERED TREATMENT OF PATIENTS WITH BORDERLINE PERSONALITY DISORDER

So far there is no treatment manual for the client-centered treatment of BPD available. A theoretical framework has been worked out, however, that specifically covers this disorder. It was first suggested by Höger (1989), who wanted to demonstrate with this taxonomy that the principles of client-centered psychotherapy, formulated by Rogers (1957), are on an abstract level and that on this level the therapist's actual behavior in reaction to a patient suffering from a particular disorder is not explicitly specified. His taxonomy covers four levels, in hierarchical order (see Table 15.2).

The correlations between these various levels obey certain laws, of which the most important is that *the postulates on one level may not contradict the postulates on the level above it.* The theory of therapy formulated by Rogers (1957, 1959) is largely on level 2. Theoretical postulates prescribing specific kinds of behavior depending on the patient's disorder would belong to levels 3 and 4.

For treating borderline patients the postulates on levels 1 and 2 are certainly highly relevant, as are most of those on level 3. Some additions would be necessary to the postulates on all three levels, or they would have to be given a different emphasis to take the special characteristics of this disorder into account. For instance, as we describe later, observing the principle of nondirectiveness (level 1) has different implications when treating patients with BPD than when treating neurotic patients; it is essential to apply this

TABLE 15.2. The Four Abstract Levels in Client-Centered Theory of Therapy

1. The level of the "therapeutic relationship" in general, as distinct from other kinds of relations (mother–child, lawyer–client, etc.)
2. The level of combined features, in client-centered therapy "unconditional positive regard," "empathic understanding," and "congruence," marking the relationship offered by the psychotherapist
3. The level of a classification of separate kinds of behavior, for instance, "client's self-exploration," "verbalization of the client's experiencing by the therapist," and the guidelines the therapist makes use of, etc.
4. The level of the actual ways the therapist and client behave in a specific observed or documented session

*Note.* Data from Höger (1989, p. 199).

principle in a modified way. One example of a treatment rule on level 4 for patients with BPD is as follows: whenever it becomes obvious that the patient is recounting an experience that reveals her/his tendency to "split," the therapist should include and refer to the "split-off" part of the experience when verbalizing the patient's experience. He/she may however only apply this rule if it does not contravene a postulate on one of the higher levels. It would be a contravention, for instance, if the therapist reminded his/her patient that she/he is just damning someone whom she/he had unconditionally admired for her moral integrity in the previous session: "You always just see half the person. Last time you thought she was marvellous and I was supposed to share your admiration and was not allowed to utter a word of criticism." With an intervention like this the therapist would of course have broken the rule on unconditional positive regard.

In what follows it is not our aim to define a complete client-centered theory on treating BPD; rather, we want to look into various aspects of such a theory. The task of systematically constructing a detailed treatment guide is a matter for future research.

We propose to look at the following points:

1. How does a borderline disorder present itself to the psychotherapist?
2. What consequences does this have for the client-centered psychotherapist?
3. What do certain borderline symptoms and behaviors mean?
4. How and when should the therapist convey to the patient that the therapist has understood her/him?
5. Are there particular issues that ought to be dealt with during therapy?
6. How should the clinician organize the therapeutic setting?

## How Does a Borderline Disorder Present Itself to the Psychotherapist?

Here is an example from a group therapy showing how patients tend to idealize or denigrate those who try to enter into close relations with them. Mr. A gets the members of the group to focus exclusively on him and his current problem throughout the whole session. For the umpteenth time he seems likely to lose his job, which he has only had for a few weeks. He does not manage to get to work on time, and therefore simply stays away, persuading the doctor to give him sick leave. The group is sympathetic, commiserating with him and trying to discover what stops him from being punctual. Mr. A obviously feels understood and calms down, so that by the end of the session his initial nervousness has vanished. In the next session Mr. A starts off by scornfully running down the whole group: nothing ever happens here except a lot of empty chat; the therapist must be mad if he thinks that one cripple can help another; the group is just a bunch of mental wrecks. After the last session he felt terrible. His symptom, a physical sensation that he is shrinking, recurred in severe form. Again the session is given over to him, though this time it is full of mutual recriminations and insulted withdrawals. When discussing the session afterward both of the therapists remarked on the barely disguised triumph with which Mr. A presented his complaints and accusations. This sequence of events, with Mr. A quite evidently benefiting from the group in one session and in the next pouring derision on its efforts, repeated itself several times.

"Typical" borderline patients—

- Idealize and denigrate us
- Avoid real contact, apparently because they are frightened of closeness and the sense of helplessness this induces in them
- React to empathic verbalizations as if they were insinuations or statements about their characters

They cannot understand themselves and do not expect others to understand them; instead they—

- Block us with their own inner emptiness and emotional void
- Become psychotic or suicidal or simply do not turn up for the sessions

## What Consequences Does This Have for the Client-Centered Psychotherapist?

The client-centered offer of a relationship with the patient is characterized by empathy, congruence, and unconditional positive regard. Our example from the group sessions has probably made it clear already: in treating borderline patients the therapist's unconditional positive regard is constantly in peril. So here is a rule to stick to: as a client-centered psychotherapist treating a borderline patient, hang on to your unconditional positive regard for all you are worth. It is not just endangered by the patients' direct attacks or idealizations but also by the fact that they often seem to ignore you, especially in group therapies, or perceive you in a way that has nothing to do with your own personality. A "person to-person" encounter seems out of the question: the patients see in the therapist someone they bring with them. Here is another example of what we mean:

One of our woman patients, who had recently completed an inpatient psychotherapy, rang me (J.E.) and complained that her mother wanted her to go back to work. She was quite desperate, since in her state she could not possibly hold down a job. I made an appointment with the patient and her mother, and started off by talking to the patient on her own. She was very angry and upset, complaining bitterly about her mother's lack of understanding of her illness. I brought the mother in and wanted to suggest that I thought her daughter needed more time before returning to work but did not have time to even finish my first sentence before the patient started to shout at me. How dare I insult her mother like this? If I were a good therapist she would have been able to work long ago. Her mother was absolutely right. The patient worked herself up into such a rage that she half demolished a chair in my room and sent all the plant pots on the windowsill crashing to the floor.

Here it is vital to realize the following: My patient found it quite impossible to acknowledge how angry she was with her mother as soon as she was in her presence. She projected this feeling onto me and assumed that I wanted to blame her mother, or in other words wanted to do something wicked which would destroy her mother. Realizing all this was essential, before I could sense the specifically borderline anguish that made her behave so violently toward me. During the episode itself I could not have pointed out to the patient what was happening. In her perturbed and confused state she was quite incapable of taking in or understanding any such suggestion, or would have thought it was yet another proof of what a bad therapist I was to even suggest that she was really angry with her mother.

In our experience there are two stages during therapy where we very often have to apply the rule: whatever you do, hang onto your unconditional positive regard. The first is at the beginning of therapy, getting the patient involved and establishing a viable relationship; the second is at the end of treatment, with its partings and farewells. For borderline patients both these phases, permitting oneself to engage in a close contact and being able to give it up again, touch areas so fraught with distress and disappointment that they have to mobilize their defenses in a way that is often very hard to bear.

There is one aspect of client-centered psychotherapy that is very well attuned to the special problems borderline patients have and facilitates the contact between therapist and patient: its nondirectiveness. As a result of what they have been through these patients have a deep fear of being manipulated and misused. One form of exploitation they particularly worry about is that the therapist really hopes their symptoms will soon vanish, confirming that he/she is a "good" therapist. So the client-centered therapist is well advised to genuinely aim at nothing more than really understanding his/her borderline client. Faced with this kind of fear once, I remarked to the patient, "I am not interested in making you better but just in helping you to understand yourself better," and the patient was quite obviously very relieved.

The principle of nondirectiveness must however be put aside more often than with neurotic patients, especially for instance when there is evidence of self-destructive behavior or during phases when the patient's grasp of reality is obviously shaky. Where expressing feelings is concerned one should adhere as far as possible to the principle of nondirectiveness. As a rule borderline patients have no difficulty in feeling their anger, but they are terrified of being overwhelmed by it and behaving in a dangerous or destructive way. This fear can become so great that they lose touch with the anger behind it and instead react in a mentally confused and disoriented way (see the example below). With these patients it is important to realize that they are fleeing from their rage and to grasp how they are doing it. In such situations any suggestion by the therapist that they should express their rage is likely to overtax them. The therapist's aim should be restricted to helping the patients register that their rage seems to have got lost and—if possible, and only tentatively—to suggest they can feel a hint of it (i.e., symbolize it correctly).

## What Do Certain Borderline Symptoms and Behaviors Mean?

There are several borderline symptoms and ways of behaving that we cannot understand simply by referring back to our own experience. These include the symptoms associated with the defense mechanism known as splitting. The therapist can barely imagine the fears that induce the patients to split off their feelings. It is therefore essential that the therapist remembers that borderline symptoms specifically are likely to recur or become more severe when the patient is faced with a disappointing situation where others would probably react by being angry or depressed, or more likely a mixture of both.

If patients talk about having impressions, feelings, reactions, or symptoms that the therapist cannot understand and that leave the therapist confused and uneasy, then as a rule the therapist can conclude that the patient is feeling exactly the same. Even if patients talk about their symptoms in a quite matter-of-fact tone, the therapist should ask whether they understand them. The therapist should also take the unintelligible parts into account as possible signs of one of the "early" defense mechanisms. If, for instance, there is any sign of splitting, it is often enough to talk about it. One can point out that the patient has other feelings as well for the person being so bitterly and ruthlessly criticized, perhaps even gentle and affectionate feelings, but they seem to have been momentarily forgotten, even though they were mentioned a few hours ago.

Here is an example: A woman patient who had been in group therapy was picked up by the police right at the end of the subway line and brought to a hospital. She still knew her name but could not work out where she was or why. Her plan had been to consult her psychiatrist, but his office lay in the opposite direction. While talking to her about her state and this episode it turned out that during her last visit to the psychiatrist she had asked him whether she could have an appointment with him once a week, rather than only once a fortnight. He had, however, more or less ignored this request and instead had handed her a list of addresses of self-help groups for mentally disturbed persons. When I asked whether she had been disappointed she replied that she could not remember feeling anything like that. On the contrary, she had blamed herself for bothering her overworked psychiatrist with such a request.

Here is a second example: A patient with a borderline disorder had fallen in love and started a relationship. He was happy and described his new girlfriend as absolutely ideal. The therapist understood his description of the woman as a sign that he was in love. A few sessions later the patient described his girlfriend in such hate-ridden and disparaging terms that the therapist had difficulties realizing that this was the same woman who had been praised to the skies. Having grasped this, and that the patient was trying to cope with being disappointed by his girlfriend, the therapist could perceive the specifically BPD form of defense. Because of his tendency to split, the patient was unable to feel his own disappointment, as that could mean he was so greedy that he demanded things that the other could not give. So he "rescued" his image of himself by completely devaluing his girlfriend. She was the wicked one.

It is a help for the therapist to remind him-/herself of these factors when trying to keep his/her unconditional positive regard intact, for otherwise the regard is likely to give way to a feeling of bewildered frustration and anger. After all the therapist had been glad—and a little bit proud—that his patient now, perhaps partly because of the therapy, could enter into a relationship that obviously did him some good.

Having noticed these splitting tendencies, it is useful to verbalize them and consider what they mean for the patient and the therapist and their relation to one another. The therapist should make an effort to talk about the "split-off" aspects of the patient's experiencing, signaling understanding perhaps as follows: "You are so disappointed that you have completely forgotten the aspects of your girlfriend which you really appreciate and love."

When dealing with the feelings that borderline patients do not permit themselves to have, it is important to realize that patients should not "learn" to have these feelings, nor should they be encouraged to express them. The first and most important step toward integrating these feelings is to point out that for some reason the appropriate emotional responses like being disappointed or angry are currently not available to the patient or are presumably so frightening that the patient feels highly alarmed. Attempting to understand what lies behind this anxiety is then a further step in the therapeutic process. Some borderline symptoms are apparently linked to these patients' shaky sense of identity, their fragile self-concept. In this respect they differ most clearly from patients with neurotic disorders. The borderliners' dislike of being alone is probably a consequence of this. If they really are alone they are often overwhelmed by a deep sense of insecurity about who they are and about whether what they feel really belongs to them. One woman patient reported that she could alleviate this sense of being unreal by going to the mirror and looking at her own face. Other patients start to ring people up or—this is more often a male variation—visit the pub.

Many borderline patients report that when they cannot feel themselves any longer or only have a dreadful sense of being utterly void, they cut themselves, often with a razor blade, because the self-inflicted pain restores their awareness that they actually exist. Hurting themselves, thinking about suicide, or actually trying to kill themselves sometimes helps to suppress the unwanted feelings lurking behind the emptiness. A woman inpatient was able to stop hacking at herself with a razor blade when she realized during therapy that she had fallen in love with the nurse on the ward.

Generally speaking, the following assumptions are helpful in understanding borderline symptoms: there are two aims behind most of the symptoms and especially the way these patients organize their relationships with others; they want to (1) be able to experience or feel themselves at all, and (2) steer clear of any suspicion that they are bad.

## How and When Can We Convey to Patients That We Have Understood Them?

Here we should like to remind you of the main task a client-centered psychotherapist has when treating a borderline patient. Before intervening in any way, therapists should ask themselves whether they can do so with unconditional positive regard. If they are certain that they respect their patient in this manner, it is of secondary importance how they convey what they have understood about the patient's inner world. They can confront the patients or explain something or point out that their perception is awry or take up a feeling or even give a transference interpretation. One very helpful approach for borderline patients, because it often comes as a great relief to them, is explaining in a more or less informative manner that feeling disappointed and being very angry or belligerent are quite natural reactions to the suffering inflicted on them. Many such patients are convinced, like Kernberg, that something in their genes makes them wicked people. More specifically we use sentences like the following ones to explain and lighten their burden:

- "Rage is the oldest feeling we humans have when we are forced to defend ourselves. It is a reaction to something bad happening to us, for instance, being deprived, not being fed when we need it, and so on."

- "One painful experience that many children go through is that their parents don't understand them. Many parents, for whatever reason, fail to notice what their children are feeling or imagine they are feeling something else. But children are not in a position to realize that they react angrily when they are misunderstood or ignored, and so instead of feeling hurt they feel wicked."

- "A little kid can't think, 'I've got parents who aren't really interested in me.' It can only register sensing, 'There's something wrong with me, otherwise my parents would love me more.'"

We cannot suggest any rules as to when to use which kind of intervention. In our experience, if a good relationship has been established, the patients themselves make sure that the issues that are relevant for them get discussed. These are often presented in the form of a complaint or an accusation; one of our former patients who was also in psychiatric care criticized me (J.E.) with the words, "You haven't even asked me how many tablets I have hoarded up again." The same patient opened the first session after a longish holiday by declaring as she was entering the room, "We're not going to do that again!"; the subject of the session was her disappointment that I had deserted her.

## Are There Certain Issues That Ought to Be Dealt with during Therapy?

We have already mentioned the three most important areas to be looked into in a borderline therapy: (1) the special defensive behavior, and in particular the exclusive goodness or badness; (2) the patients' fear of emotions, above all of rage and aggressiveness, which is the outcome of profound disappointment; and (3) psychotic experiences, above all dissociation, which indicate how frail their sense of self is. In addition (4) we have found it necessary and in the long term helpful if the patients "learn" in the course of therapy to "look at their parents" (i.e., to gain a realistic picture of them as real individuals). When talking about the parents the therapist must carefully guard him-/herself and the patient from giving them the blame for the patient's problems. Even if the parents were in a certain sense responsible, this is not a subject to be dealt with in the patient's therapy. The goal is rather to assemble an all-around picture of them, including those aspects that caused the suffering, that is, as complete and realistic a picture of them as possible.

In fact it is rarely necessary for therapists to deliberately tackle any of these issues. It is usually enough if they realize how important they are and are prepared to go into them with unconditional positive regard whenever the patients bring them up.

## How Should We Organize the Therapeutic Setting?

In many respects we are far less strict about the therapeutic setting with borderline patients than we are with neurotics. Here are three examples:

1. We are not against borderlne patients making use of other therapeutic offers while they are in therapy with us. By this we do not just mean psychiatric care, which is the rule because of the medication most of these patients require, but also other kinds of psychotherapeutic treatment. Our reasoning is that the patients should have a chance to widen their range and undergo other experiences, which they can compare with those had with us, and possibly prefer them without us rejecting them. This attitude is based on Margaret S. Mahler's (1975) hypothesis, which we have found confirmed again and again, that the difficulties many borderline patients have originate in the individuation/separation phase.

2. For similar reasons we try to get in touch with a patient who has twice missed a session without excusing her-/himself.

3. We always tell neurotic patients in time when we are going away. We tell borderline patients in addition exactly where we are going and what we plan to do there, that is, have a holiday or go to a conference. This is to prevent the patients feeling that we have deserted them and that they might be the reason, that because they are so hard to cope with we have to recover from them in a secret retreat. It also seems to calm borderline patients if they know exactly where their therapist is. Nevertheless, in the many years of working with them we have never been rung up by a borderline patient while on holiday, let alone been visited by one.

Here finally are some remarks on the setting. Because of these patients' problems with ending therapy, we have found it helpful to set firm time limits, especially for the groups. These are furthermore invariably closed groups, so that all the participants leave at the same time. As far as frequency is concerned, one session a week is not enough; we have found that meeting twice weekly is a good workable arrangement for groups and individual therapies. Treatment is likely to last from between 2 and 6 years. This does not mean, however, that the patients need two sessions a week over the whole period; often after a year they can be seen once a week or even less. We never exclude the possibility that a patient who has finished treatment, broken it off, or gone to another therapist may return to us if she/he wants to.

## WHAT IS THE LONG-TERM PROGNOSIS FOR PATIENTS WITH BORDERLINE PERSONALITY DISORDER?

Many years ago a youngish patient who had discovered that she fulfilled all the criteria for BPD anxiously enquired whether she was now bound to be afflicted with this borderline condition for the rest of her life. That was in the early 1980s. In those days we were in no position to give a clear, empirically backed answer to this question. In the meantime, however, a number of empirical studies have been carried out worldwide into the long-term development of this disorder. One can distinguish between medium-term follow-ups, on average 5–7 years after treatment began (Pope, Jonas, Hudson, Cohen, & Gunderson, 1983; Perry, 1985, 1988; Modestin & Villiger, 1989; Kullgren & Armelius, 1990; Hoke, Lavori, & Perry, 1992; Links, Mitton, & Steiner, 1990; Links, Heslegrave, Mitton, van Renkum, & Patrick, 1995), and long-term follow-ups, after 15 years (McGlashan, 1986; Plakun, Burkhardt, & Muller, 1985; Stone, Hurt, & Stone, 1987; Paris, Brown, & Nowlis, 1987). The long-term follow-ups are, however, all only retrospective. It is difficult to compare the results of the separate studies with one another, as there are wide differences in the methods used, the kind and length of treatment, the severity of the disorder, and so on. Generally speaking, however, one can conclude from all the results so far that in the long term the psychosocial prognosis for a patient with BPD is better than for patients with psychotic disorders and slightly worse than for patients with neurotic disorders.

The results of a study in our institute (Eckert & Wuchner, 1996) confirm this generalization. Here in brief are some of the main findings of this investigation, which included 14 borderline patients who took part in client-centered group therapy. This outpatient therapy group met twice a week; most of the patients had just finished treatment as psychiatric inpatients. The groups were closed and limited to 100 sessions. Each group consisted of seven to nine patients with a variety of diagnoses; in addition to a maximum of three or four borderline patients, each group included patients with other diagnoses suited to group therapy.

The BPD diagnosis was established via clinical interviews and the Rorschach test. The patients were examined at the beginning and the end of group therapy by means of the Diagnostic Interview for Borderline Patients (DIB; Gunderson, Kolb, & Austin, 1981) and other diagnostic measures. A further examination using the same instruments took place 2½ years after the end of group therapy, so that the whole time of investigation covered on average 4½ years. We compared our borderline patients with patients diagnosed as suffering from (neurotic) depression and schizophrenia. Figure 15.1 shows how the borderline symptoms developed as measured on the DIB.

Before treatment began 93% of the borderline patients fulfilled the criteria laid down in the DIB (global score = 7 on a scale with a range from 0 to 10) for the presence of BPD; after treatment only 14% fulfilled the criteria. The mean value in the DIB total declined significantly within 4 years from $M = 8.3$ to $M = 5.4$. Before treatment began the depressive and schizophrenic patients hardly showed any specifically borderline symptoms, and at follow-up there was only a slight reduction in them. As far as their impaired professional and social lives were concerned, the borderline patients showed marked

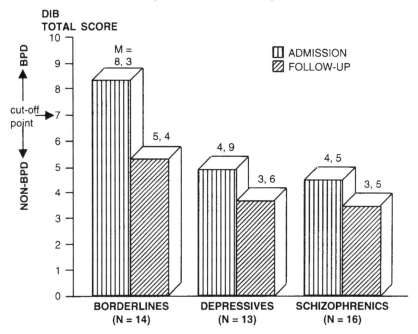

**FIGURE 15.1.** Changes in borderline specific symptoms (DIB rated, range 0–10; 7 points are needed for the diagnosis BPD) from pretreatment to follow-up in borderline patients compared with depressive and schizophrenic patients.

improvements at follow-up compared with their situation at the outset. The majority of changes took place during therapy; thereafter, in the follow-up period, there were no or only very small additional positive changes. There was no deterioration in any of the areas examined during the follow-up period; that is, the "gains" achieved during group therapy were either "maintained" or "augmented." Our study cannot unequivocally prove precisely how much the client-centered group therapy contributed to the positive change in the patients, because we could not compare the changes achieved with the changes in untreated borderline patients. We share with all borderline researchers the problem of finding an adequate control group. The borderline patients who come to a psychiatric institution for treatment are as a rule so acutely in need of therapy that, for ethical reasons, one cannot assign them to an own-control group and let them—as the design of our study would have required—wait a whole year before their treatment begins.

We should like to close by recalling the aforementioned borderline patient who anxiously asked whether she was going to be afflicted with this disorder for the rest of her life. Our results allow us to reply as follows: if borderline patients can permit themselves to get deeply involved in psychotherapeutic treatment, they have a good chance of being diagnosed as nonborderline after 3 or 4 years.

## REFERENCES

American Psychiatric Association. (1994). *Diagnostic and statistical manual of mental disorders* (4th ed.). Washington, DC: APA Books.

Aronson, T. A. (1989). A critical review of psychotherapeutic treatments of the borderline personality: Historical trends and future directions. *Journal of Nervous and Mental Disease, 177,* 511–528.

Biermann-Ratjen, E.-M. (1989). Zur Notwendigkeit einer Entwicklungpsychologie für Gesprächspsychotherapeuten aus dem personenzentrierten Konzept für die Zukunft der klientenzentrierten Psychotherapie. In R. Sachse & J. Howe (Eds.), *Zur Zukunft der klientenzentrierten Psychotherapie* (pp. 102–125). Heidelberg: Asanger.

Biermann-Ratjen, E.-M. (1990). Identifizierung: Ein Beitrag zu einem Modell der Entwicklung der gesunden und kranken Persönlichkeit. *GwG-Zeitschrift, 78,* 31–35.

Biermann-Ratjen, E.-M. (1993). Abschliessende Bemerkungen. In J. Eckert, D. Höger, & H. Linster (Eds.), *Die Entwicklung der Person und ihre Störung* (pp. 99–120). Cologne: GwG-Verlag.

Biermann-Ratjen, E.-M. (1996). On the way to a client-centered psychopathology. In R. Hutterer, G. Pawlowsky, P. F. Schmid, & R. Stipsits (Eds.), *Client-centered and experiential psychotherapy: A paradigm in motion* (pp. 11–24). Frankfurt am Main: Lang.

Biermann-Ratjen, E.-M., Eckert, J., & Schwartz, H.-J. (1995). *Gesprächspsychotherapie: Verändern durch Verstehen* (7th rev. & expanded ed.). Stuttgart: Kohlhammer.

Bohart, A. C. (1990). A cognitive client-centered perspective on borderline personality development. In G. Lietaer, J. Rombauts, & R. Van Balen (Eds.), *Client-centered and experiential psychotherapy in the nineties* (pp. 599–621). Leuven, Belgium: Leuven University Press.

Eckert, J., & Wuchner, M. (1996). Long-term development of borderline personality disorder. In R. Hutterer, G. Pawlowsky, P. F. Schmid, & R. Stipsits (Eds.), *Client-centered and experiential psychotherapy: A paradigm in motion* (pp. 11–24). Frankfurt am Main: Lang.

Gunderson, J. G., Kolb, J., & Austin, V. (1981). The Diagnostic Interview for Borderline Patients. *American Journal of Psychiatry, 138,* 896–903.

Höger, D. (1989). Klientenzentrierte Psychotherapie: Ein Breitbandkonzept mit Zukunft. In R. Sachse & J. Howe (Eds.), *Zur Zukunft der klientenzentrierten Psychotherapie* (pp. 51–63). Heidelberg: Asanger.

Hoke, L. A., Lavori, P. W., & Perry, J. C. (1992). Mood and global functioning in borderline personality disorder: Individual regression models for longitudinal measurements. *Journal of Psychiatric Research, 26,* 1–16.

Kernberg, O. F. (1975). Borderline conditions and pathological narcissism. New York: Aronson.

Kernberg, O. F., Selzer, M. A., Koenigsberg, H. W., Carr, A. C., & Appelbaum, A. H. (1989). *Psychodynamic psychotherapy of borderline patients.* New York: Basic Books. [German ed. (1993): *Psychodynamische Therapie bei Borderline-Patienten.* Bern: Huber.]

Kullgren, G., & Armelius, B. A. (1990). The concept of personality organization: A long-term comparative follow-up study with special reference to borderline personality organization. *Journal of Personality Disorders, 4,* 203–212.

Links, P. S., Heslegrave, R. J., Mitton, J. E., van Renkum, R., & Patrick, J. (1995). Borderline personality disorder and substance abuse: Consequences of comorbidity. *Canadian Journal of Psychiatry, 40,* 9–14.

Links, P. S., Mitton, J. E., & Steiner, M. (1990). Predicting outcome for borderline personality disorder. *Comprehensive Psychiatry, 31,* 490–498.

Mahler, M. S. (1975). Die Bedeutung des Loslösungs- und Individuationsprozesses für die Beurteilung von Borderline-Phänomenen. *Psyche, 29,* 1078–1095.

McGlashan, T. H. (1986). The Chestnut Lodge follow-up study: III. Long-term outcome of borderline personalities. *Archives of General Psychiatry, 43,* 20–30.

Modestin, J., & Villiger, C. (1989). Follow-up study on borderline versus non-borderline personality disorders. *Journal of Personality Disorders, 3,* 236–244.

Paris, J., Brown, R., & Nowlis, D. (1987). Long-term follow-up of borderline patients in a general hospital. *Comprehensive Psychiatry, 28,* 530–535.

Perry, J. C. (1985). Depression in borderline personality disorder: Lifetime prevalence at interviews and longitudinal course of symptoms. *American Journal of Psychiatry, 142,* 15–21.

Perry, J. C. (1988). A prospective study of life stress, defenses, psychotic symptoms and depression in borderline and antisocial personality disorders and bipolar type II affective disorder. *Journal of Personality Disorders, 2*(1), 49–59.

Plakun, E. M., Burkhardt, P. E., & Muller, J. P. (1985). 14-year follow-up of borderline and schizotypal personality disorders. *Comprehensive Psychiatry, 26,* 448–455.

Pope, H. G., Jonas, J. M., Hudson, J. I., Cohen, B. M., & Gunderson, J. G. (1983). The validity of DSM-III borderline personality disorder. *Archives of General Psychiatry, 40,* 23–30.

Rogers, C. R. (1957). The necessary and sufficient conditions of the therapeutic personality change. *Journal of Consulting Psychology, 21,* 95–103.

Rogers, C. R. (1959). A theory of therapy, personality and interpersonal relationships as developed in the client-centered framework. In S. Koch (Ed.), *Psychology: A study of science: Vol. III. Formulations of the person and the social context* (pp.184–256). New York: McGraw-Hill.

Rohde-Dachser, C. R. (1995). *Das Borderline-Syndrom.* (5th rev. & expanded ed.). Bern: Huber.

Searles, H. F. (1958). Positive feelings in the relationship between the schizophrenic and his mother. *International Journal of Psycho-analysis, 39,* 569–585.

Stern, D. N. (1985). *The interpersonal world of the infant.* New York: Basic Books.

Stone, M. H., Hurt, S. W., & Stone, D. K. (1987). The PI 500: Long-term follow-up of borderline inpatients meeting DSM-III criteria: I. Global outcome. *Journal of Personality Disorders, 1,* 291–298.

Swildens, H. (1990). Client-centered psychotherapy for patients with borderline symptoms. In G. Lietaer, J. Rombauts, & R. Van Balen (Eds.), *Client-centered and experiential psychotherapy in the nineties* (pp. 623–644). Leuven, Belgium: Leuven University Press.

Wolberg, A. R. (1973). *The borderline patient.* New York: International Medical Book Corp.

# 16

\*\*\*\*\*

# A Client-Centered Approach
# to Therapeutic Work
# with Dissociated
# and Fragile Process

## Margaret S. Warner

*In recent years*, a number of client-centered therapists at the Chicago Counseling and Psychotherapy Center have done intensive work with clients experiencing dissociative identity disorders. During therapy these clients manifest distinctive alternate personality states and often come to experience previously blocked memories of intensive childhood sexual or physical abuse. Given their histories of abusive experiences with authority figures, these clients are often particularly sensitive to issues of domination and control in psychotherapy. In our experience, they respond particularly well to a client-centered style of therapy that allows high levels of client control over the content, style, and speed of the therapeutic process.

I believe that an extended description of dissociated process as we have observed it in client-centered therapy can be valuable for a number of reasons. Dissociated process is one of three styles of processing (along with fragile and psychotic process) that we have frequently found in clients whose experience is often difficult to handle or overwhelming for psychotherapists. I believe that therapists are much more likely to be effective with these clients if they have an understanding of common ways that dissociated process is experienced by these clients. In addition, a client-directed style of work with dissociative identity disorders offers an alternative to the highly structured, directive styles of therapy advocated in most of the clinical literature. This style may be more easily integrated into the working styles of therapists who ordinarily follow more relational, nonintrusive styles of psychotherapeutic work.

The client-centered style of working has the added advantage that it is less subject to many of the criticisms commonly lodged against therapists working with dissociative disorders that therapists have iatrogenically created the syndrome through their strong use of interpretation, hypnosis, and confrontation of "resistance" to the diagnosis. A number of memory researchers have suggested that intense, ongoing interpretation and confrontation is particularly likely to be associated with the creation of false memories (Brown, 1995).[1] By observing a more client-directed therapy process, we can consider reasons for accepting or doubting the validity of client memories in the absence of some of these confounding factors.

To explore these issues, I will give a brief overview of dissociative processes related to early trauma and describe ways that we have worked with these experiences within a client-centered style of therapy, with particular emphasis on the ways that fragile and dissociated process often interrelate in client experience. I will then briefly review the controversy over dissociative identity disorders in the psychological literature. Finally, I will consider my reasons for believing in the overall validity of the dissociated processes and retrieved memories reported by my clients.

## DISTINCTIVE CHARACTERISTICS OF DISSOCIATED PARTS

Clients who have suffered from early trauma often find that aspects of their experience are subjectively experienced as autonomous and out of their control. Therapists and clients differ as to whether to call the more person-like clusters of dissociated experiences "personalities" or "parts" or "ego states."[2] Clearly experiences of dissociated parts differ significantly from the full everyday personalities of clients. Yet, they are a great deal more person-like than are ordinary mood states.

While a dissociated part is fully present in a person's awareness, that part is likely to experience itself as having an autonomous existence and life history separate from that of the host personality or that of other parts. Dissociated parts have the ability to alter perceptions much the way a person in a trance might. For example, while a part is present, a client looking in the mirror may see herself with the characteristics of that part—as older or younger, fatter or thinner, or of a different age or sex. One client on leaving our session experienced herself as a young man driving a Jaguar to an unknown destination. Parts may be able to feel no pain under the most excruciating circumstances or create sensations with no external cause.

Along with the capacity to alter perceptions, dissociated parts often lack the sense of reality testing that ordinarily would cause them to experience such perceptions as strange. Parts are quite untroubled by the idea that there are several of them in one body, that they were born when the client was a particular age, or that they exist in some part of the client's body (such as the right side). They often believe that they could kill the client without killing themselves. Parts often think quite concretely, believing that their feelings could literally contaminate and harm the therapist or that angry thoughts could make the therapist's plane crash.

Along with the ability to alter perceptions, parts have quite amazing abilities to generate physiological changes in the client's body. Clinically demonstrable signs of illness may disappear within hours, only to reappear at another time or in another location. For example, one client had an infection in her left hand that had moved to the right hand by the time of her next medical exam a few days later, much to the consternation of her doctors.

## THE DEVELOPMENT
## OF TRAUMA-DRIVEN DISSOCIATION

Our clients' accounts of their experiences in combination with the general literature on dissociative identity disorders allow us to construct an understanding of the origin and functioning of trauma-driven dissociation.[3]

The clients we have seen who have experienced dissociative parts virtually all came to remember experiences of sexual or physical trauma before the age of seven. At such early ages children have high levels of openness to imagination and hypnotic suggestibility.[4] Faced with overwhelming trauma and lacking the more complex ways of coping with experiences available to older children, our clients seem to have stumbled on dissociation as a solution. One client, for example, found that when she stared at dots on her bedspread she could separate herself out from the terror and anguish of being raped by her father. Some clients describe experiencing themselves as out of their bodies and watching the events from the ceiling.

Understandably, dissociation under these circumstances is extremely reinforcing. Children go from an overwhelming state of anguish to a lack of intense pain and an ability to put the whole thing out of their minds the next day. This capacity makes family life seem tolerable and, for some, allows the illusion that they have a normal, happy family life. Clients seem to take a larger lesson from the apparent effectiveness of these early dissociation experiences—that emotional pain is destructive and that the way to live successfully is to make painful experiences disappear.

Such early childhood dissociation seldom seems to stop with amnesia or emotional separation from the experience within a unified personality, as is typical of adult posttraumatic stress disorders. Children almost always divide the dissociated aspects of their experiences into a number of compartments that are separate from each other. I suspect that this happens because young children have a number of intense reactions that seem irreconcilable with each other and they do not yet have the mental capacities to integrate such contradictions.

Typically our clients describe having felt helplessness, terror, pain, and anguish that were so intense that they felt that they might die from those feelings. In this they simultaneously felt afraid of dying and wished that they could die. They felt intense rage and wished that they could do violence to the perpetrator. Still, they wished that they could hold onto the times when their parents seemed loving or nurturing.

In the helpless part of their feelings they were terrified of the violence of their angry feelings. From the angry part of their feelings, they felt disgust and shame at their reactions of helplessness and a sense that such experiences would threaten survival. In their wish that they could hold onto some normal life, they wished that both the angry and the helpless, anguished reactions would disappear. Probably as a result of these contradictions, a number of different clusters of experience separated out within their dissociated experiences. These clusters of experience came to have a very distinctive sort of "person-like" experience of themselves, each with its own feelings, history, and way of looking at the world.

A number of dissociated parts typically take on self-abusive or suicidal qualities. These impulses seem to arise when the pain of dissociated memories threatens to return. Typically, though not always, this anguish is held by a young-child part who is terrified and alone and wishes someone would come help. (Angry abusive parts are also frightened children and have their own disturbing memories that they may be trying to get away from.)

In either case, when memories threaten to return, one or more parts would rather die than let that happen. I suspect that clients stumble on the fact that a wide number of self-destructive behaviors are effective in containing memories. By adulthood clients are likely to be engaged in eating disorders, impulses to cut themselves, substance abuse, suicidal ideation, and/or various compulsive sexual, athletic, or work behaviors. They often hear disparaging voices that tell them that they are worthless or press them to cut themselves or take pills. Some clients keep these behaviors quite hidden from themselves and others. Others present to therapists with an astonishing array of out-of-control, seemingly impulsive behaviors. As a result, they are often mistakenly diagnosed as borderline or schizophrenic and treated within symptom-specific inpatient programs.

Clients often have one or more parts that take on qualities of the perpetrator—wanting to dominate and harm others, or being attracted to sadistic or masochistic sexual experiences. One woman commented that she felt so awful being a helpless victim that she preferred seeing herself as an active participant, feeling that she was her father's real "wife" and that she was superior to her mother.

These parts have often concluded that emotional connection leaves them vulnerable to being violated and manipulated—as they were by their abusers—and should be avoided at all costs. They have often drawn drastic conclusions about the relation of power, vulnerability and ultimate well-being, believing that people who have the most power and the fewest out-of-control feelings are the ones who succeed in life. This anticonnection stance often puts them severely at odds with child parts who have desperate longings for help and comfort from nurturing others.

## CLIENT-CENTERED THERAPY WITH DISSOCIATIVE DISORDERS

We have found that when therapists understand dissociative process and remain empathically connected with clients, a natural process tends to develop in which dissociated memories and parts emerge on their own. Once this process is established in the therapeutic relationship, clients seem to have a finely attuned sense of timing, allowing just as much dissociated material into consciousness at any given time as they can handle without total loss of day-to-day functioning. And they seem to sense the order in which they are able to tolerate working on particular memories and life issues.

The process of regaining memories almost always feels chaotic and painful to clients. Clients often wish that they could forget about the experience and return to their former lives, however restricted or symptomatic. Yet, they also seem to sense intuitively that the process is important and that they need to stay with it if their lives are to have any sense of vitality or wholeness in the future. While some clients stop therapeutic work, most find that they are unable and unwilling to pull away from the process once memories begin to emerge in an empathic environment.

The work that we are doing with clients who experience dissociation follows classic client-centered principles. As is true with many other client groups, we have found that therapeutic relationships grounded in empathy, authenticity, and prizing of clients tend to foster latent capacities for self-directed change and that other more directive techniques can easily inhibit the development of such self-directed change processes.

Given the particularly intense wishes and fears of clients having dissociative experiences, I find that the balance between therapeutic effectiveness and ineffectiveness is often tipped by the accuracy and sensitivity of the therapist's empathy. While basic empathic skills are essential, I believe that empathic understanding is greatly enhanced when therapists have some background understanding of dissociative processes as commonly experienced by clients. And I think that particular empathic sensitivity needs to be developed for communicating understanding to clients who experience several personality parts that operate independently, since understanding expressed to one part may feel like a disparagement or a threat to another part.

### Initial Client Presentation in Therapy

In my experience, very few clients come to therapy describing dissociative experiences in ways that are obvious to therapists who aren't experienced in work with dissociation.[5] Some will immediately show drastic puzzling mood shifts in therapy sessions or even talk about separate personalities. Most clients, however, begin by describing more commonplace symptoms. They may discuss relationship issues, work blocks, global anxiety, depression, self-destructive impulses, or eating disorders. Sometimes they describe troubled or incestuous family backgrounds; sometimes they describe memories of idyllic families that are virtually problem free.

Some clients do a considerable amount of therapeutic work without addressing the dissociation at all. They may make indirect use of therapeutic techniques that encourage work with ego states—such as Gestalt therapy, psychodrama, or focusing processes—without acknowledging the degree of their dissociative experiences in the process. Or they may work on current life problems. They often seem to make great progress for a while but then hit a plateau in which problems seem puzzlingly intractable and their behaviors seem to be perversely contradictory.

I think that these clients come to a point at which they can't progress further without remembering and processing overwhelming memories of early childhood trauma. And they can't connect with these issues without acknowledging dissociative aspects of their experiences to themselves and to their therapists. In this sense, it is often a sign of progress in therapy when clients become more "multiple-like." As memories start to press more urgently to the surface, clients are likely to become more obviously fragmented and aware of dissociated parts that are trying desperately to keep the experience in control.

For example, one advanced graduate student spent years in a seemingly productive analytically oriented therapy. She knew that she had memories of being molested by her uncle as a teenager, but she had no feelings attached to the memories. She suddenly found that she was having intensive suicidal impulses, was losing track of hours at a time at work, and was sometimes finding herself feeling like a 5-year-old unsure of how to get home. For a while she frequently said that she knew that there was something that she needed to know but that she didn't want to know it. One evening she felt particularly frightened and went home with a friend. Once there she shifted into a vivid flashback in which she remembered her uncle raping her while her father looked on. The experience was enormously painful, but she said that she also felt great relief in finally knowing.

When clients begin to trust their therapists more they are likely to begin to describe some of the various oddnesses occurring in their experience or allow themselves to manifest parts in the therapist's presence. This level of trust may come within weeks or only after years of work with a therapist.

Since clients are often afraid that they will be rejected or labeled as crazy if they talk about such experiences, they may begin by presenting dissociated experiences in ways that are oblique or seemingly casual to see how the therapist will react. Dissociated experiences are often foreign enough to therapists that they may miss what clients are saying altogether or assume that their clients are speaking metaphorically.

One client of mine was switching in sessions and felt hurt that I didn't sense what was going on. While in her everyday self she didn't want to be touched at all, she had switched during several sessions into a very vulnerable part and wished that I knew that she wanted me to come and sit next to her and hold her hand. She even tried to draw a picture for me of how her experiences felt to her, though she didn't explain what the picture was about. For several months she kept saying, "I've laid out a puzzle. You have to put it together." Only while I was away on summer vacation did it occur to me that she might be trying to tell me that she had been having dissociative experiences in our sessions. After I returned she commented that it was both a relief and a little bit frightening to her how well I now understood what she was saying to me.

## Client Experiences of Dissociated Parts

Generally, parts seem to emerge when trauma memories are pressing to the surface. This can happen when some life experience, such as going to a violent movie or seeing a child being hurt, stimulates feelings related to the original trauma. Similarly, clients may have memories triggered in current relationships that have abusive elements. On the other hand, clients may find that the memories begin to press to the surface when they are becoming emotionally healthy in many other ways. Clients who have been making progress in therapy often begin to sense that the memories need to be dealt with for them to become whole.

Parts tend to experience *themselves* as having a continuous history of all the times they have been "out" and times they have been aware of the experiences of other parts. However, the host personality—that part of the client who is most in contact with day-to-day reality—may experience other parts in more or less fragmentary ways at any given moment. Parts vary both in their knowledge of the existence of other parts and in their understanding of the sorts of feelings and thoughts that motivate other parts.

Some clients go for years with very little awareness of the parts. To stay away from part experiences, though, they generally need to lead quite restricted lives. At times, clients don't experience parts directly but are aware of various disowned thoughts, actions, or feelings. At other times clients experience parts as presences in consciousness without having the parts take over control of their overall personality. Clients may then sense the parts as personalities with distinctive intentions, thoughts, feelings, and memories, and may feel threatened or pressured by such parts to act in ways they wouldn't otherwise act. Often, when parts emerge in consciousness, previously puzzling feelings and behaviors come to make more sense. The dissociated parts often follow unusual logics, but these logics tend to be quite consistent and often aimed at protecting the client in some way.

At certain points clients may "switch" and dissociated parts take over control of the client's consciousness and behavior. This can happen dramatically with a named other personality. At other times the switch can be more subtle, with the client sliding into another frame of mind without identifying it to outsiders. When clients switch, they often can't remember what happened afterward.

Clients typically have parts that try to intervene to keep switching from being too obvious to outsiders. If behavior begins to get out of control, the person may say she/he is feeling sick and leave or invent some other cover story. Blatantly obvious switching in front of strangers or acquaintances often indicates that the client is extremely overwhelmed and can no longer keep her-/himself from being flooded by traumatic memories.

## Connecting with Dissociated Parts

I have found a number of quite simple responses helpful when I am not sure whether a client might be dissociating. These include the following: sensitizing myself to the possibility of dissociation from outside clues; listening concretely to client expressions that might easily be assumed to be metaphoric; welcoming parts explicitly; inquiring about trauma when acting-out behaviors escalate; and explaining dissociation when asked by clients. All of these responses have the underlying aim of making it easy for clients to speak of dissociated experiences without advocating or pressuring them to do so. I will describe each of these responses briefly.

I make a mental note whenever clients report anything about their life experiences that might be consistent with dissociation. These include any incest experiences in the immediate or extended family, a history of self-abusive, impulsive, or substance-abusing behavior, reported memory lapses, nightmares, headaches or odd states of consciousness, and demeaning or suicidally oriented voices. I try not to assume that a client is dissociating, but if a number of these signs manifest themselves, I begin to listen closely to client communication that might refer to dissociative experiences.

When clients describe experiences that are odd, disconnected, or divided into parts, I am likely to let the client know that I have heard them, expressing my understanding in almost the same words that the client used. In doing this, I am trying to reflect in a way that doesn't make a prejudgment as to whether particular comments are meant literally or metaphorically. So, if a client says, "I feel that I'm only here with my head and like my body is in some whole other place," I'm likely to say, "So it does feel like your head is here and the rest of your body is somewhere else." Paraphrasing or loose reflection that would work perfectly well under other circumstances is often experienced by clients as an unwillingness or inability to understand. For example, a therapist might unintentionally miss the "parts" aspect of the communication by saying, "You're not quite here yet" or "It's hard to get started today."

Communicating an openness to dissociative experiences is particularly delicate when clients describe experiencing monstrous presences in consciousness or disconnected impulses to cut or harm themselves. Clients are likely to express the wish that the therapist would help them to get rid of these experiences. I have found that if I simply express my understanding that the client wants help in making these experiences go away, the persecuting parts often feel that I want them destroyed. They are then likely to escalate their threatening actions while remaining out of awareness. One such client ended up in the hospital after serious threats to drink poison. Later, when I became aware that parts were operating, that personality commented, "That was the first time I ever tried to talk to you, and you wouldn't listen to me and I ended up being taken to a hospital in an ambulance."

Given these experiences, I now try to say something to indicate that the part would be welcomed by me whenever I think that a part may be present in the client's experience. Again, I try to say this in a way that doesn't press the client into dissociative experiences if none are present or push the client to talk about things she/he doesn't want to share. So, I might say something like the following: "I know that you are afraid of the impulses to cut yourself, and I don't want you to be physically hurt in any way. But I also wonder whether there may be some part of you that has reasons for wanting to do that."

Such welcoming statements often make no sense to the client at the time. She might say, "How can you say that? What could be good about cutting myself?" I don't press the issue or try to clarify it much further than saying, "I don't know if its true of you. It's just been my experience that when people want to hurt themselves, there is sometimes a part of them that has reasons for feeling that way." If a persecuting part is present, no matter how outwardly menacing, it is likely to feel scared, lonely, and misunderstood inside. The idea that I might be able to understand is very tempting, though also frightening since the client has experienced betrayal so many times in the past.

If persecuting parts are present, this amount of understanding often takes the urgency out of their need to act on their abusive impulses. Once they feel that they are welcome, they are likely to emerge more clearly—if not at that moment, then sometime in the next few sessions. One such part, which carried the client's rage, said to me, "I was the only one left around when the abuse was happening. All the rest of them left me alone to handle it. We wouldn't have survived if it wasn't for me. I don't understand why they're all so mad at me."

Ironically, persecuting parts often feel lonely and misunderstood in the difficulties that they face. They often come to care a lot about whether the therapist values and understands their position even while denying that this is the case. For example, I have found that when I go on vacation it is often persecuting parts (who have just begun to trust me against their better judgment) who react the most strongly to being left for that period of time. When persecuting parts aren't present I have found that open-ended welcoming comments pass fairly harmlessly, leading clients to explore different sides of their feelings about the self-abusive impulses.

If the client is flooded with self-destructive impulses but isn't talking about memories pressing, I may say that I wonder if there are some experiences coming up that are upsetting and hard to handle to some parts of her/him. This seems to be helpful even if the client doesn't talk about the experiences explicitly. For example, a client of mine was having very strong impulses to take pills after the session. When I asked if experiences might be coming up that were upsetting, she checked with the part that wanted to take pills and then said that, yes, he was having memories but she wasn't ready to know them and was afraid that he might try to bring them out. In the process of talking about this her need to harm herself subsided.

Clients who are experiencing upsurges of dissociative experiences are often afraid that they are having a psychotic break or that they will be seen as crazy by others. This fear is exacerbated by the terror many incest survivors have that they somehow caused the trauma to happen or that they are fundamentally and irretrievably damaged as a result of the trauma. If clients sense that I am able to connect to their dissociatively related experiences, they often ask what it is that I think is going on with them. Under these circumstances, I am likely to say that I don't know for certain but that their experiences are similar to those of people that I have known who had extremely painful experiences early in life. I will often explain that dissociation is a protective coping mechanism somewhat like self-hypnosis that is common to young children undergoing trauma. I may note that, in my experience, the emergence of dissociative symptoms often indicates that as an adult the person feels strong enough to handle experiences that were too overwhelming to be handled as a child. Many clients are relieved to know that I don't think of their symptoms as indicating a fundamental or irretrievable defect in their mental functioning.

## Therapeutic Work with Dissociated Parts

In general, I don't believe that therapists need to press clients to connect with dissociated experiences. The experiences press themselves on the client from the inside. Clients are living with an intense conflict of opposing impulses. Child parts who have been left alone with traumatic experiences desperately wish they could reveal them and get help. Persecuting parts feel that any connection with those experiences is likely to destroy the client and anyone else who is in contact with her.

In fact, in an empathic environment a rhythm tends to develop between the different sides of the client's feelings. As memories get more intense, child parts may emerge who want to talk to the therapist but feel that they can't. At the same time, clients may feel an onslaught of symptoms as well as self-destructive or socially deviant impulses, usually aimed at stopping the child parts and their associated memories from emerging. When persecuting parts emerge, they may talk a lot about why it is important not to trust the therapist or others too much, why feelings and memories are a bad thing, why death feels like a good thing. It is easy for the therapist to see all of these negative thoughts as resistance to change and therapeutic progress.

I have found, however, that if I just stay with the various thoughts and feelings of persecuting and deviant parts, their need to act tends to disappear or be containable by the client. And such clients ultimately let themselves connect to as much of the memories that have been pressing on them as they can handle at that time.

I have come to respect the fact that clients have a refined sense of timing in this process and that all of the parts have valuable roles to play. Typically, the persecuting parts are trying to keep memories from flooding the client and in fact offer the only means the client has of slowing the process down. These parts also need time to consider whether trusting people or connecting with experiences is a good idea, given the client's life experiences. Child parts are pressing for connectedness and healing that can only come by reconnecting with the experiences that have been cut off.

The most effective ways of connecting or working with parts differ a great deal from client to client. I have found that clients know a great deal about what will work for them. They are often reluctant to speak because of the fears and concerns different dissociated parts have about each other. And they often wish that they could bypass the therapeutic situation altogether by ignoring the past or by finding a solution that would get the pain over instantaneously. However, over time, their own experiences tend to convince them that they need to process early trauma memories.

At some times clients feel more of a sense of control when they experience "parts" in consciousness without their taking over the person's everyday personality; at other times clients feel the need to switch into a part or find themselves unable to stop the process. I do not feel the need to take a position on any of this unless the client asks for some particular kind of help. Useful processing seems to happen in all of these modes.

One client found that she connected with different parts when she looked in different directions. She found a frightened child part when she looked down at the floor and an angry monster part when she looked up at the ceiling. Another found that she had vivid spatial images when she focused on the middle of her body. So, for example, she saw a trap door on a stage with a face peeking out. When she opened the door farther in her mind, the face of a girl part became visible and emerged into her consciousness. Some clients experience parts most vividly in dreams, only occasionally switching into them in daytime situations. Others can only connect with particular parts in particular physical positions, such as lying on the right side. Some can connect through certain modalities such as art or writing or music, but not speech.

Many therapeutic techniques and ways of understanding personality change may be useful to clients experiencing dissociation. I prefer, however, to ask for my client's ideas first and to bring up my own ideas as tentative suggestions that the client may or may not want to pursue. A number of clients have particularly liked learning imaging techniques that moderate the intensity of dissociative experiences between sessions or at the end of sessions. One method that often works is to ask all the parts to imagine quiet spaces that they could go to by themselves, and then ask them to go to those spaces after a backward count of 10. If the experiences of one part are particularly distressing for another part, that part may wish to imagine a vacation place that he/she can go to while the other part is working. Again, the therapist can suggest that the part go to that place after a backward count of 10. Both of these techniques are only likely to work if the parts involved are agreeable to the idea. But, if the client is interested, she/he is likely to have a remarkable facility with this kind of consciousness-altering imagery.

Clients undergoing dissociative experiences are struggling to control highly intense and volatile experiences. At the same time, they have typically had very aberrant experiences of nurturing and control from parental figures in their lives. As a result, they often alternate between extreme unassertiveness, with the conviction that they cannot ask for the simplest consideration from others, and a demanding expectation of help that is far beyond that ordinarily offered in therapy or in intimate relationships in general.

I have found that a moderate level of flexibility is often extremely helpful to clients. Alterations of the length or timing or format of sessions can often facilitate the client's ability to handle intense experiences. And the knowledge that some flexibility is available can foster the client's sense of being personally valued in the therapeutic relationship.

There are, however, great dangers for both the client and the therapist if the therapist becomes overextended. If a client feels that the therapist has given an excessive amount, she/he may feel guilty and burdened—and she/he may feel inhibited from expressing the full range of negative feelings that inevitably come up.

Therapists may feel moved by their clients' situations in a crisis and extend themselves unrealistically without realizing that they will not be able to keep up that level of involvement on an ongoing basis. Once therapists have overextended themselves, they are likely to be particularly vulnerable to feeling wounded by further client demands and angry claims of entitlement. Therapists can easily work themselves into a situation in which they feel that they have to terminate therapeutic relationships altogether.

Clients often alternate between regaining memories and integrating the new material into their day-to-day lives. Memories will press for a while with the accompanying onslaught of uncomfortable and self-destructive feelings. Once that piece of memory has returned, the client often feels relief and a wish to return to normal living, sometimes hoping that that is the end of the dissociated experiences.

The return of a memory often brings new feelings and capacities into play, and the clients may need some time to get used to them and to learn how to integrate them into their lives. A client who had been an outsider found that she was freer to confide experiences and now had friends. She got several job promotions; men began to be interested in dating her. She began to feel anger and sadness and physical pain, where all of these had previously been relegated to dissociated parts.

## Fragile Process and Dissociated Parts

Dissociated parts often manifest a style of processing experience that I have described elsewhere (Warner, 1991) as "fragile." Dissociated parts that have a fragile style of processing tend to experience core issues at very low or high levels of intensity. They tend to have difficulty starting and stopping experiences that are personally significant or emotionally connected. And they are likely to have difficulty taking in the point of view of another person while remaining in contact with such experiences. For example, a client may talk circumstantially for most of a therapy hour and only connect with an underlying feeling of rage at the very end. Yet at this point she may feel unable to turn the rage off in a way that would allow her to return to work. She may then spend hours walking in the park trying to handle the intensity of the feeling. The client may be able to talk about feelings of rage at the therapist and very much want them understood and affirmed. Yet, therapist comments to explain the situation or disagree with the client will be felt as attempts by the therapist to annihilate the experience.

I believe that fragile process tends to develop when early childhood experiences have not been received empathically and, if such experiences are overwhelmingly painful, soothed and comforted to some degree. Certainly the lack of such empathic holding and soothing is common within abusive families.

When clients have learned to dissociate to protect themselves from being flooded by traumatic feelings, they begin to separate out whole clusters of experience from learning experiences in the rest of their day-to-day lives. They use dissociation as a substitute for more ordinary styles of processing experience, and by doing this they seem to freeze the development of emotional skills relating to those clusters of experience. If, for example, from the age of four a person has shifted into a dissociated part whenever pain or anger have passed a certain threshold of intensity, the person's ability to hold such experiences in attention and process them in more ordinary ways won't have had the chance to develop much beyond those of that 4-year-old.

Clients who experience a dissociated process, then, seem particularly likely to experience fragile process within some or all of their parts; sometimes they experience fragile process in their everyday personalities as well. The intensity of fragile process seems to relate to the age and severity of traumatic experiences and the degree of empathic failure in surrounding adults.

Empathic understanding responses are often the only sorts of responses people can receive while in the middle of fragile process without feeling traumatized or disconnected from their experience. The ongoing presence of a soothing, empathic person is often essential to the person's ability to stay connected without feeling overwhelmed. In a certain sense, clients in the middle of fragile process are asking if their way of experiencing themselves at that moment has a right to exist in the world. Any misnaming of the experience or suggestion that they look at the experience in a different way is experienced as an answer of "no" to the question.

## Therapeutic Interaction with Fragile Process

Ideally, therapy with adults who have a fragile style of processing creates the kind of empathic holding that was missing in the clients' early childhood experiences. If the therapist stays empathically connected to significant client experiences, the clients are likely to feel the satisfaction that comes from staying with their experiences in an accepting way. Initially this tends to be a very ambivalent sort of pleasure, since the experiences themselves are often painful and the client is likely to be convinced that they are shameful and likely to result in harm to themselves and others.

Clients may feel the need to test therapists in various ways before trusting that the therapists can relate to their experience or believing that their experience can have any value. They may be afraid that expressing their experience will make them vulnerable to manipulation and control by the therapist or that their experience has the power to overwhelm and harm the therapist. Over time, however, clients are likely to find that their reactions make more sense than they thought and that seemingly inexorable feelings go through various sorts of positive change and resolution.

Comments, interpretations, or questions are often experienced as violating to clients in the middle of fragile process since they can't take in the therapist's point without annihilating their own experience of the moment. For example, a client may say that she feels upset when she thinks that she has to come to therapy sessions and the therapist may ask why she feels that she has to come. The client may be just starting to sense that she can hold her upset feeling and to believe that she is all right in the process. Under those circumstances, the therapist's question is likely to be experienced as a message that the client's experiences are all wrong and that she has no right to have them. Yet, if the client expresses anger at the therapist, the therapist is likely to feel puzzled and annoyed by the client's reaction.

While clients are beginning to hold and process fragile experiences in therapy they are likely to feel very reliant on the therapist. At this stage, the empathic presence of the therapist is essential to clients' ability to hold experiences without feeling traumatized. It is as if the therapist held an oxygen mask for clients, who spend the rest of the week struggling to be able to breathe. Quite sensibly, clients may hate to leave sessions and resent the time that they have to spend out of contact with the therapist. Gradually, though, clients come to be able to hold their experience for longer and longer periods of time between sessions. Often, having several sessions a week lets them bridge between sessions without losing their sense of connectedness. In this in-between phase clients can often reconnect with their experience by calling up the image of the therapist in various ways. Brief phone contact, hearing tape recordings of the therapist's voice, holding an object that belongs to the therapist, or sitting outside of the therapist's office may help recall the therapy experience.

As the therapy progresses, clients become increasingly able to hold intense feelings in awareness and to work through them. Successive layers of trauma memories are remembered and processed, becoming integrated into the everyday consciousness of the client. As a result, both the desire and the need to use dissociation as a means to manage the intensity of experience tends to disappear.

## THE CONTROVERSY OVER DISSOCIATIVE IDENTITY DISORDERS

The dissociative identity disorders have received extensive attention—both positive and negative—in the psychological literature in recent years. The intensity of the debate is partially attributable to the fact that the "alters" or "multiple personalities" characteristic of dissociative identity disorders often only become clearly visible during the process of psychotherapy. Initially clients are likely to present with a bewildering variety of dissociative and nondissociative symptoms that could be seen as indicative of other diagnoses such as schizophrenia, anxiety disorders, depression, or borderline personality disorder. A substantial group of therapists believe that these clients are manifesting a dissociative style of coping with early trauma. Others are skeptical of this way of understanding the phenomenon.

Research results are suggestive but inconclusive on both sides of this debate. Numerous studies document a relationship between early childhood sexual and physical abuse and a wide range of adult symptoms including dissociative states (for summaries of this literature, see Zelikovsky & Lynn, 1994). A dissociative disorders inventory has been developed that reliably separates clients with dissociative identity disorders from those clients in other diagnostic categories (see Steinberg, 1993; Steinberg, Rounsaville, & Cicchetti, 1990; and Ross, 1995). A very high percentage of these clients come to remember incidents of severe sexual and physical abuse in early childhood during dissociatively oriented therapy (Horevitz & Loewenstein, 1994, pp. 289–290). If even a significant proportion of these memories are valid, they suggest a strong etiological connection between severe early sexual and physical abuse and adult dissociative disorders.

In psychotherapy with therapists who believe in the syndrome, clients tend to shift fairly rapidly into clear presentations of alternate personalities with the particular trance-like qualities characteristic of dissociation. These personalities virtually always manifest rigid, mutually contradictory ideas about the best way to handle overwhelming experiences of abuse. For therapists who work with dissociative identity disorders, the syndrome represents a conceptual breakthrough, offering ways of helping large numbers of clients whose life-crippling difficulties have previously had very poor prognoses in psychiatric treatment. Colin Ross (1989) declares that

> When I am assessing a patient with features of chronic trauma disorder and can contact preexisting personalities, I feel good because I know what to do and have an effective treatment to offer. . . . I think that it's a fact that for chronic trauma patients without MPD [multiple personality disorder], psychiatry has little to offer other than trails of medication and supportive therapy. (p. 203)

While many therapists report positive results in treating dissociative identity disorders, outcome research is very limited and suffers from a lack of rigorous controls. This lack of research data is not surprising given the fact that treatment tends to be long and complex and the fact that renewed interest in dissociative disorders is relatively recent (for a brief history of dissociative theories in clinical psychology, see Putnam, 1989, pp. 26–44). The largest number of client outcomes have been presented by Kluft and Ross. Kluft (1984), in reviewing 123 cases treated by himself or by other therapists, reported that 83 (or 67.5%) reached stable integration, most in less than 3 years of treatment. Ross (1989, pp. 197–203), in reviewing the treatment records of 22 clients seen at the Winnipeg Dissociative Disorders Clinic, estimates stable integration will be reached and maintained by 54.5–72.7% of their clients. Ross (1989) notes that "a 70 percent response rate is as good as any treatment for any complex disorder in psychiatry, be the treatment biological, psychotherapeutic, or behavioral. MPD, I believe is as common as schizophrenia and more treatable" (p. 203).

Those who doubt the validity of the disorder suggest that the characteristic syndromes of personalities and trauma memories are largely iatrogenic (see, e.g., Belli & Loftus, 1994; Tillman, Nash, & Lerner, 1994; Frankel, 1994; Ganaway, 1994). They point out that memory is a complex and fallible process under the best of circumstances. Theorists from all schools of thought agree that dissociative identity disorder clients are particularly adept at moving into trance-like experiences. Many of the most widely accepted therapeutic techniques for working with dissociative disorders involve pressing clients to accept the reality of their dissociative disorder, asking for alter personalities to emerge, and using a range of hypnotic techniques during the therapy process (Horevitz & Loewenstein, 1994). Skeptics, then, question whether many of the memories that emerge are artifacts of the trance process itself. Belli and Loftus (1994) declare that

> given the attributional source of memories, there simply is no reliable means to correctly judge when a memory is based on reality and when it is not.

> In our view, the practice by some therapists of encouraging adult clients to recover memories of childhood abuse is creating the very real danger that child abuse incidents are being misreported. . . . If everyone is a victim, then no one is. (p. 429)

Much of the critique of work with dissociation has focused on therapists who use extraordinary methods such as interviewing with hypnosis or Amytal Sodium (amobarbital sodium), strongly advocating that clients accept a dissociative diagnosis or pressing clients to come up with clearer memories. Brown (1995) notes that while under laboratory conditions subjects may produce misinformation as to peripheral details, people tend to be correct in their memories of the main aspects of personal events of importance. He notes that the only substantial research evidence for falsifying the central aspects of personal memories relates to circumstances of intense and leading questioning, which can create "interrogatory suggestion" (pp. 10–12). As a result, he suggests that "less authoritarian, egalitarian therapists . . . are likely to reduce memory confabulation in therapy."

## THE VALIDITY OF DISSOCIATED EXPERIENCES

The concerns raised by skeptics are not trivial. However, I continue to think that dissociatively oriented therapeutic work is essential to the emotional recovery of many clients who have suffered early trauma. I believe that false memories are the exception rather than the norm, particularly when less confrontive and interpretive styles of therapy are used.

Clients I have worked with for substantial periods of time who showed the distinctive dissociative clusters of "alters" have all come to remember severe sexual or physical trauma before the age of seven. Similar patterns have emerged in the clients of therapists with whom I have consulted. Connection with memories through the experience of the "alters" has seemed to be essential to enable these clients to work through the trauma and to produce an overall improvement of their ability to function in their current lives. I have found their dissociative experiences convincing for a number of reasons:

Clients who have worked through these sorts of traumatic memories have tended to get better. Their lives have become less constricted; they function with an increased emotional range; their relationships become more productive and stable; their work lives become more successful. This is a gradual process with many ups and downs. Of course, a client's initial connection with dissociated parts and traumatic memories can make her/his life more painful and overtly symptomatic, and not all clients continue with the therapy process. But, as work proceeds, clients who have been unable to sustain friendships make deep and lasting connections. Clients who have been underemployed get promotions. Clients with a limited range of personal emotion become comfortable with anger, sadness, and pain.

I have generally found that when clients connect with dissociated parts, aspects of their experience that have seemed disconnected and incomprehensible over long periods of time come into a much more live process. This occurs in two ways. First, actions that seemed totally disconnected with bodily felt experiencing become emotionally grounded as clients connect with "parts" experiences. Thus, a client who has been performing angry actions will feel the anger when connecting to a "part." And, in the process, situations in the client's lives that have seemed perversely stuck and unmoving begin to go through changes that are therapeutically productive. Feelings and actions that are initially only experienced by parts tend to spontaneously reintegrate into the person's regular life narrative in a more reality-oriented form. Secondly, actions that seemed out of control or perverse come to be experienced as owned, motivated actions—initially with somewhat unusual, dissociative-type logics associated with them. (For example, instead of saying, "My hands suddenly turned the steering wheel and the car went off the road," the person might say, "the enforcer is very angry that I told you his name and feels that I should be punished, so he turned the wheel." Once such events are experienced as motivated actions, they come to be much more readily engaged in therapy and clients lose much of their tendency to act on them. Ultimately, such feelings and thoughts tend to become integrated into a single, more reality-oriented narrative. For example, at a later time the person might say, "I used to feel so afraid of the pain that I would want to drive into a wall just to make it stop."

I have been impressed by the number of memories that emerged in work with dissociated parts that have been directly or indirectly confirmed by others. For example, a woman who recovered memories of being raped by her uncle when she was a young child was told by her aunt that she had recently discovered that he had been molesting his own daughter. A client who was having feelings of horror associated with dissociated parts commented that she had a "regular" memory of wanting to play "torture" with her friends in kindergarten. She asked me if that was usual for a 5-year-old child. A client who recovered a memory of being tied up and taunted by neighborhood children had that memory confirmed in a conversation with her brother.

In spite of the level of overall validation I have received for client memories, the laboratory research on memory has convinced me that it is possible for clients to misremember or unintentionally fabricate a belief in events that didn't actually happen. (And, as with any disability, a small number of people will intentionally pretend to suffer from the disorder in the hopes of gaining sympathetic attention.) When memories come up for which there is no external validation, I can only stay with my clients experience as they decide for themselves how to weigh their validity.

I am struck by the fact that therapists at the Chicago Counseling and Psychotherapy Center have diagnosed and long worked with the distinctive syndrome of "alters" and traumatic memories using a client-directed style that doesn't employ the kinds of directed questioning or confrontation that

Brown and others see as likely to elicit false memories. In this sense, a client-centered style of therapy seems to offer an approach that is effective in recovering and reworking trauma memories while minimizing the likelihood that false memories will be induced in the process. And the client-centered approach, which fosters a relatively equal, person-to-person therapeutic relationship and leaves the primary control over core therapeutic decision making in clients' hands, is often particularly appreciated by clients who have been abused by previous authority figures in their lives.

## NOTES

1. In my descriptions of dissociated process I have been helped by client-centered therapists who have shared their experiences with me over time. I am particularly indebted to Barbara Roy, Laurel Jonas, Kevin Krychka, and Robert Oppenheimer. Details of client situations described in this paper have been altered to protect client confidentiality.

2. For the purposes of this chapter, I use the terms "part," "dissociated part," and "personality" interchangeably in referring to dissociated states derived from early childhood trauma.

3. Our overall understanding of dissociative phenomena is quite similar to that of more directively oriented therapists, such as Kluft (1985, 1993), Putnam (1989), or Braun (1985). These phenomena do, however, present themselves in significantly different ways in a client-directed therapeutic process.

4. Despite the trance-like qualities of dissociated states, investigators have found variable levels of correlation between hypnotizability and dissociation as measured by the Dissociative Experiences Scale (DES). E. B. Carlson (1994, pp. 46–49) reports moderately strong correlations in several studies, but believes that the scales are measuring related, but distinct phenomena. Horevitz and Loewenstein (1994, pp. 439–440) suggest that dissociative capacity may be more related to a genetically based ability to segregate and idiosyncratically encode experience into separated psychological or psychobiological processes with great fluidity in identity than to hypnotizability per se.

5. The majority of my experience and that of my colleagues is with voluntary outpatient treatment. Typical client presentation may be different in involuntary, institutional settings.

## REFERENCES

Belli, R. F., & Loftus, E. F. (1994). Recovering memories of childhood abuse: A source monitoring perspective. In S. J. Lynn & J. W. Rhue (Eds.), *Dissociation: Clinical and theoretical perspectives*. New York: Guilford Press.

Braun, B. G. (Ed.). (1985). *Treatment of multiple personality disorder*. Washington, DC: American Psychiatric Press.

Brown, D. (1995). Pseudomemories: The standard of science and the standard of care in treatment. *American Journal of Clinical Hypnosis*, 37(3), 1–24.

Carlson, E. B. (1994). Studying the interaction between physical and psychological states with the Dissociative Experiences Scale. In D. Spiegel (Ed.), *Disso-*

*ciation: Culture, mind and body*. Washington, DC: American Psychiatric Press.

Frankel, F. (1994). Dissociation in hysteria and hypnosis: A concept aggrandized. In S. J. Lynn & J. W. Rhue (Eds.), *Dissociation: Clinical and theoretical perspectives*. New York: Guilford Press.

Ganaway, G. K. (1994). Transference and countertransference shaping influences on dissociative syndromes. In S. J. Lynn & J. W. Rhue (Eds.), *Dissociation: Clinical and theoretical perspectives*. New York: Guilford Press.

Horevitz, R., & Loewenstein, R. J. (1994). The rational treatment of multiple personality disorder. In S. J. Lynn & J. W. Rhue (Eds.), *Dissociation: Clinical and theoretical perspectives*. New York: Guilford Press.

Kluft, R. P. (1984). Treatment of multiple personality disorder. *Psychiatric Clinics of North America, 1*, 9–29.

Kluft, R. P. (Ed.). (1985). *Childhood antecedents of multiple personality disorder*. Washington, DC: American Psychiatric Press.

Kluft, R. P., & Fine, C. G. (Eds.). (1993). *Clinical perspectives on multiple personality disorder*. Washington, DC: American Psychiatric Press.

Putnam, F. W. (1989). *Diagnosis and treatment of multiple personality disorder*. New York: Guilford Press.

Ross, C. (1989). *Multiple personality disorder*. New York: Wiley.

Ross, C. (1995). The Validity and Reliability of Dissociative Identity Disorder. In L. M. Cohen, J. N. Berzoff, & M. R. Elin (Eds.), *Dissociative disorder: Theoretical and treatment controversies*. Northvale, NJ: Jason Aronson Inc.

Steinberg, M. (1993). *Structured Clinical Interview for DSM-IV Dissociative Disorders (SCID-D)*. Washington, DC: American Psychiatric Press.

Steinberg, M., Rounsaville, B., & Cicchetti, D. V. (1990). The structured clinical interview for DSM III-R disorders: Preliminary report on a new diagnostic instrument. *American Journal of Psychiatry, 147*, 76–82.

Tillman, J., Nash, M., & Lerner, P. (1994). Does trauma cause dissociative pathology? In S. J. Lynn & J. W. Rhue (Eds.), *Dissociation: Clinical and theoretical perspectives*. New York: Guilford Press.

Warner, M. S. (1991). Fragile process. In L. Fusek (Ed.), *New directions in client-centered therapy: Practice with difficult client populations* (Monograph Series I). Chicago: Chicago Counseling and Psychotherapy Center.

Zelikovsky, N., & Lynn, S. J. (1994). The aftereffects and assessment of physical and psychological abuse. In S. J. Lynn & J. W. Rhue (Eds.), *Dissociation: Clinical and theoretical perspectives*. New York: Guilford Press.

# 17

*****

# Pre-Therapy and Pre-Symbolic Experiencing
## EVOLUTIONS IN PERSON-CENTERED/ EXPERIENTIAL APPROACHES TO PSYCHOTIC EXPERIENCE

**Garry Prouty**

## A BRIEF HISTORY

In person-centered treatment populations, schizophrenia shows the least therapeutic effect (Greenberg, Elliott, & Lietaer, 1994). Also, it is well known that Carl R. Rogers did not believe person-centered therapy was suitable for mentally retarded clients (Ruedrich & Menolascino, 1984).

Person-centered explorations of schizophrenia began with the work of Shlien (1961), who describes the disorganization of the psychotic self-structure. Starting with the "impossible life," he outlines three phases: self-defense, self-denial, and self-negation. Rogers, Gendlin, Kiesler, and Truax (1967) describe the major findings of the Wisconsin Project: (1) clients perceived low levels of the "therapeutic attitudes" regardless of reality; (2) experiencing did not improve as a function of these "attitudes"; (3) gains were measured with clients who successfully experienced the therapist "attitudes." Gendlin (1967) describes these clients as lacking "self-propelled process" and as characteristically rejecting the therapist. He proposes the sharing of congruent experiencing as a solution. Gendlin (1970) conceptualizes the schizophrenic psychosis as the absence of experiencing. Hinterkopf and Brunswick (1975, 1981) successfully taught clients to utilize focusing and reflection with each other, resulting in successful outcomes. Teusch, Beyerle, Lange, Schenk, and Stadtmüller (1983; also Teusch, 1990) describe improved outcomes combining therapy with medications.

Person-centered therapy (PCT) with retarded clients has been almost nonexistent due to Rogers's (1942) belief that these clients lacked the autonomy and introspective skills necessary for therapy. A few European papers have appeared that describe PCT with retarded persons (Peters, 1981, 1986, 1992; Badelt, 1990; Pörtner, 1988).

## THE THEORETICAL PROBLEMATICS

Classical person-centered/experiential psychotherapy contains theoretical problematics that affect clinical practice with schizophrenic and retarded populations. First, Rogers's theory of therapy describes "psychological contact" as the first condition of a therapeutic relationship (Rogers, 1957). Prouty (1990) observes (1) that contact is a gratuitous assumption in regressed, psychotic populations; (2) that Rogers fails to provide a theoretical description of "psychological contact"; and (3) that Rogers fails to provide a clinical method for impaired "psychological contact." These limitations necessitate the development of a theory and method of psychological contact for clients who are too *contact impaired* for a therapeutic relationship.

Gendlin (1964) forms the experiential concept of "structure bound" to describe hallucinatory experiencing. Experiencing is structure bound when (1) it is perceived "as such" by the client; (2) when it is isolated, that is, not in the felt functioning of the organism; and (3) when it is rigid, that is, not in experiential process. Gendlin also utilizes the adjectives "static" and "repetitious." This *pre-process structure* yields the problem of how to develop a *process structure* with hallucinating clients. Pre-symbolic processing is a theoretical and practice description that solves the structure bound problematic.

## PART I: PRE-THERAPY

Pre-therapy is an evolution in person-centered psychotherapy. It evolves from Rogers's (1959) concept of "psychological contact" as the first and necessary condition of a therapeutic relationship, and Perls's (1969) concept of "contact as an ego function." Pre-therapy is described as a theory of psychological contact. The result of this fusion is the hypothesis that psychological contact is the necessary function, or *pre-condition*, for a therapeutic relationship. Pre-therapy develops or restores the psychological contact *necessary* for psychotherapy with *contact-impaired* clients. This approach has proved relevant to psychotic and retarded dual-diagnosed populations, thereby expanding the general range of humanistic–experiential therapy (Prouty, 1976, 1995, in press; Prouty & Kubiak, 1988; Van Werde, 1989, 1990; Prouty & Cronwall, 1990; Prouty, Van Werde, & Pörtner, 1998; Van Werde & Prouty, 1992).

## A Concrete Phenomenology

Pre-therapy is a "pointing to the concrete" (Buber, 1964, p. 547). It is a concrete response to the extraordinarily concrete level of client experiencing and expression that is characteristic of schizophrenic and retarded persons (Prouty, 1994).

### The Concrete Attitude

A. Gelb and K. Goldstein (see Gurwitsch, 1966) describe the "concrete attitude" of brain-damaged clients. Normal clients experienced multiple shades of a color as the same color (categorical attitude). Brain-damaged soldiers experienced the multiple shades as different colors. They did not categorize essence; they were stimulus bound. As a result, they manifested a "concrete attitude." Research also provided similar data from schizophrenic clients (Arieti, 1955). Pre-therapy represents an extraordinary concrete response to extraordinary concrete cognition of retarded and psychotic clients.

### The Concrete Phenomenon

The concrete phenomenon is labeled "as itself." It is a description of the properties of the phenomenon as "naturalistic," "self-indicative," and "de-symbolized." The concept "naturalistic" refers to experiencing the phenomenon exactly as it appears *naturally* in consciousness (Farber, 1959, 1967). The concept "self-indicative" describes the phenomenon as meaning itself, referring to itself, and implying itself (Sartre, 1956). The term "desymbolized" refers to the idea that something can be self-given only if it is *not* mediated by symbols. Philosophy is the continual desymbolization of the world (Scheler, 1953). These concepts are *guidelines* that will, I hope, help focus the therapist on the literalness of client experiencing and expression.

## Theoretical Structure

Pre-therapy emerges from Rogers's concept of "psychological contact" as the first condition of a therapeutic relationship (Rogers, 1959, p. 251) and Perls's concept of "contact as an ego function" (Perls, 1969, p. 14). Pre-therapy is a theory of psychological contact (Prouty, 1990). As such it describes therapist's responses (contact reflections), client psychological functions (contact functions), and emergent measurable behaviors (contact behaviors).

### Contact Reflections

According to Rogers (1966), reflection conveys nondirectivness, empathy, and unconditional positive regard. Gendlin (1968) conceives reflection as the facilitation of the *experiencing process*. Pre-therapy describes reflections as the development or restoration of psychological contact. This is carried out by five very literal and concrete responses within the context of an *empathic* and *receiving* attitude toward the client's pre-expressive levels of communication and behavior:

1. *Situational reflections* (SR). Situational reflections have the theoretical function of developing the client's contact with a situation, environment, or milieu. A simple example of SR is "John is rolling the ball." This facilitates reality contact.

2. *Facial reflections* (FR). Facial reflections help provide the client's contact with pre-expressive affect. Clients often exhibit flattened affect due to psychosocial isolation, institutionalization, and overmedication (Reiss, 1994). They do not experience their feelings with a sense of self. An example of FR is "John looks mad." This provides affective contact.

3. *Word-for-word reflections* (WWR). Word-for-word reflections help develop client communicative contact. Many of these clients, because of schizophrenic communicative mechanisms or brain damage, express themselves in incoherent ways. Often, there are streams of incoherence with tiny islands of coherence—for example, "unintelligible vocal sound," "unintelligible vocal sound," "house," "unintelligible vocal sound," "tree," "unintelligible vocal sound," "unintelligible vocal sound," "car." The therapist would reflect, separately, and *word for word*, "house, tree, car." Sometimes emotional tones are reflected. This helps develop communicative contact.

4. *Body reflections* (BR). Psychotic or retarded dual-diagnosed clients often express themselves through "bodying." Examples are catatonia, echopraxia, or other forms of bizarre behavior. The therapist may use BR such as "Your body is stiff" or "Your arm is in the air." Occasionally, therapists may use their own bodies as empathic expressions.

5. *Reiterative reflections* (RR). Reiterative reflections embody the principal of recontact. If one of the contact reflections is successful in producing a response, then repeat the reflection. This strengthens the contact and carries the client deeper into the experiencing process.

Tempo and spatiality are also important considerations in pre-therapy. Therapists may overreflect or underreflect, depending on the client. Hyperactive and manic clients might require faster responses; depressed and withdrawn clients might need a slower tempo. Hallucinatory clients often require consideration of spatiality since hallucinations can be three dimensional (Havens, 1962).

## Contact Functions

Contact functions are an expansion of Perls's (1969, p. 14) concept of "contact as an ego function." They are conceived as awareness functions involving the *world, self, or other* (Merleau-Ponty, 1962, p. 60). These awareness functions are defined as follows:

- *Reality contact* is the awareness of people, places, things, or events.
- *Affective contact* is the awareness of moods, feelings, and emotions.
- *Communicative contact* is the symbolization of reality and affect to others.

Pre-therapy is the use of contact reflections to facilitate the contact functions. Contact reflections develop the awareness of the world, self, and others. The following vignette is an example of developing reality, affective, and communicative contact. The client, Dorothy, is a chronic schizophrenic custodial patient.

Dorothy is an old woman who is one of the more regressed women on X ward. She was mumbling something (as she usually did). This time I could hear certain words in her confusion. I reflected only the words I could clearly understand. After about 10 minutes, I could hear a complete sentence:

CLIENT: Come with me.

THERAPIST: [WWR] Come with me. (*Dorothy led me to the corner of the dayroom. We stood there silently for what seemed to be a very long time. Since I couldn't communicate with her, I watched her body movements and closely reflected these.*)

CLIENT: (*Dorothy put her hand on the wall.*) Cold.

THERAPIST: [WW/BR] (*I put my hand on the wall and repeated the word.*) Cold. (*Dorothy had been holding my hand all along; but when I reflected her, she would tighten her grip. She would begin to mumble word fragments. I was careful to reflect only the words I could understand. What she was saying began to make sense.*)

CLIENT: I don't know what this is anymore. (*Touching the wall* [Reality contact].) The walls and chairs don't mean anything anymore [existential autism].

THERAPIST: [WW/BR] (*Touching the wall.*) You don't know what this is anymore. The chairs and walls don't mean anything to you anymore.

CLIENT: (*Dorothy began to cry* [Affective contact]. *After a while she began to talk again. This time she spoke clearly* [Communicative contact].) I don't like it here. I'm so tired . . . so tired.

THERAPIST: [WWR] (*As I gently touched her arm, this time it was I who tightened my grip on her hand. I reflected*) You're tired, so tired.

CLIENT: (*The patient smiled and told me to sit in a chair directly in front of her and began to braid my hair.*)

## Contact Behaviors

Contact reflections facilitate the contact functions resulting in the emergence of contact behaviors. The contact behaviors are the measurable results of pre-therapy. They can be utilized for scale constructions and represent the therapeutic consequences of pre-therapy:

- *Reality contact* is operationalized as the verbalization of people, places, things, and events.
- *Affective contact* is operationalized as the verbal, facial, or bodily expression of affect.
- *Communicative contact* is designated as the client's verbalization of words or sentences.

Pilot studies of pre-therapy have developed measures of significant differences, construct validity, and reliability (Hinterkopf, Prouty, & Brunswick, 1979; De Vre, 1992; Prouty, 1994). Utilizing a different measuring scheme, Dinacci (1994, 1997) found significant increases in communication with chronic and functionally retarded schizophrenic patients.

Contact reflections, functions, and behaviors are the essential structures of pre-therapy.

## Applications

### Catatonia

Prouty and Kubiak (1988) describe the application of pre-therapy to a catatonic schizophrenic client. The client was a 22-year-old Caucasian male who had been hospitalized several times.

The client was one of 13 children. His parents were farmers of Polish ethnicity. His mother had been hospitalized several times for schizophrenic problems.

Family observation revealed at least one sibling, although not hospitalized, displaying psychotic symptoms. The family brought the client to the United States for evaluation. A preliminary observation confirmed that the client was potentially responsive to pre-therapy.

According to psychiatric documents, the client had been described as "mute," "autistic," "catatonic," "making no eye contact," "exhibiting trance-like behavior," "stuporous," "confused," "not establishing rapport," "delusional," "paranoid," and finally "experiencing severe thought blocking." He had been diagnosed variously as "manic–depressive," "hysterical reaction," "hebephrenic schizophrenic," "paranoid schizophrenic," "catatonic schizophrenic," "profound schizophrenic," "schizophrenic, affective type." He had received six electroshock treatments, as well as numerous chemical interventions including trifluoperazine, trifluoperazine dihydrochloride, diazapam, imipramine, chlorpromazine, clomipramine, phenothiazine, fluphenazine dihydrochloride, and haloperidol.

The client was returned to his home for several months while arrangements for residential care and legal details were arranged. My associate therapist arrived and found that the client, kept at home for several months, had deteriorated into psychosis. The parents had not rehospitalized him. He was in a severe catatonic state, having withdrawn to the lower portion of the three-story home. He did not eat meals with the family, only creeping out at night to use the family refrigerator. He had lost considerable weight and his feet were blue from being cramped and stiffened due to his lack of movement and circulation.

This vignette describes segments of a 12-hour process that illustrates the application of contact reflections, the successful resolution of the catatonic state, and the development of communicative contact (without medication).

The patient was sitting on a long couch, very rigid, with arms outstretched and even with his shoulders. His eyes were straight ahead, his face was mask-like, and his hands and feet were blue-gray. The therapist sat on the opposite side of the couch giving no eye contact to the patient. Reflections were given 5 to 10 minutes apart:

**Segment I** (approximately 2:00 P.M.)

THERAPIST: [SR] I can hear the children playing.

THERAPIST: [SR] It is very cool down here.

THERAPIST: [SR] I can hear people talking in the kitchen.

THERAPIST: [SR] I'm sitting with you in the lower level of your house.

THERAPIST: [SR] I can hear the dog barking.

THERAPIST: [BR] Your body is very rigid.

THERAPIST: [BR] You are sitting very still.

THERAPIST: [BR] You are looking straight ahead.

THERAPIST: [BR] You are sitting on the couch in a very upright position.

THERAPIST: [BR] Your body isn't moving. Your arms are in the air.

CLIENT: (*No response—no movement.*)

**Segment II** (approximately 3:30 P.M.)

[The therapist brought a chair and sat in it directly in front of the patient and mirrored his body exactly as she saw it.]

THERAPIST: [BR] Your body is very rigid. You are sitting on the couch and not moving.

[Approximately 15–20 minutes later]

THERAPIST: I can no longer hold my arms outstretched. My arms are tired.

CLIENT: (*No response—no movement.*)

THERAPIST: [BR] Your body is very stiff.

THERAPIST: [BR] Your arms are outstretched.

THERAPIST: [BR] Your body isn't moving.

CLIENT: (*Put his hands on his head as if to hold his head, and spoke in a barely audible whisper.*) My head hurts me when my father speaks.

THERAPIST: [WWR] My head hurts me when my father speaks.

THERAPIST: [BR] (*Therapist put her hands as if to hold her head.*)

THERAPIST: RR/WW My head hurts when my father speaks.

CLIENT: (*Continued to hold head for 2–3 hours.*)

**Segment III** (approximately 8:00 P.M.)

THERAPIST: [SR] It's evening. We are in the lower level of your home.

THERAPIST: [BR] Your body is very rigid.

THERAPIST: [BR] Your hands are holding your head.

THERAPIST: [RR/WW] My head hurts when my father speaks.

CLIENT: (*Immediately dropped his hands to his knees and looked directly into therapist's eyes.*)

THERAPIST: [BR] You've taken you hands from your head and placed them on your knees. You are looking right into my eyes.

CLIENT: (*Sat motionless for hours.*)

THERAPIST: [RR/BR] You dropped your hands from your head to your knees.

THERAPIST: [SR] You are looking straight into my eyes.

CLIENT: (*Immediately, he talked in a barely audible whisper.*) Priests are devils.

THERAPIST: [WWR] Priests are devils.

THERAPIST: [BR] Your hands are on your knees.

THERAPIST: [SR] You are looking right into my eyes.

THERAPIST: [BR] Your body is very rigid.

CLIENT: (*He talked in a barely audible whisper.*) My brothers can't forgive me.

THERAPIST: [WWR] My brothers can't forgive me.

CLIENT: (*Sat motionless for approximately an hour.*)

**Segment IV** (approximately 1:45 A.M.)

THERAPIST: [SR] It is very quiet.

THERAPIST: [SR] You are in the lower level of the house.

THERAPIST: [SR] It is evening.

THERAPIST: [BR] Your body is very rigid.

CLIENT: (*Immediately, in slow motion, put his hand over his heart and talked.*) My heart is wooden.

THERAPIST: [BR/WW] (*In slow motion, put her hand over her heart and talked.*) My heart is wooden.

CLIENT: (*Feet started to move.*)

THERAPIST: [BR] Your feet are starting to move.

CLIENT: (*More eye movement.*)

The therapist took the patient's hand and lifted him to stand. They began to walk. The patient walked with the therapist around the farm and in a *normal conversational mode* spoke about the different animals. He brought the therapist to newborn puppies and lifted one to hold. The client had good eye contact. The client continued to maintain communicative contact over the next 4 days and was able to transfer planes and negotiate customs on the way to the United States. The client was able to sign himself into the residential treatment facility where he underwent classical person-centered/experiential psychotherapy.

This vignette illustrates the function of pre-therapy, which is to restore the client's psychological contact enabling treatment. Very clearly, this client's reality and communicative contact were improved sufficiently to enter psychotherapy.

## Newer Developments

Newer developments have occurred as pre-therapy has been practiced by therapists in different settings with different client populations.

*The Pre-Expressive Self.* Pre-therapy develops contact with the pre-expressive self. This is the central intuition of the approach. The pre-expressive self is a *meta-theoretical* construct that organizes several types of evidence. First, actual pre-therapy case studies illustrate the client's struggle from a pre-expressive to an expressive level. Secondly, statistical data (Hinterkopf et al., 1979; De Vre, 1992; Prouty, 1990, 1994; Dinacci, 1994, 1995) reveal a continuum from a pre-expressive to a more fully expressive state. Third, clinical observations of psychotic clients indicate a semiotic structure of pre-expressivity. Psychotic clients make statements that are without direct context or reference, thereby appearing "without reality," ergo, psychotically meaningless. These statements often contain the expressive potentials for reality that are manifested later in therapy (Prouty & Kubiak, 1988). The psychoanalytic concept of regression simply does not illuminate the possibility of expressive potentials. The concept of psychotic regression is descriptive, not therapeutic. Fourth, clinical anecdotes (Prouty, 1994) describe withdrawn and psychologically isolated clients who suddenly move from a noncontactful, pre-expressive state into full contact and expressivity. Although this shift is sudden, it still reveals the same pattern of movement from a pre-expressive to an expressive state. These anecdotes illustrate the presence of a buried self that experiences contact and suddenly emerges.

All of this requires that therapist attitudes include an empathy for the client's efforts at moving from the pre-expressive to the expressive state. This is particularly true if the self-formative tendency is actualized in a therapeutic relationship. The movement from the pre-expressive self to the expressive self is a form of self-actualization for these clients. What is involved is the presence of an underlying "pre-expressive self" that is eclipsed by regression, autism, retardation, psychosis, dementia, communications disorders, and the like. This must be the primary empathic sensibility of the therapist. Pre-therapy facilitates the pre-expressive self to the full existential selfhood of psychological contact with the *world, self, or other.*

*Pre-Therapy as a Ward Milieu.*  Van Werde (1992, 1994) has developed a psychiatric ward milieu based on pre-therapy. His fundamental purpose is to strengthen patient contact functions through the interpersonal processes of a psychiatric ward staff. This is not individual psychotherapy, but rather a milieu therapy. Staff members apply the contact reflections during the everyday ward interactions and structures, that is, ward meetings, perception therapy, work therapy, movement therapy, and spontaneous occurrences in ward life. This provides the client with a contact milieu that strengthens the client's contact with the world, self, or other, thereby providing an anti-psychotic antidote on a psychological level.

## Other Applications

Roy (1991) describes the application of pre-therapy to multiple personality clients with alternate self-structures. Such alternates often manifest themselves in halting, primitive symbolizations through the face, body, situation, or words. Roy would make full psychological contact with the alternates by the use of contact reflection, thereby contributing to integration.

Retardation professionals report additional uses of pre-therapy. First, the contact reflections can be used as recreational therapy for profoundly retarded clients in prevocational and vocational settings. It is reported that clients really enjoy the "human contact." Secondly, parents of profoundly retarded clients report "human satisfaction" for themselves and their children when contact reflections are used. This approach allows parents and children to have psychological contact that normally wouldn't have been present.

Also, it has been found that contact reflections can be used to resolve psychotic episodes during a psychodrama (Prouty, 1994). These techniques help put a psychodrama client in reality contact if a psychotic episode occurs within the therapeutic process.

## PART II: PRE-SYMBOLIC EXPERIENCING

Pre-symbolic experiencing (Prouty, 1977, 1983, 1991; Prouty & Pietrzak, 1988) is a theoretical description of the structure and processing of the schizophrenic hallucination. It arises from a problematic in Gendlin's (1964) conception of the "structure bound" hallucination. Gendlin conceives the hallucination as structure bound, meaning that the hallucinations is perceived literally "as such" by the client. Secondly, it is described as "isolated," meaning that the hallucination is not in the felt functioning of the organism. Thirdly, it is described as "rigid," that is, not in experiential process. The difficulty is that this describes the hallucination as a *nonprocess structure*. The problematic is how to conceive the hallucination as a *process structure*.

### An Epistemic Shift

The reconceptualizing of the hallucination as a process structure requires an epistemic shift from phenomenology to symbology. This first necessitates a basic distinction between the symbol and the phenomenon. Whitehead (1927) describes the symbol as an experience that implies another experience. Sartre (1956), in sharp contrast, defines the phenomenon as an experience that implies itself. The symbol is *a* implies *b* and the phenomenon is *a* implies *a*. This is a sharp epistemic distinction in describing the structure of the hallucination. We are moving from a phenomenological to a *symbolic* description.

### Symbols and Motivation

Cassirer (1955) describes *Homo sapiens* as "an animal symbolicum" (a symbolic animal). The vast superstructure of culture, including language, philosophy, science, art, communications, etc., are thought of as "symbolization." Human beings and their culture are conceived as symbolic. Suzanne K. Langer (1961, pp. 46–47) evolves this conception further by describing the human brain as a "transformer" that changes "the current of experience into symbols." This metaphor allows us to think of human organisms as motivated to symbolize experience.

### Symbolic Structures

Humans symbolize their experience at different levels of abstractness and concreteness. Hans Reichenbach (see Szasz, 1961) describes a continuum of abstractness/concreteness for symbols. The "metasymbol" is an extremely abstract symbol, as in the scientific formulation $E = Mc^2$. This has nothing to do with direct experience. On a somewhat less abstract level is "object language." For example, the word "stone" arbitrarily refers to the physical object. On a more basic level, a concrete experience can *stand for* a concrete experience. Clouds can stand for rain. This is called an "indexical sign." Even more concretely experienced is the "iconic sign." The iconic sign is a duplicate of the referent. Photos, TV images, radio broadcasts, etc., are literal copies of the referent—actual duplicates.

## The Pre-Symbol

Even more concretely manifest is the "pre-symbol" (Prouty, 1994). This primitive expression is characterized as "It cannot be clarified by something else" and "It is inseparable from what it symbolizes" (Jaspers, 1971, p. 124). The pre-symbol is the structure of the hallucination as distinct from its processing; that is, the hallucination is itself a pre-symbol. It is an extraordinarily concrete form of human expression.

## The Pre-Symbolic Hallucinatory Structure

The term "pre-symbol" refers to the literal and conceptualized properties of the hallucinatory image (Prouty, 1986). It is described as "expressive," "phenomenological," and "symbolic."

### Expressive

Describing the hallucination as expressive refers to its motivational quality or "self-intentional" nature. As already noted (Langer, 1961, pp. 46–47), the human brain has been described as a "transformer" that changes "the current of experience into symbols." This metaphor allows us to think of the hallucination as the transformation of life experience into image form.

### Phenomenological

As a phenomenological structure, the hallucinatory image can be described as "self-indicating." It is experienced as real, and as such it means itself. The hallucinatory image is "self-indicative." The image means itself. The image refers to itself. Experience *A* implies experience *A*. The image means itself as itself.

### Symbolic

As a symbolic structure, the hallucination is described as "self-referential." As a symbol, it is an experience that implies another experience. The image implies an "originary" experience—the image implies its origins, refers to its origins. Experience *A* implies experience *B*. The image means itself within itself.

## The Hypothesis

The self-intentional, self-indicative, and self-referential descriptions of the hallucinatory image become hypotheses. Do these properties actually occur? Can they be detected in the hallucinatory experience? Prouty (1994) provides a clinical description that substantiates these assertions.

## The Client

The client, a Caucasian male, age 19, was diagnosed as moderately retarded (Stanford–Binet IQ = 65). He was from working class origins. There was no mental illness in the family of origin, nor had the client been diagnosed or treated for mental illness; that is, *he was not receiving any medications* for psychosis. He was a day client in a vocational rehabilitation workshop for the mentally retarded. He was referred to therapy with the present author because of severe withdrawal and noncommunicativeness. In addition, the client behaved as though he was very frightened. He was exhibiting severe shaking and trembling at his work station and during his bus ride to the facility. At home, he hardly ever talked with his parents, and he never socialized with neighborhood peers.

During the early phases of therapy, the client expressed almost nothing and made very little contact with the therapist. He was very frightened during the sessions and could barely tolerate being in the same room. Gradually, with the aid of contact reflections, the client accepted minimal relationship and expressed himself in a minimal way.

Eventually, it became clear the client was terrorized by hallucinations that were constantly present to him.

The following description provides an account of pre-symbolic process. It provides an outline of hallucinatory "movement" and its subsequent resolution about its origins. The first phase describes a purple, demonic, evil appearance that just "hangs there" above the client. The second phase describes an orange, square image with anger "in it." This has a profound frightening effect on the client. The third phase presents a woman with orange hair and green eyes. She is both pretty and helpful—also mean and bad. It also contains the active recapturing of a real-life experience in which the retarded client is beaten by a nun because he did not understand his school lessons.

### Phase I: Purple Demon

CLIENT: It's very evil, this thing. What it wants to do is to rip me apart, you know. It's very evil . . . and it's very evil, this thing. It wants to rip me apart, but it's very evil, this thing. That's why I don't want anything to do with it. I'm tempted by it, you know. It's so small, but it has so much strength and it wants to rip me apart, you know. It wants to drive me into the past. It wants . . . it wants to make the past come back, and I don't want the past to come back like it did a long time ago. It's over with, you know. It's not coming back anymore. The past doesn't come back, it's over with already.

THERAPIST: It's evil and strong. It wants the past to come back.

CLIENT: This evil thing is a picture. It's a purple picture that hangs there. It just hangs and I can see it. I can see it. . . the picture, you know. It's purple, it's very dark. It's very dark. So I can see it and I don't like it. I don't like it at all. It's very dark.

THERAPIST: It's a dark purple picture and you don't like it.

CLIENT: And . . . it's very tempted and I don't want to be tempted by it. It's very small. It's very evil, you know . . . that's all . . . (*brief pause*). It just hangs there. It don't do nothing. It's very evil. It's tempted. I'm tempted by it and it's very evil, you know. It's just like a picture. A purple picture. It just stays there. It just stays there, you know, the picture . . . it don't do nothing, it's evil, you know. I don't like it at all. It's not good and this thing, whatever it is . . . *It's in the past and it's very strong, the past* . . . and it's over with and it's not coming back anymore. The past doesn't come back and this is like now. It ain't the past, you know. It's over with, and I don't want to be tempted by it anymore. Yeh, Yeh . . . it's very evil, very evil and very strong and has a lot of strength to it.

THERAPIST: It's evil and it's in the past. It's strong and it hangs there. You don't want to be tempted by it.

CLIENT: This thing, you know . . . this thing has a very lot of strength to it. It's evil, you know, this thing has a very lot of strength to it. It's evil. It's not good, and that's why it's not good at all. It's very evil, you know. I don't like it. It's very evil, this thing (*pained laughter*). It's over with. It's the past and it's not coming back anymore. It's over with a long time ago, you know. It's not going to come back anymore. I used to talk about the trees and the flowers, grass, and it's all over with. It's not coming back anymore. It's something else, the picture. The purple picture just hangs there. It's evil. No?

THERAPIST: The purple picture just hangs there. It's evil and you don't like it.

CLIENT: *The past, it came from the past*, and the past is over with. It's not coming back anymore, you know.

THERAPIST: It comes from the past.

CLIENT: It's a picture. It's just a picture. A big purple picture. It just hangs there . . . (*brief pause*). I don't think it will rip me apart. I think it's very strong, but it ain't going to rip me apart, I don't think it will rip me apart at all, no.

THERAPIST: It's a big purple picture. It won't rip you apart.

CLIENT: This thing is getting big and large. It's very big and large. It wants to get me. I won't let it. It's evil. It's like a demon, a bad demon. It wants to chop me all up. I won't let it chop me all up because it's bad. Very bad (*loud sobs*). Just a temptation, like any other temptation. A temptation is a temptation. You shouldn't be tempted by it, and you know I want to pull away from it. I don't want to go by it . . .

THERAPIST: It's big and large and evil. It wants to chop you. It's very tempting.

CLIENT: It's very bad and it's very destructive. It ain't good at all by it. It's like a bad demon, like a . . . like a demon devil or something. Like a demon devil and I don't care for it too much. You know, at all. I . . . I don't like it too much, no. I don't like it at all, this thing. It's very bad and very evil, you know. It ain't no good. It's very bad. It's with the past, and it's not going to come back anymore. It's over with, you know, and talking about the trees and the flowers and grass and that's over. I mean, it's not coming back, but this is right now, I mean.

THERAPIST: It's bad and destructive, like a demon devil. It's evil and with the past.

CLIENT: It's not coming back, but this is right here now. I can feel it, you know. It's like air. It's up above me. It's very up above and I can feel . . . almost touch it, you know. It's so close, very close. It's like a demon, you know, demon devil or something. "Ho, ho, hoing" and all like that, you know . . . very bad, very bad. It forces me, pressing, very pressing on me . . . it's very pressing, it forces, a lot of force to it and it wants to grab me, you know. It wants to grab me. The feeling wants to grab me. The feeling wants to grab me.

THERAPIST: It's very close and it wants to grab you.

CLIENT: The feeling . . . the feeling . . . ah, it's in the picture. The feeling is in the picture. Yes, it's there and I can see it. I don't like it. It's over with, you know. It's like the past and it's not coming back anymore. It's over. It's just the trees and flowers and grass and that old . . . and it's not coming back.

Phase I describes a purple demonic image that just "hangs there." The client experiences it as evil and powerful. The image is considered destructive and wants to "rip me [the client] apart."

This phase contains the structural property of being *self-intentional* (transformation of life experience into images). The client experiences: "It wants to drive me into the past." "*It wants . . . to make the past come back,* and I don't want the past to come back like it did a long time ago." "It's over with, you know." "It's not coming back anymore." "The past doesn't come back, it's over already." *"It's in the past and it's very strong."* "The past and it's over with and it's not coming back anymore." "The past doesn't come back and this is like now." "It ain't the past, you know." "It's over with and I don't want to be tempted by it." "It's the past and it's not coming back anymore."

As illustrated by this example, self-intentional means the expressive transformation of real-life past experiences into images.

## Phase II: Orange Square Hate

CLIENT: It's orange, the color's in a square. It's an orange color that's square and it hates me. And it don't even like me. It hates me.

THERAPIST: It's orange and it's square and it hates you.

CLIENT: It hates me a lot, you know, and it scares. I get scared because of that. I get scared because it hates me.

THERAPIST: It's orange and it's square and you get scared a lot.

CLIENT: And because it's orange that scares me and I get scared of the bad hating.

THERAPIST: The orange and bad hating scare you a lot. That hate scares you.

CLIENT: I get scared because of that. I get scared a lot. I get scared of the orange thing. It's orange.

THERAPIST: You get scared of the orange thing.

CLIENT: Big orange, square thing. It's square and it's orange and I hate it. It don't like me because it hates me. It hates me and I get scared and I get excited over it too. I get very excited.

THERAPIST: You get very excited.

CLIENT: It's exciting, I'm excited over it too. I do, I do. I get excited over it a lot. What? (*Audio hallucination.*) I get scared a lot about it. It makes noises. It makes noises.

THERAPIST: It's orange and it makes noises.

CLIENT: It makes noises . . . It hates me. It also gets me excited. It gets me excited. It does, it gets me very excited a lot. I get, I get, I get very excited over it. I do, I do. I do. There's so much hate and it scares me and it makes me uncomfortable. It does. And it's *real* . . . it's *real*, it is.

THERAPIST: It's real.

CLIENT: It is, it's very *real*.

THERAPIST: You point to it. It's over on your side. You see it.

CLIENT: I see it. Over there, over there.

THERAPIST: It's over there (*pointing*).

CLIENT: It makes sounds too.

Phase II has an image which is orange, square, and has hate in it. The client is very frightened of it. Phase II contains *self-indicating* structural properties (experience as real, a phenomenon; it implies itself). The client's process is as follows: "*and it's real . . . , it is.*" "*It is, it's very real.*" "*I see it.*" "*Over there.*" "*Over there.*" "*It makes sounds too.*"

## Phase III: Mean Lady

CLIENT: Yeah, well. Yeah, I would. I would. She's . . . I don't know. There we go. What? What? (*Audio hallucination.*)

THERAPIST: Okay, let's talk about what you see.

CLIENT: Well, she ain't real, you know, and she ain't real, you know. What? (*Audio hallucination.*) Ha (*sob*). She has orange hair and yellow eyes.

THERAPIST: She has orange hair and yellow eyes.

CLIENT: She's very pretty. She's very pretty. She loves getting mean when I am bad. She could get . . . she's mean, you know.

THERAPIST: She's pretty.

CLIENT: She's also mean too. She can be mean if I'm bad. The possibility of the mean scares me. It does scare me a lot over that.

THERAPIST: She's pretty and mean.

CLIENT: She is. She is. No, really she is. Really she is—with yellow eyes and orange hair. Boy! That scares me. That scares me a lot. That scares me a lot . . . Yeah, both the meanness and the . . . What? (*Audio hallucination.*) Yeah. Aah, I can see it, and I don't even want to see it. It's over with, and it's not coming back anymore. I can even see it.

THERAPIST: You can see it.

CLIENT: Yeah, that scares me. Yeah, it does. I think about it. I think it scares me.

THERAPIST: When you think about it, that scares you.

CLIENT: I get scared. I don't want to think about it. I got it. I got it.

THERAPIST: You don't want to think about it, but you got it.

CLIENT: I got it. It's orange, you know. That's helping, she's helping.

THERAPIST: She's helping.

CLIENT: She scares me though, she scares me, but as long as I'm good, but as long as I'm good, I am . . . she's a friend.

THERAPIST: As long as you're good, she's a friend.

CLIENT: But she's scary.

THERAPIST: She's scary.

CLIENT: Scary. Yellow eyes, orange hair she has, she does. Reminds me of a dragon, you know. Her eyes are like that.

THERAPIST: Her eyes are like a dragon.

CLIENT: Almost, you know, like a dragon . . . Her eyes are like a dragon . . . She's strong . . . She's strong, I'm weak. And I'm good, but she's also mean. She can be mean, too, see? And I'm good, if I'm good and I am. I really am, but she's all . . . she's very mean. She can be mean . . . and it scares me.

THERAPIST: She's mean and that scares you.

CLIENT: She looks over me. She watches over me, but she has eyes like a dragon . . . Right. That's like a dragon, and then she scares me and I get scared.

At this point, the client appeared upset and wanted the tape recorder turned off. Over the next two sessions the image processed into a nun who (had) beaten the retarded client because he did not understand his school lessons.

Phase III contains an image of a woman that the client describes as pretty, mean, and scary. She has orange hair and yellow eyes. This also deeply frightens the client. The significant theoretical observation on this phase is its processing to its "originary" experience. The client recaptures a real memory of being beaten by a nun who punished him for incomplete lessons. This phase illustrates the *self-referential* property of hallucinations; that is, it symbolizes an experience within itself. It refers to an "originating" event (the nun).

## SUMMARY

This chapter describes two sets of theory and practice for schizophrenic and mentally retarded clients. The first is pre-therapy. The second is pre-symbolics.

Pre-therapy is an evolution in Rogers's theory of psychotherapy. Rogers's first condition of psychotherapy is *psychological contact*. Rogers fails to define psychological contact and does not describe a technique to restore it when it is impaired. Pre-therapy is a theory of psychological contact. At the level of practice, it is described as *contact reflections*. At the level of internal psychological functioning, it is described as *contact functions*. The level of behavioral measurement is defined as *contact behaviors*. Pre-therapy develops or restores the psychological contact necessary for treatment. Pilot studies have provided beginning evidence for construct validity, reliability, and significant movement in predicted directions.

Pre-symbolics is an evolution in experiential theory and practice. Gendlin describes the hallucination as *structure bound*, which essentially means the experience of the hallucinations is *not in process*. The problematic becomes how to move the *nonprocess structure into a process structure*. This involves a shift in the epistemological basis from phenomenology to symbology. The *pre-symbol* describes the structure and the properties of the hallucination. The term *self-intentional* refers to the expressive motivational aspects of the hallucination. The term *self-indicating* refers to its phenomenological properties. The term *self-referential* refers to its symbolic nature. The language of pre-symbolics has dual properties of being symbolic and phenomenological. Case histories demonstrate the existence of these properties and the shift from a nonprocess to a process structure.

The methodologies and case histories presented in this chapter, will, I hope, encourage the reader to view psychotic clients as pre-expressive human beings. Hallucinations need not be alarming to the therapist; rather, they should be seen as an opportunity to restore the self.

# REFERENCES

Arieti, S. (1955). *Interpretation of schizophrenia* (p. 213). New York: Brunner.

Badelt, I. (1990). Client-centered psychotherapy with mentally handicapped adults. In G. Lietaer, J. Rombauds, & R. Van Balen (Eds.), *Client-centered and experiential psychotherapy in the nineties* (pp. 671–681). Leuven, Belgium: Leuven University Press.

Buber, M. (1964). Phenomenological analysis of existence versus pointing to the concrete. In M. Friedman (Ed.), *The worlds of existentialism* (pp. 547–549). New York: Random House.

Cassirer, E. (1955). Man: An animal symbolicum. In D. Runes (Ed.), *Treasury of philosophy* (pp. 227–229). New York: Philosophical Library.

De Vre, R. (1992). *Prouty's pre-therapie*. Master's thesis, Department of Psychology, University of Ghent, Ghent, Belgium.

Dinacci, A. (1994). Colloquio pre-terapeuticó: *Legge e psiche. Rivista di Psicolgia Giurdica*, 2(3/4), 24–32.

Dinacci, A. (1995). *Experimental research on the psychological treatment of schizophrenic clients with Garry Prouty's pre-therapy and innovative developments*. Unpublished manuscript.

Dinacci, A. (1997). Ricera Sperimentale Sul Trattamento Psicologico De Pazienti Schizofrenic con La Pre-terapia di G. Prouty. *Psicologia Della Persona* II(4), III–VIII.

Farber, M. (1959). *Naturalism and subjectivism*. New York: State University of New York Press.

Farber, M. (1967). *Phenomenology and existence* (pp. 14–27). New York: Harper & Row.

Gendlin, E. T. (1964). A theory of personality change. In P. Worchel & D. Byrne (Eds.), *Personality Change* (pp. 102–148). New York: Wiley.

Gendlin, E. T. (1967). Therapeutic procedure in dealing with schizophrenics. In C. R. Rogers (Ed.), *The therapeutic relationship and its impact: A study of psychotherapy with schizophrenics* (pp. 369–400). Madison: University of Wisconsin Press.

Gendlin, E. T. (1968). The experiential response. In E. Hammer (Ed.), *Use of inter-pretation in treatment* (pp. 208–228). New York: Grune & Stratton.

Gendlin, E. T. (1970). Research in psychotherapy with schizophrenic patients and the nature of that illness. In J. T. Hart & T. M. Tomlinson (Eds.), *New directions in client-centered therapy* (pp. 280–291). Boston: Houghton Mifflin.

Greenberg, L. S., Elliott, R., & Lietaer, G. (1994). Research on experiential psychoterapies. In A. Bergin & S. L. Garfield (Eds.), *Handbook of Psychotherapy and Behavior Change* (4th ed., pp. 509–539). New York: Wiley.

Gurwitsch, A. (1966). Gelb–Goldstein's concept of "concrete" and "categorical" attitude and the phenomenology of ideation. In *Studies in phenomenology and psychology* (pp. 359–384). Evanston, IL: Northwestern University Press.

Havens, L. (1962). The placement and movement of hallucinations in space, phenomenology and theory. *International Journal of Psychoanalysis, 43,* 426–435.

Hinterkopf, E., & Brunswick, L. (1975). Teaching therapeutic skills to mental patients. *Psychotherapy: Theory, Research & Practice, 12*(1), 8–12.

Hinterkopf, E., & Brunswick, L. (1981). Teaching mental patients to use client-centered and experiential skills with each other. *Psychotherapy: Theory, Research & Practice, 18*(3), 394.

Hinterkopf, E., Prouty, G., & Brunswick, L. (1979). A pilot study of pre-therapy method applied to chronic schizophrenic patients. *Psychosocial Rehabilitation Journal, 3*(Fall), 11–19.

Jaspers, K. (1971). *Philosophy* (Vol. 3). Chicago: University of Chicago Press.

Langer, S. K. (1961). *Philosophy in a New Key* (pp. 46–49). New York: Mentor Books.

Merleau-Ponty, M. (1962). *Phenomenology of perception.* New York: Routledge & Kegan Paul.

Perls, F. S. (1969). *Ego, hunger and aggression.* New York: Random House.

Peters, H. (1981). Luisterend helpen: Poging tot een beter omgaan met de zwakzinnige medemens. [Helping to listen: An attempt at better contact with mentally retarded fellow humans. (Private translation.)] Lochem/Poperinge, The Netherlands/Belgium: De Tijdstroom.

Peters, H. (1986). Client-centered benaderingswijzen in de zwakzinnigerzorg. [Client-centered approaches in the care of the mentally retarded. (Private translation.)] In R. Van Balen, M. Leijssen, & G. Lietaer (Eds.), *Droom en werkelijkheid in client-centered psychotherapie* (pp. 205–220). Amersfoort, The Netherlands/Leuven, Belgium: Acco.

Peters, H. (1992). *Psychotherapie bij geestelijk gehandicpaten.* Amsterdam: Swets & Zeitlinger.

Pörtner, M. (1988). *Client-centered therapy with mentally retarded persons.* Paper presented at the International Conference on Client-Centered/Experiential Therapy, Leuven Catholic University, Leuven, Belgium.

Prouty, G. (1976). Pre-therapy, a method of treating pre-expressive psychotic and retarded patients. *Psychotherapy: Theory, Research and Practice, 13*(Fall), 290–294.

Prouty, G. (1977). Protosymbolic method: A phenomenological treatment of schizophrenic hallucinations. *International Journal of Mental Imagery, 1*(2), 339–342.

Prouty, G. (1983). Hallucinatory contact: A phenomenological treatment of schizophrenics. *Journal of Communication Therapy, 2*(1), 99–103.

Prouty, G. (1986). The pre-symbolic structure and therapeutic transformation of hallucinations. In M. Wolpin, J. Shorr, & L. Kreuger, (Eds.), *Imagery* (Vol. 4, pp. 99–106). New York: Plenum.

Prouty, G. (1990). Pre-therapy: A theoretical evolution in the person-centered/experiential psychotherapy of schizophrenia and retardation. In G. Lietaer, J. Rombauts, & R. Van Balen (Eds.), *Client-centered and experiential psychotherapy in the nineties* (pp. 645–658). Leuven, Belgium: Leuven University Press.

Prouty, G. (1991). The pre-symbolic structure and processing of schizophrenic hallucinations: The problematic of a non-process structure. In L. Fusek (Ed.), *New directions in client-centered therapy: Practice with difficult client populations* (pp. 1–18). Chicago: Chicago Counseling Center.

Prouty, G. (1994). *Theoretical evolutions in person-centered/experiential psychotherapy: Applications to schizophrenic and retarded psychoses.* Westport, CT: Praeger (Greenwood).

Prouty, G. (1995). Pre-therapy: An overview. *Chinese Mental Health Journal, 9*(5), 223–225.

Prouty, G. (in press). Pre-therapy: A treatment for the psychotic retarded. In *The handbook of treatment of mental illness and behavior disorder in children and adults with mental retardation.* Washington, DC: American Psychiatric Association.

Prouty, G., & Cronwall, M. (1990). Psychotherapy with a depressed mentally retarded adult: An application of pre-therapy. In A. Dosen & F. Menolascino (Eds.), *Depression in mentally retarded children and adults* (pp. 281–293). Leiden, The Netherlands: Logon.

Prouty, G., & Kubiak, M. (1988). The development of communicative contact with a catatonic schizophrenic. *Journal of Communication Therapy, 4*(1), 13–20.

Prouty, G., & Pietrzak, S. (1988). Pre-therapy method applied to persons experiencing hallucinatory images. *Person-Centered Review, 3*(4), 426–441.

Prouty, G., Van Werde, D., & Pörtner, M. (1998). *Prä-Therapie.* Stuttgart: Klett-Cotta.

Reiss, S. (1994). *Handbook of challenging behavior: Mental health aspects of mental retardation.* Worthington, OH: IDS Publishing Corp.

Rogers, C. R. (1942). *Counseling and psychotherapy.* New York: Houghton-Mifflin.

Rogers, C. R. (1957). The necessary and sufficient conditions of therapeutic personality change. *Journal of Consulting Psychology, 21*(2), 95–103.

Rogers, C. R. (1959). A theory of therapy, personality, and interpersonal relationships as developed in the client-centered framework. In S. Koch (Ed.), *Psychology: A study of a science* (Vol. III). New York: McGraw-Hill.

Rogers, C. R. (1966). Client-centered therapy. In S. Arieti (Ed.), *American handbook of psychiatry* (Vol. 3, pp. 183–200). New York: Basic Books.

Rogers, C. R., Gendlin, E. T., Kiesler, D. J., & Truax, C. B. (1967). The findings in brief. In C. R. Rogers (Ed.), *The therapeutic relationship and its impact: A study of psychotherapy with schizophrenics* (pp. 73–93). Madison: University of Wisconsin Press.

Roy, B. C. (1991). A client-centered approach to multiple personality and dissociative process. In L. Fusek (Ed.), *New directions in client-centered therapy: Practice with difficult client populations* (pp. 18–40). Chicago: Chicago Counseling and Psychotherapy Research Center.

Ruedrich, S., & Menolascino, F. (1984). Dual diagnosis: An overview. In F. Menolascino & J. Stark (Eds.), *Handbook of mental illness in the mentally retarded* (pp. 45–82). New York: Plenum.

Sartre, J.-P. (1956). *Being and nothingness.* New York: Washington Square Press.

Scheler, M. (1953). Phenomenology and the theory of cognition. In J. Wild (Ed.), *Selected philosophical essays* (p. 143). Evanston, IL: Northwestern University Press.

Shlien, J. M. (1961). A client-centered approach to schizophrenia: A first approximation. In A. Burton (Ed.), *Psychotherapy of the psychoses* (pp. 285–317). New York: Basic Books.

Szasz, T. S. (1961). *The myth of mental illness* (pp. 115–116). New York: Hoeber.

Teusch, L. (1990). Positive effects and limitations of client-centered therapy with schizophrenic patients. In G. Lietaer, J. Rombauts, & R. Van Balen (Eds.), *Client-centered and experiential psychotherapy in the nineties* (pp. 637–644). Leuven, Belgium: Leuven University Press.

Teusch, L., Beyerle, U., Lange, H. U., Schenk, G. K., & Stadtmüller, G. (1983). The client-centered approach to schizophrenic patients. In W. R. Minsel & W. Herff (Eds.), *Research in psychotherapeutic approaches* (pp. 140–148). Frankfort am Main: Lang.

Van Werde, D. (1989). Restauratie van het psychologisch contact bij acute psychose. *Tijdschrift voor Psychotherapie, 5,* 271–279.

Van Werde, D. (1990, May 3 & 4). Psychotherapy with a retarded schizo-affective woman: An application of Prouty's pre-therapy. In A. Dosen, A. Van Gennep, & G. Zwanikken (Eds.), *Treatment of mental illness and behavioral disorder in the mentally retarded: Proceedings of an international congress* (pp. 469–477). Amsterdam: Logon.

Van Werde, D. (1992). Contact-faciliterend werk op een afdeling psychosenzorg: Een vertaling van Prouty's pre-therapie. *Vereniging voor Rogeriaanse Therapie, 4,* 3–20.

Van Werde, D. (1994). Dealing with the possibility of psychotic content in a seemingly congruent communication. In D. Mearns (Ed.), *Developing person-centered counseling* (pp. 125–128). London: Sage.

Van Werde, D., & Prouty, G. (1992). Het herstellen van het psychologisch contact bij een schizofrene jonge vrouw, een toepassing van pre-therapie. *Tijdschrift Klinische Psychologie, 22*(4), 269–280.

Whitehead, A. N. (1927). *Symbolism.* New York: Capricorn Books.

# 18

*****

# Psychopathology According to the Differential Incongruence Model

## Gert-Walter Speierer

*A differential view* of incongruence (Speierer, 1994) allows one to reintegrate client-centered therapy into the mainstream of clinical and counseling psychology, with diagnosis and assessment as integrative parts of therapeutic action (Speierer, 1996a, 1996b). The differential incongruence model (DIM) is a diagnostic tool to document, evaluate, and compare psychopathology, therapeutic processes, and results of patients specifically with respect to incongruence and congruence. Treatment in client-centered therapy is redefined by this model as a therapy of incongruence. The aims of therapy are expanded to include not only the experiencing of congruence or at least less incongruence experiencing but also better coping with incongruence, as well as larger incongruence tolerance.

## A BROADENED VIEW OF THE CONCEPTS OF ACTUALIZATION AND OF CONGRUENCE
### On the Actualization Tendency

The DIM proposes that the healthy self-actualization tendency is not omnipresent nor absolute. It is assumed that in certain psychopathological conditions actualization may be temporarily blocked, as in acute states of crisis reactions and some acute states of psychoses. The actualization tendency may be irreversibly blocked or lacking or even replaced by somatopsychic malfunctioning and handicaps that can inevitably lead to a fatal end of the patient without directive active intervention.

Therefore the nondirectivity principle is also viewed as not absolute. Consequently the DIM postulates and allows one not only to "facilitate" but also at times to actively create and promote conditions for healthy self- and personality development. Under the aforementioned circumstances the DIM legitimizes temporarily or continuously introducing therapeutic interventions that go beyond Rogers's (1957) necessary and sufficient conditions of psycho-therapeutic personality change. Promoting therapeutic experiences of congruence, reducing incongruence experiencing, and developing strategies of incongruence coping and incongruence tolerance as aims of therapy mean not only to "unfreeze" and mobilize a still existing healthy actualization tendency; when necessary therapeutic interventions must also be available to compensate a deficient actualization and to stop "actualization" that is detrimental to the patient.

## Rogers's Definition of Congruence

Originally, the term "congruence" was introduced by Rogers (1961) to describe a person when "the feelings the person is experiencing are available to him, available to his awareness, and he is able to live these feelings, be them and communicate them, if appropriate" (p. 61).

## Necessary Additions

This definition of a congruent self seems too reductive. The congruent self seems to be reduced to the consonant identification, the conscious availability, expression, and communication of those feelings, which have their origin in the self-actualization of the human organism. More comprehensively congruence can be defined as the experiencing of compatibility between *all* possible current emotional, cognitive, and physical experiences that are subjectively important experiences and the self. Congruence is further extended here to include notions of congruence as agreement, compatibility, conformity, consonance, and peaceful coexistence. The DIM distinguishes between self-congruence, on the one hand, and congruence between experience and self, on the other. The self is seen as composed of inherited dispositional, social-communicatively mediated and life-event-determined parts. Self-congruence is the experienced compatibility between these parts of the self. Thus, self-congruence means experienced consonance or compatibility between the dispositional organismic evaluation, the social-communicatively mediated introjected conditions of worth and the personal values of the person, which go along with his or her constructs of life experience. Congruence between ideal self and real self would be only one example of self-congruence.

Congruence between experience and self means that the individuals' evaluations of those parts of their experiencing that they are currently aware of are congruent with their present self at a given moment. However, experience refers not only to the self but also to the social environment, to the society, or to the situation. Healthy congruence therefore includes not only evaluation of the person's own behaviors as self-acceptable but likewise those of significant others and the social and nonsocial aspects of the situation.

As to the person's experiencing of the dispositional, social-communicative, and life-event-formed parts of the self and the subjectively meaningful world, congruence is also assumed to be possible when an individual willingly chooses to live up to the values of one or two of the self-components and thereby relativizes or ignores the demands of the other one or two for a certain amount of time.

The extended definition of congruence recognizes the coexistence of experiences that are congruent with some parts of the self and incongruent with other parts of the self. These incongruent experiences are not necessarily pathogenic. For example, the present experience of a person can, for a certain amount of time, be incongruent with his or her organismic maxims of being (e.g., maintenance of the species and having children without psychopathogenic consequences). This can happen when this experience is congruent with current personal life experiences or life planning constructs, for example, conditions that may at present be optimal for a person's career. The person can then decide to renounce having children or a family life without becoming ill. Later, having experienced personal satisfaction through work, he/she may choose to have a family and children.

The ability to experience congruence, that is, the capacity to evaluate experiences self-congruently, is essential if a person is to stay psychically healthy. The most important attitude that promotes congruence is incongruence tolerance. Incongruence tolerance enables an individual to accept self-incongruent experiences. It allows a person to recognize the unresolvable contradictions of his/her existence and to accept them without becoming "crazy." Furthermore, incongruence tolerance protects an individual against pathogenic consequences that may result from the psychophysical activity and stress associated with experiencing incongruence. Moreover, it can eventually promote an individual's creativity. Incongruence tolerance serves to maintain and develop the healthy self. Thus, the promotion of incongruence tolerance is an important part of psychotherapeutic work.

The ability to experience congruence and incongruence tolerance optimally develops in a social climate of social interpersonal communication, including body contact, the exchange of feelings, common activities, and nonverbal or paraverbal and especially meaningful verbal communication. Verbal communication plays a predominant role because it is the basis of a differentiated, accurate, and intersubjective objective symbolization of experiences, of the self, and of situations. Furthermore, it is the basis for the forming of concepts. Therefore, speech is the precondition of a differentiated development of a healthy self and personality. The social-communicative parts of the ability to experience congruence and incongruence tolerance result first from an evaluation, by significant others, of the person's actualization, and then from an evaluation of the other dynamic and structural aspects of the person. The evaluation by these significant persons and later the society must be compatible with the individual's evaluation of the self and the environment. Only then can these evaluations be integrated into the self-concept as congruent. This, in turn, gives rise to self-assurance and self-worth (pride) in a positive sense and to a good conscience. When the significant persons value the activities of a child congruently to his/her organismic valuing, they not only promote feelings of self-worth but also autonomy. The child's own activities then become a source of self-regard, self-worth, and self-reliance. Children become their own significant persons. The mutual reinforcements of self-assurance and autonomous activities can already be observed in the first year of life. In other words, the parents' unconditional positive regard fulfills the child's basic need to be loved and accepted. It is congruent with the organismic evaluation or the organismic valuing process of the child. It promotes an environment in which the child's self-concept and self-actualization develop and unfold. Thus, the child's behaviors and experiences mutually reinfore each other.

## The Congruence Dynamic in Healthy Persons

The congruence dynamic can be summarized as follows: Psychically healthy persons or successfully treated patients have predominately self-congruent experiences. However, they are not free from experiencing incongruence. Their sources of incongruence are primarily social-communicative ones. They are conscious of them as introjects of worth and unattainable ideals of perfection and being. By mainly using cognitive strategies, they can limit and relativize incongruencies within the total realm of experiencing. Thus, they are able to tolerate them (incongruence tolerance). Such individuals can in part compensate incongruence and reduce it actively. Thinking, feeling, and acting in a flexible manner allow the healthy person to resolve incongruence. The healthy individual can use incongruence as an impetus for change. Incongruence can mobilize the individual's creative abilities. As a result, the self can move toward self-actualization.

## A DIFFERENTIAL INCONGRUENCE THEORY OF PSYCHIC DISORDER

### Incongruence: The Central Theoretical Construct

Psychopathological processes (which are amenable to psychotherapy) are determined by conscious incongruencies that, at least, are at the edge of awareness. The incongruence theory of psychic disorders is based upon work done by Rogers (1959a).

The accentuated significance of incongruence in patients does not imply that incongruencies are only experienced by sick persons. In an empirical analysis, for example, Gess (1992) compared the frequencies and the intensity of self-incongruent experiences in 74 patients with coronary heart disease and 108 medical students. He found the frequency of self-incongruent experiences was not statistically different in either group. However, the intensity of experienced incongruence was significantly higher ($p < .001$) in the group of the patients. As a consequence of this investigation it can be assumed that incongruence only becomes pathological when it surmounts an individually tolerable critical level and when it is accompanied by the experienced inability to change, diminish, or tolerate it. It should be noted that not every psychic disorder is caused by incongruence and accompanied by self-incongruent experiences. However, it is postulated that psychic disorders without consciously experienced incongruence cannot be successfully treated by psychotherapy. Like congruence, incongruence is also a quality of experiencing. The experiencing of incongruence results when the present self (the amalgam of organismic evaluation, conditions of worth, life experience, and life planning constructs) is endangered by current experiences of which the self is only slightly aware. These experiences must be of a quality and intensity that the self can neither tolerate nor ignore.

The last definition of incongruence authored by Rogers can be found in a contribution to the *Comprehensive Textbook of Psychiatry*: "Incongruence is the discrepancy that can come to exist between the experiencing of the organism and the concept of self" (Rogers & Sanford, 1985, p. 1382). Thus, persons whose illness can be traced to psychological factors are not able to congruently experience personally meaningful parts of their experiences of the past, present, or imagined future. In other words, they cannot congruently integrate them into their actual self. They cannot make them tolerable or self-acceptable. Instead, they suffer from the incongruence between their experiences and their self. Their self is thereby questioned, devaluated, endangered, falsified, or destroyed. The more experiences endanger the self as a whole, the more likely the experienced incongruence will be a nonconflict incongruence, that is, without experiencing conflict but rather with the experiencing of personal strain or distress.

Also according to Rogers, it can be assumed that incongruence exists not only between experiences *and* the self but also *within* the self because of the human ability to self-reflect, self-question, self-experience, and self-evaluate. Rogers writes about incongruence without actually using the term in his *Counseling and Psychotherapy* (1942): "The individual is under a degree of tension, arising from incompatible personal desires or from the conflict of social and environmental demands with individual needs" (p. 76).

If one accepts that incompatible personal desires are located within the self-concept, and if one accepts that also social and environmental demands may be introjected in a person's self-concept, then it is likely that incongruence has its origin within the self-concept. Furthermore, the parts of the self may be experienced as incongruent and thereby cause psychopathological symptoms as the result of the person's self-experiencing. At this point, the experienced incongruence will most likely be a conflict incongruence.

The DIM allows one to describe a person's psychopathology by differentiating and weighting the interaction of possible inherited dispositional, social-communicatively mediated, and life-event-determined sources and aspects of the self that lead to incongruence. Depending on its predominant dispositional, social-communicative, and/or life-event-determined sources, different therapeutic options are more likely to alleviate or resolve the incongruence.

The experiencing of incongruence itself causes an uneasy psychophysiological strain. It manifests itself often but not exclusively as anxiety feelings, which were originally described by Rogers and Sanford (1985, p. 1382): "The client is experiencing at least a vague incongruence, which causes him to be anxious."

Therefore it can be postulated that symptoms other than anxiety also are consequences and equivalents of incongruence. According to the DIM this includes, for example, feelings of depression, anger, shame, and guilt, as well as a large variety of psychosomatic symptoms, excessive vegetative reactions, and pain. The phenomenological description of incongruence experiencing and the incongruence equivalents as well as the qualitative and quantitative operationalizations of the incongruence phenomena can be seen to a certain extent in the first stages of the original process conception of psychotherapy (Rogers, 1961, p. 125ff.) or later in the process scales (Rogers, 1959b; Tomlinson & Hart, 1962, 1970). In a quantitative and qualitative analysis of psychotherapy transcripts of 27 patients who were suffering, according to the international classification of psychic disorders (ICD-10; see World Health Organization, 1991), from mixed neurotic, stress, somatoform, and other disorders with psychological and behavioral factors, we found a common rank order of 10 categories of incongruence symptoms and incongruence equivalents. We termed it the "general incongruence dynamic." It includes the following categories: (1) inadequate control of self and behavior, overwhelming and excessive reactions; (2) subjective illness theory —person-related internal versus external hypotheses of causation; (3) consciously experienced incongruence/incompatibility of experiences with self-concept; (4) negative self-evaluation, poor self-confidence, and self-pity; (5) insufficiency, lack of achievement, and stress intolerance; (6) generalized negative evaluation of experiences and body symptoms; (7) a feeling of not being understood by significant others and fears of rejection or negative criticism by many people; (8) restriction of behavior, experience, and experiencing; (9) unattainable self-ideals; and (10) stress by nonorganismic conditions of worth (Speierer, 1994, p. 92ff.).

## From the Rogerian Uniformity Assumption to a Differential–Etiological and Multietiological View

Three alternate forms and sources of incongruence are postulated. The social-communicative incongruence results from deficits in social-communicative conditions and experiences. Rogers and most supporters of client-centered therapy deal exclusively with this form of incongruence in their conception of psychic disorders. However, the DIM relativizes social-communicative incongruence by assuming the existence of two other forms and sources of incongruence: (1) the sources of dispositional incongruence are not of a social-communicative nature but are either inherited, inborn, or primarily bio-neuropsychologically determined; (2) the sources of life-event-determined incongruence are either socially or nonsocially mediated life events. The three sources of incongruence may interact differently in the pathology of a sick person. Rogers apparently rejected not only the medical model of psychic illness but also the medical model's etiological view. He did not make use of the medical results that favor a differential and multietiological theory of psychic disorders. He maintained a uniformity assumption, namely, that only a social-communicative handicap of the self-actualization tendency can be the source of incongruence and psychic disorders. Accordingly, he postulated the neutralization of human self-alienation through the reconciliation of the natural healthy self-actualization tendency with its social and societal limits by a self that becomes increasingly autonomous. Similarly, he viewed unconditional positive regard, congruence, and empathic understanding to be the necessary (and sufficient) conditions for psychotherapy with clients experiencing at least a vague incongruence and perceiving the therapist's attitudes (see Rogers & Sanford, 1985).

The etiological and therapeutic uniformity assumptions have since been refuted for a multitude of persons with psychic disorders. The DIM was developed in part as an alternative model. The etiological view of the DIM answers two reciprocally related questions that have not been adequately resolved or discussed in the client-centered literature:

First, why and under which conditions can one expect client-centered therapy options to provide optimal therapeutic results in persons with differently classified psychic disorders according to international classifications of diseases? The DIM postulates optimal results in persons with psychic disorders who suffer from incongruence due to social-communicative sources and when a disorder is maintained by inter- and intrapersonal forms of communication that enhance incongruence.

Second, why and under which conditions is client-centered psychotherapy only partially effective or not effective? (1) The DIM claims that client-centered psychotherapy is not effective when persons with psychic disorders experience incongruence that is not largely social-communicatively determined but that is predominantly determined dispositionally or by life events of a nonsocial nature. (2) The DIM maintains that client-centered standard therapy in terms of the three attitudes will be ineffective in persons whose organismic actualization tendency is disturbed. This is possible when the healthy self-developmental and self-healing potentials of a person are lacking because of temporal or permanent bioneuropsychological malfunctions. In the worst case, the biopositive actualization is replaced by autodestructive malfunctioning of the organism. (3) Client-centered psycho-therapy cannot be effective in persons with psychic disorders without incongruence. (4) It also does not work in disorders with compensated incongruence. The persons then may notice an incongruence, but they do not suffer from it. They successfully use cognitive as well as behavioral strategies to cope with it, tolerate it, or compensate it. From an expert view a person may have a fear of heights, but "the patient" is not motivated for therapy because he/she has chosen not to encounter fearful experiences in mountain climbing and instead is enjoying holidays at sea. (5) An exclusively communicative and relational client-centered therapy is not optimally effective or is ineffective in persons with disorders stemming from life events that enduringly surmount a healthy person's strategies to cope with incongruence. Examples are incurable bodily illness, torture, and natural catastrophes like earthquakes and man-made ones like war.

## Dispositional Incongruence

The notion of dispositional incongruence is important because it shows the limits of communicative psychotherapy with respect to Rogers's basic assumptions. The dispositional incongruence results from inherited or constitutional biological deficits of congruence ability. In the literature these biological sources of psychopathology are addressed, for example, as biological vulnerability, proneness to stress, or presumed biochemical malfunctioning (Koehler & Dahme, 1996).

In order to achieve congruence between personally significant parts of the experiences and the self and/or of a deficit of incongruence tolerance, there must be an ability to tolerate self-incongruent experiences to a degree that is necessary for psychic health (see above). The dispositional parts of experiencing incongruence can be seen as personality traits. Their magnitude and individual range of change are different from person to person. They belong to the organismic biopsychophysiological inventory of a person. The dispositional parts of congruence ability and incongruence tolerance are assumed to develop independently from social-communicative experiences!

Dispositional incongruence can change during an individual's life through *noncommunicative* experiences like aging, bodily mutilation, and psycho-physical illness processes. Dispositional incongruence can also appear during an illness and can become manifest in the beginning of enduring psychic disorders, for example, in acute stages of depressive and/or hallucinatory psychoses. Disorders involving dispositional incongruence require treatment of the organism's main symptoms, usually in the form of medical and not by social-communicative psychotherapy.

*Four variations of dispositional incongruence* are described within the DIM. The *first variation of dispositional incongruence* can be observed in persons who are *not* able to do the following because of bioneuropsychological deficits: (1) they consciously perceive their organismic actualizations and their social and nonsocial environment; (2) they conceptualize their organismic actualizations as experiences; and (3) they form a self-concept beyond the organismic evaluation processes and develop a self-reflecting personality. Whether their psychophysical patterns and behaviors can be interpreted as states of congruence or incongruence, however, depends on the intactness of their organismic self, which consists of organismic actualization and organismic evaluation. If there is an intact organismic self, incongruence can arise without the ability to consciously symbolize experience from within the self, within the person, or outside the person. However, these persons do not suffer from incongruence that is bound to the ability to consciously symbolize experience because of their deficits of perception, experience, or symbolization. The psychotherapeutic inaccessibility of the disorders of persons with inborn or acquired personality deficits can be understood within the DIM. According to ICD-10, these disorders are classified as organic, including symptomatic disorders, and as deficits of intelligence or mental retardation (F7). Therefore, psychic disorders without conscious incongruence experiencing are recognized within the DIM. Persons with psychic disorders but without conscious incongruence experiencing are considered to be outside the realm of client-centered therapy, defined as the psychotherapy of incongruence.

In a *second variation of dispositional incongruence*, a self-concept has been formed. The behaviors due to organismic actualization tendency can be perceived, reflected, and conceptualized as experiences. However, they cannot be evaluated as below the organism's incongruence tolerance and hence as congruent by organismic evaluation. (Organismic evaluation is assumed as an inborn ability to evaluate experiences according to the organism's basic needs.) So organismic activation, for example, vegetative arousal, as well as cognitive, emotional, and muscular behaviors that belong to the individual's inborn program to act and react, can become an enduring source of incongruence. The resulting organismic stress can come to awareness, for example, as anxiety or body symptoms. This variation of dispositional incongruence also is incompatible with psychic health. Psychic and psychophysical forms of suffering, which are often accompanied by diminished social functioning, develop chronically or sometimes end up being fatal.

According to ICD-10 classification, persons with these disturbances are often classified as *patients with somatoform disorders* (F45) within the subgroups somatization disorder (F45.0) and hypochondriacal disorder (F45.2). Persons with these disorders often consider their experience with former, present, and future significant others "sufficient" or "satisfying" with respect to their basic needs of being unconditionally valued, empathetically understood, and congruently encountered. Negatively evaluated experiences of a social-communicative nature (which are incongruent to their actual self) are always present, just as they are in the life of healthy individuals, and are also compensated for, more or less.

However, persons with these disorders suffer from incongruence experiencing that is *not related to social-communicative sources*. For example, they have long-lasting fears of suffering from an undiscovered or deadly illness. They may suffer from minor skin irritations on parts of the body, of which they are ashamed. They feel changing body symptoms as a menace to their existence that can never be successfully alleviated either by medical or psychological help. They may have a negative self-evaluation due to their own external appearance. They may also experience unexplainable fatigue, faintness, aches in the head and limbs, feelings of total exhaustion, sleeping disorders, and the inability to relax in combination with depressive, dysthymic, and anxiety feelings.

In spite of some similarities in the predominantly bodily symptoms and complaints, these disorders are not to be erroneously classified as "psychosomatic disorders," which in the ICD-10 classification are labeled as *disorders with psychological and behavioral factors* (F54). According to our empirial data (Speierer, 1994), these psychosomatic patients suffer much more from social-communicative incongruence and therefore have a much better prognosis, when they are treated with client-centered therapy (as, among others, Sachse, 1995, has convincingly demonstrated; see also Sachse, Chapter 13, this volume).

Instead, persons with somatoform disorders suffer from self-incongruent experiences that rely much more on the individual's marked attention and perception of his/her own body than on deficient social-communicative experiences. Psychotherapy can only alleviate this incongruence to a small extent, if at all. Brief personal contact on a regular basis may have some positive results when these persons suffer from their condition as well as from social isolation over a long period of time. To date, there has been no evidence of successful client-centered therapy with these patients.

Speierer (1994, pp. 318–350) analyzed three transcripts taken from initial sessions of patients with somatoform disorders ($N = 2$) and hypochondria ($N = 1$) using his categories of incongruence analysis. Vegetative hyperreactivity and hypersensitivity to their own body sphere were found to be the dispositional sources of the incongruence in these patients. Social communicative sources of incongruence were lacking or not recognized. Life events that caused incongruence were severe bodily illness or the death of significant others. Disturbances from the patients' own body sphere were the most self-incongruent experiences. They were aggravated by a self-ideal in which bodily health and strength were highly valued. Two of the patients dropped out of therapy. One patient finished client-centered therapy after 22 one-hour sessions in an agreement with his therapist. Transcripts of his therapy were also evaluated. The results demonstrated that the most limiting factor of this client-centered incongruence therapy was an unchanging subjective illness theory of self-incongruent suffering as being caused by organic factors (here an infection of the intestine). In addition to participating in psychotherapy sessions, the patient received medication. Often, he self-congruently attributed the alleviation of his symptoms to the injections and pills he had been prescribed. The client-centered therapy was able to help this patient only to a certain—but small—degree. First, he was accepted as a suffering person by the therapist. Second, psychophysical relations were explained to him in a nonoffending way and were described as normal phenomena, having nothing to do with "insanity." Through the acceptance of the patient's bodily symptoms in the context of all his actual experiences, the symptoms became slightly more self-congruent. Once this was achieved, the patient wished to end psychotherapy. Three years after the end of his psychotherapy, the patient stated that the therapy had helped him. However, he was still convinced that there were organic reasons for his continually changing condition.

A *third variation of dispositional incongruence* is characterized by disorders with disturbed processing of information from the body sphere, cognitive, emotional, and motoric actualization, and disturbed perceptions of the social and nonsocial environment as well as of the self-concept, which is endangered by intrapersonal and outside experiences. Such incongruencies can be found in patients with psychotic disorders. According to the ICD-10 classification the disorders belong to the groups of schizophrenia and schizophrenic and delusional disturbances (F2) and to certain groups of affective disorders, especially manic episodes (F30) and bipolar affective disorders with psychotic symptoms (F31). Patients with other affective disorders like depressive episodes without psychotic symptoms (F32.0, F32.1, F32.2) and enduring affective disorders like dysthymia (F34.1) have been treated successfully by client-centered psychotherapy (Elliott et al., 1990; Speierer, 1994, pp. 236–259). However, their psychotherapeutic success is dependent on the absence of the aforementioned type of dispositional incongruence and its symptoms.

For example, a person with an acute delusional state (say, in schizophrenia) might be extremely anxious (as an illustration I use Rogers's leading symptom of incongruence). The "cause" of the anxiety may be the incongruence between the person's delusional experience of being poisoned by a significant other or by everybody in his environment, on the one hand, and his self who wants to stay alive, on the other. Or the cause of his anxiety may be the incongruence between a part of the self, which tells him to commit suicide, and another part, which says that committing suicide is the worst possible sin. In both states, the person suffers from incongruence: in the first, he attributes the source of incongruence experiencing outside of his self; in the second, he may locate subjectively and clearly the deadly danger within the self.

According to current medical knowledge, the terrifying incongruence experiences of these states most likely have their origin in a *disposition* to develop acute schizophrenia spontaneously or under certain circumstances, which are not completely known. The failure to recognize this dispositional incongruence (or, as I have also termed it, *disorder-bound* dispositional incongruence) may have detrimental consequences for the patient. An appropriate drug treatment may need to be taken into consideration.

*Incongruence here is not an inability but a dispositionally disturbed ability to realistically symbolize and evaluate experience, either from within the self, within the person, or from outside the person in awareness.* The intensive suffering of these persons and their characteristic psychic and body symptoms can be understood within the DIM as the consequence of disorder-bound dispositional incongruence. It is not caused by social-communicative experiences. However, it changes the person's social-communicative behavior, social-communicative experiences and evaluation.

Moreover, other persons often react to these psychotic patients negatively and with low or no positive regard, congruence, and empathy. The disorder-bound dispositional incongruence of patients with psychotic disorders, therefore, cannot be treated successfully by client-centered communicative psychotherapy. This form of incongruence disappears when the psychotic symptoms recover spontaneously or by means of antipsychotic medication. However, *client-centered psychotherapy has been shown to be helpful in the treatment of these patients after acute phases of their disorder* (Rogers, Gendlin, Kiesler, & Truax, 1967; Truax, 1970; Mann, 1976; Rank, Stephan, Grüss, Weise, & Weise, 1986; Teusch, 1986; Swildens, 1988; Prouty, 1990; Binder & Binder, 1991).

By means of the differential view of incongruence, the results on client-centered therapy with schizophrenic patients can now be rigorously understood: Offering a therapeutic relationship with unconditional regard, empathic understanding, and congruence does not help the patients to work on their incongruence during the disorder's acute stages, because incongruence is then predominantly determined dispositionally. However, psychotherapy can help near the end of and after the acute stages of the illness and in the subacute phases of the illness. The best results of client-centered psychotherapy can be seen in those patients whose incongruence is then more determined by social-communicative experiences and life events in which significant others and their behaviors are involved. Psychotherapy, however, does not help much when incongruence experiencing again results from dispositional sources in the form of residual phenomena like delusionary contents. Optimal treatment involves a multimodal therapeutic plan, including specific information about the illness, information as well as training for coping with daily requirements, and taking disorder-specific medications. As Gaebel (1986) has stated, the life-event-determined parts of incongruence of chronic schizophrenic patients can only be alleviated to a small extent by client-centered psychotherapy. What is most needed is social-psychiatric care, social casework, and vocational rehabilitative measures, as well as suitable posibilities for living, working, and leisure activities. In addition, help is often needed for the patients' partners who take care for them. Persons with schizophrenia at times may not suffer at all from either dispositional, social-communicative, or life-event-determined incongruence. Their incongruence too can be compensated by strategies of coping with incongruence, which are not different from those in healthy persons.

A *fourth variation of dispositional incongruence* consists of disturbed or missing links between the experience of the organismic actualization and the organismically formed, social-communicatively formed, and life-event-formed parts of the self, as well as of reduced conscious congruence and/or incongruence experiencing. This form of dispositional incongruence can be found in persons with antisocial personality disorders (F60.2) and in persons with self-mutilating behaviors (or, according to ICD-10, factitious disorder, F68.1). Within the DIM the impulsive actions of the antisocial disorder are explained as follows: Actions and self seem to be independent. As a result, the person does not experience his/her antisocial behavior toward another person as self-incongruent. When, however, the person evaluates the antisocial behavior, it may be experienced as incongruent to societal values that his/her own self accepts but not as incongruent with the other two parts of the self, his/her organismic evaluation and life-experiencing constructs. Thus, the person may accept the fact that his/her deed has to be punished but also believes that his/her act was justified and so would do it again, because the other person had provoked him/her.

Using the DIM, it is possible to explain why these persons do not respond well to social communicative psychotherapy. The few reports on client-centered therapy with these persons (see Swildens & de Haas, 1991) illustrate these difficulties.

Again, persons classified according to ICD-10 as having antisocial personality disorder or factitious disorder should be differentiated from persons with borderline personality disorder (F60.31). There are a few recent studies showing that this borderline group can be treated with client-centered therapy on a long-term basis with more or less stable success (Eckert & Wuchner, 1996). Our group has not done research with such persons, and therefore we do not yet have data as to the different and specific determinants of their incongruence experiencing. (See Eckert & Biermann-Ratjen, Chapter 15, this volume.)

## Social Communicative Incongruence

Though the DIM relativizes, differentiates, and supplements the idea of an exclusive social-communicative genesis of psychic disorders, the social-communicative sources of suffering still remain very important nonetheless. The DIM claims that the beginning and development of social-communicative incongruence is important not only in early childhood but also throughout the whole life history. This incongruence is marked by deficient social-communicative relational experiences with significant others. According to the expanded incongruence definition of the DIM, an inability to reach congruence and reduced incongruence tolerance can also result from social-communicative experiences. As the conditions and disorders resulting from social-communicative incongruence have been comprehensively described in the client-centered psychotherapy literature, they will not be further elaborated upon in this chapter.

## Life-Event Determined Incongruence

Within the DIM, the third form of incongruence is seen as a result of stressing life events. These strike persons with or without a dispositional background of pathological stress reactions. Life events can additionally gain their psychopathological power because of their social-communicative nature and consequences. Incongruence of this type elicited by life experiences can be viewed and dealt with as social-communicative incongruence and can be treated sucessfully with client-centered therapy. But incongruence caused by stressing life experiences can also arise without social-communicative sources, for example, in victims of natural catastrophes like earthquakes or of man-made disasters like airliner crashes. Societal changes that significantly restrict the personal essentials of life are also sources of this form of incongruence (e.g., job loss, body mutilations caused by accidents, or chronic and acute illnesses).

This form of incongruence can be found in disturbances that are classified according to ICD-10 in the group of stress reactions and disorders of adaptation (F43). The differential view of the psychopathology of these disorders allows us to differentiate the dispositionally, social-communicatively, and life-event determined parts of the incongruence that the patients are experiencing. According to the results of the incongruence analysis, different therapy options including client-centered psychotherapy can be offered in such cases.

For example, excessive physiological reactions with a strong dispositional background resulting in tension headaches may be a very significant self-incongruent experience in an enduringly stressful life situation—like having lost one's job due to the closing of one's firm. Client-centered incongruence therapy may then first communicatively help the patient to understand his/her self-incompatible bodily symptoms as also dispositionally determined personal reactions to stress. To reduce them, a relaxation training in combination with biofeedback might be offered. An additional social-communicative therapy focus might be to understand the incongruence the patient is also experiencing because of having lost his/her job. Here, the meaning of work to the self has to be considered and may have to be changed. Further, the individual's resources in terms of incongruence tolerance and congruence ability, including incongruence-coping strategies, may be mobilized and improved. But the genuine source of this person's incongruence—the loss of the job—should never be neglected. Thus, the "causal" therapeutic suggestion here would be to seek vocational counseling and to contact an employment agency in order to optimize the patient's chances of getting a new job.

Bodily handicaps and chronic illnesses are increasingly seen as subjects of psychological intervention and thus deserve special attention. Psychotherapy should only be used after the patient has been subjected to the appropriate medical treatment and/or rehabilitation program. The nonsocial origin of the incongruence of these persons is the reason for this strategy. When a person is born or faced with a bodily handicap or chronic illness early in life, these conditions can impede the unfolding of an originally existent ability to congruence and even destroy it when significant others reject such persons. Thus, the chances to reach a satisfying, self-congruent arrangement with the handicap or illness are not good. In such a case, medical treatment, rehabilitation, *and* additional social-communicative psychotherapy focusing on the patient's self-esteem, self-confidence, self-respect, and remaining capacities for autonomy may help the patient's self to tolerate her/his handicaps without further risk of psychopathology.

When these disorders begin later in life, they can surmount a congruence ability and incongruence tolerance that had earlier been sufficient for psychic health. For example, when a person loses an arm in an accident, she may experience incongruence that results in a long-lasting depression. The severity of the incongruence suffering depends on how much the actual self is endangered by the loss of the limb. If it can be correctly assumed that the organismic part of the self contains a body image, the loss may result in an incongruence. The "phantom pain" that has been frequently recorded in the literature could then be viewed also as a result of this incongruence. As to the parts of the patient's self that contain his social-communicative experiences and life-experiencing-constructs, she will experience more incongruence, the more she views the loss of her arm as reducing her chances to be the person she wants to be in her personally important areas of life, for example, with respect to familial, vocational, and leisure activities. The therapeutic reduction of the incongruence experiencing and its symptomatic equivalents—here the depression—may be sufficiently achieved without psychotherapeutic help after medical treatment and rehabilitation. This may most likely be done through restoring the arm's impeded functions with the help of a suitable prosthesis. If this is not adequate, psychotherapeutic help may become necessary. One option may also be to help the patient change her self-concept in order to reduce incongruence. Another therapeutic option would be to help the patient to realize her compensatory resources and develop and train her abilities to regain self-congruent experiences that were formerly provided by having and using the arm. A third therapeutic option would be to strengthen incongruence tolerance and the aforementioned strategies to cope with incongruence.

In some persons who suffer from self-incongruent experiences because of an incurable and/or terminal illness like malignant tumors, a psychotherapeutic option would be to reduce this incongruence by encouraging the patients not to focus on the reality of their illness, at least for a time. Instead, they should engage in activities and act as if the illness were not present. As a last option, coping strategies that may transcend psychological thinking into the transpersonal realm (e.g., through various forms of spiritual meditation) may open possibilities of an alternative psychotherapy for these patients.

## NONINDICATIONS AND CONTRAINDICATIONS

The redefinition of client-centered therapy as incongruence therapy and the differential view of incongruence have enabled us to recognize the limitations of the traditional therapeutic concept of client-centered therapy and to formulate necessary adaptations for some types of incongruence, as has been shown above. Now some nonindications and contraindications can be described as well.

The DIM acknowledges that there are patients who do not suffer from incongruence (see above). In these disorders client-centered therapy is *not indicated*, for its three therapeutic conditions aim at the reduction of incongruence to reactivate or promote healthy personal growth. The patients are not motivated for therapeutic aims like changing their self or their experiences for more congruence in the relations between self and experience. The international classification of psychic disorders (ICD-10) specifies the relevant aspects of the symptomatology of these disorders as ego syntonic (World Health Organization, 1991). Ego-syntonic symptoms are described among others in manic episodes (F30) and some personality disorders (F60). Note, however, that ego-syntonic symptoms are not present in every person with these disorders nor at all stages, so the lack of incongruence experiencing can only be assessed by an individual incongruence analysis (Speierer, 1996a, 1996b).

With the acknowledgment of nonsocial-communicative sources of incongruence in dispositional incongruence and partly in life-event-determined incongruence, there are patients who may suffer from extreme incongruence but who nevertheless will not profit from social-communicative incongruence therapy. Instead, they deteriorate when the therapist tries to focus empathically and congruently on the contents of their incongruent experiencing. In these conditions client-centered standard verbalizations are *contraindicated*. Verbally focusing on contents that for certain patients mean a real danger to life—even with an unconditional positive regarding, empathically understanding, and congruent therapist—might force such patients into more incongruence and more suffering. Because of the nature of their disorder, they can neither clear a space for working on the meaning of their experience nor can they perceive the therapist's endeavors as helpful. According to the ICD-10 these are mainly patients with ego-dystonic symptoms in *acute* delusional schizophrenic psychoses (F20), depressive disorders with psychotic symptoms (F31.5, F32.3, F33.3), and acute reactions to severe stress and adjustment disorders (F43.0). Again, it should be noted that these types of dispositional and life-event-determined incongruence do not always, nor at all stages of these disorders, dominate the incongruence experiencing in every person with these disorders. So, as mentioned above, only by an individual incongruence analysis can one assess the indicators of dispositional and nonsocially mediated life-event-determined incongruence as the criterion of a temporary contraindication. Client-centered therapy with these persons therefore includes abstaining at least temporarily from verbally and non-verbally working on the patients' incongruence, as well as refraining from offering a too close or not sufficiently structured relationship. Instead, it is necessary in such cases to make use of other therapeutic options like the more structured and directive communicatie, noncommunicative, and pharmaceutical strategies of social, psychological, and medical crisis intervention.

## REFERENCES

Binder, U., & Binder, H. J. (1991). *Studien zu einer störungsspezifischen klientenzentrierten Psychotherapie*. Eschborn, Germany: Klotz.

Eckert, J., & Wuchner, M. (1996). Long-term development of borderline personality disorder. In R. Hutterer, G. Pawlowsky, P. F. Schmid, & R. Stipsits (Eds.), *Client-centered and experiential psychotherapy* (pp. 213–233). Frankfurt am Main: Lang.

Elliott, R., Clark, C., Kemeny, V., Wexler, M., Mack, C., & Brinkerhoff, J. (1990). The impact of experiential therapy on depression: The first ten cases. In G. Lietaer, J. Rombauts, & R. van Balen (Eds.), *Client-centered and experiential psychotherapy in the nineties* (pp. 549–577). Leuven, Belgium: Leuven University Press.

Gaebel, W. (1986). Die Bedeutung von psychiatrischer Diagnose und Indikation in der Gesprächspsychotherapie. *Zeitschrift für personenzentrierte Psychologie und Psychotherapie, 4*, 399–408.

Gess, L. (1992). *Inkongruenz in Selbstaussagen bei Koronarpatienten und Medizinstudenten*. Medical dissertation, University of Regensburg, Germany.

Koehler, Th., & Dahme, B. (1996). Psychobiologische Grundlagen der Psychotherapie. In W. Senf & M. Broda (Eds.), *Praxis der Psychotherapie* (pp. 242–249). Stuttgart: Thieme.

Mann, F. (1976, September 28–October 4). Die Anwendung klientenzentrierter Konzepte in der heutigen Psychiatrie. In P. Jankowski, D. Tscheulin, H.-J. Fietkau, & F. Mann (Eds.), *Klientenzentrierte Psychotherapie heute: Bericht über den 1. Europäisch Kongress für Gesprächspsychotherapie in Würzburg* (pp. 253–259). Göttingen: Hogrefe.

Prouty, G. F. (1990). Pre-therapy: A theoretical evolution in the person-centered/experiential psychotherapy of schizophrenia and retardation. In G. Lietaer, J. Rombauts, & R. van Balen (Eds.), *Client-centered and experiential psychotherapy in the nineties* (pp. 645–658). Leuven, Belgium: University Press.

Rank, K., Stephan, A., Grüss, U., Weise, H., & Weise, K. (1986). Gesprächspsychotherapie als Basiskonzept der psychiatrischen Grundversorgung. *Zeitschrift für personenzentrierte Psychologie und Psychotherapie, 5*(4), 379–390.

Rogers, C. R. (1942). *Counseling and psychotherapy*. Boston: Houghton Mifflin.

Rogers, C. R. (1957). The necessary and sufficient conditions of therapeutic personality change. *Journal of Consulting Psychology, 21,* 95–102.

Rogers, C. R. (1959a). A theory of therapy, personality, and interpersonal relationships, as developed in the client-centered framework. In S. Koch (Ed.), *Psychology: A study of a science* (Vol. III, pp. 184–256). New York: McGraw-Hill.

Rogers, C. R. (1959b). A tentative scale for the measurement of process in psychotherapy. In *Research in psychotherapy* (Proceedings of a Conference of the American Psychological Association, Washington, DC, 1958). Washington, DC: American Psychological Association.

Rogers, C. R. (1961). *On becoming a person.* Boston: Houghton Mifflin.

Rogers, C. R., Gendlin, G. T., Kiesler, D. V., & Truax, C. B. (1967). *The therapeutic relationship and its impact: A study of psychotherapy with schizophrenics.* Madison: University of Wisconsin Press.

Rogers, C. R., & Sanford, R. C. (1985). Client-centered psychotherapy. In H. J. Kaplan & B. Sadock (Eds.), *Comprehensive textbook of psychiatry* (Vol. 2, pp. 1374–1388). Baltimore: Williams & Wilkins.

Sachse, R. (1995). *Der psychosomatische Patient in der Praxis.* Stuttgart: Kohlhammer.

Speierer, G.-W. (1994). Das differentielle Inkongruenzmodell (DIM). *Handbuch der Gesprächspsychotherapie als Inkongruenzbehandlung.* Geneva: Who Books.

Speierer, G.-W. (1996a). Client-centered psychotherapy according to the differential incongruence model (DIM). In R. Hutterer, G. Pawlowsky, P. F. Schmid, & R. Stipsits (Eds.), *Client-centered and experiential psychotherapy* (pp. 299–311). Frankfurt am Main: Lang.

Speierer, G.-W. (1996b). The differential incongruence model as a basis of specific and integrative options in counseling and psychotherapy. In U. Esser, H. Pabst, & G.-W. Speierer (Eds.), *The power of the person-centered approach* (pp. 23–32). Cologne: GwG-Verlag.

Swildens, H. (1988). *Procesgerichte gesprekstherapie.* Amersfoort, The Netherlands/Leuven, Belgium: Acco Press. [German translation (1991): *Prozessorientierte Gesprächspsychotherapie.* Cologne: GwG-Verlag.]

Swildens, H., & de Haas, O. P. (1991). Prozessorientierte Gesprächspsychotherapie bei Klienten mit psychopathischen Verhaltensstörungen. In H. Swildens (Ed.), *Prozessorientierte Gesprächspsychotherapie* (pp. 219–237). Cologne: GwG-Verlag.

Teusch, L. (1986). Gesprächspsychotherapie schizophrener Patienten. *Zeitschrift für personenzentrierte Psychologie und Psychotherapie, 5,* 391–398.

Tomlinson, T. M., & Hart, J. T. (1962). A validation study of the process scale. *Journal of Counseling Psychology, 26,* 74–78.

Tomlinson, T. M., & Hart, J. T. (1970). A validation study of the process scale. In J. T. Hart & T. M. Tomlinson (Eds.), New *directions in client-centered therapy* (pp. 206–213). Boston: Houghton Mifflin.

Truax, C. B. (1970). Effects of client-centered psychotherapy with schizophrenic patients: Nine years pre-therapy and nine years posttherapy hospitalization. *Journal of Consulting and Clinical Psychology, 3,* 417–422.

World Health Organization. (1991). Mental and behavioral disorders (including disorders of psychological development): Clinical descriptions and diagnostic guidelines. Chap. V (F) in *WHO: Tenth revision of the international classification of diseases.* Geneva: Author.

# 19

*****

# Diagnosing in the Here and Now
## *A GESTALT THERAPY APPROACH*

**Joseph Melnick**
**Sonia March Nevis**

*Experience is messy.* It is continuous, disorganized, shapeless, chaotic, and overlapping. Gestalt therapy rests on the fundamental assumption that we, as humans, are predisposed to organize this experience in order to make meaning.

Gestalt therapy borrows this assumption from Gestalt psychology's theory of perception, which postulates that we create a figure (organization) out of the ground (experience). We do this by scanning, evaluating, and assessing our internal and external environments. Formal diagnosis is the attachment of a specific form of meaning (labeling) to a recurrent pattern of figure/ground formation of an individual.

This chapter explores formal diagnosis (DSM-IV; American Psychiatric Association, 1994) from the theoretical perspective of Gestalt therapy. The Gestalt therapy "experience cycle" (Polster & Polster, 1973; Zinker, 1977) will be presented as the basis of a diagnostic system (see Figure 19.1). Specific diagnostic formulations from DSM-IV (borderline, specific phobia, histrionic, and posttraumatic stress syndrome) will be analyzed, and intervention strategies will be articulated.

## WHAT IS DIAGNOSIS?

Diagnosis is first and foremost a descriptive statement that articulates what is being noticed in the present. Yet it also means going beyond the present, implying a pattern as well as a prediction, no matter how minimal. In addition, diagnosis may or may not include a concept of causality. Thus, to diagnose is to attempt to enlarge the picture, to move from what is observable now to what is habitual. It includes a schema not only of what is to be observed but of the patterns and configurations into which our observations are organized.

Gestalt theory does not imply a system of cause. Gestalt therapists believe in causation, but they perceive it as inherently unknowable. Aligned with both systems (Kraus, 1989; Huckabay, 1992) and field theory (Parlett, 1991, 1993) perspectives, they are aware that the number of influences that impinge on any given system is so vast that a full and meaningful description of cause is improbable, if not impossible.

As indicated previously, Gestalt therapists believe that one constantly derives meaning after first organizing unorganized experience. Gestaltists believe that how one organizes what one observes is the fundamental process of meaning making, and that it is unique to each individual (including each patient and diagnostician) and to each situation. Therefore, there can be no absolutely correct diagnosis.

Despite this strongly held belief, there are several compelling reasons for diagnosing in a more formal, narrow, and systematic manner:

First, diagnosis gives one a map and describes possibilities of how a person can evolve. Therefore, the therapist benefits from a structure, that is, a compass to help organize the information and provide clues to a direction to navigate through the vast field of data.

Second, the process of diagnosing allows the therapist to control anxiety. By removing her-/himself from the data, the therapist may remain calm while waiting for a figure to emerge. Thus, the process of diagnosing is grounding and keeps the therapist from jumping precipitously into the infinite while waiting. Simply stated, it gives one something to do.

A third reason to diagnose in a more formal way is that by linking Gestalt theory to other systems of diagnosis, a vast array of research and theory opens to the clinician. Furthermore, it is efficient in that the therapist can make predictions without having to wait each time for the data to emerge from immediate experience.

Fourth, Gestalt therapists in particular need to be grounded in a wider perspective that includes the future and particularly the past. However, although Gestalt therapists explore the patient's past, this exploration is of a different nature: "We explore phenomenologically in order to understand, not believing that the past caused the present" (Yontef, 1988, p. 22).

Finally, fifth, diagnosing prevents the Gestalt therapist from becoming isolated from others with different theoretical orientations. Consequently, Gestalt theorists, even while debating issues concerning process versus structure, still use traditional diagnostic labels such as schizophrenia, narcissism, and borderline personality disorder (From, 1984; Tobin, 1985). Thus, although the use of diagnostic categories may not be totally congruent with our theory, we still employ them in communicating with others.

## HOW DOES GESTALT THERAPY
## DIFFER FROM OTHER SYSTEMS?

Gestalt diagnosis is gleaned essentially from the moment, and this provides the key to intervention, interpersonal process, and change. Because of this viewpoint, it is important to reiterate at the outset that Gestalt theory, informed by field theory, includes the therapist in the assessment process and thus makes the therapist part of the diagnosis.

This implies not only that the therapist influences what is seen but also that what is seen evokes reactions in the therapist that help create a unique systemic experience. When making a formal diagnostic statement the Gestalt therapist is making a choice to deal with only one part of the organism–environment equation, as if the clinician and environmental components could be frozen and the patient isolated from the interaction. Although this perspective is admittedly limited and incomplete, it is fairly consistent with the way people experience and interpret the world.

In diagnosing, the Gestalt therapist focuses on process and pattern making in the here and now and does not label individuals in terms of long-term, ongoing, and fixed characteristics. Gestalt therapists pay attention to blocks in one's process (i.e., avoidance or distortion of awareness or contact) and describe them as disturbances or neurotic self-regulation—projection, confluence, retroflection, retrojection, and deflection (Polster & Polster, 1973). By locating these psychological processes in the here and now, Gestalt therapy takes a therapeutically optimistic stance that is more likely to support change in people who might otherwise be restricted by the more traditional, historical, and permanent diagnostic categories. By locating diagnostic categories in the here and now, one remains open to seeing possibilities and noticing clues to new meanings and changes in the patient. The negative implication of this philosophical approach is that the therapist may fail to recognize or acknowledge, as the more traditional diagnostician might, the degree to which people's patterns of behavior are acontextual—more a function of habits and intrapsychic traits.

Consistent with the here-and-now focus on change is the Gestalt tendency to diagnose with verbs and not nouns. Seeing the world in an active and therefore potentially changing way, the clinician chooses words that emphasize behavior. Thus, the description is of "obsessing" rather than "obsessive." Once a noun is used, the person and not just the behavior is characterized, and a bit of hope is lost, for the diagnosis is not only a description of the moment but also a subtle prediction of the future. Therefore, Gestalt therapy's approach to identifying behavior patterns as opposed to character deficiencies has served as an appropriate and optimistic counterpoint to Freudian determinism.

Because of Gestalt therapy's process orientation, the individual is seen as continually moving through an overlapping series of experiences that are organized into beginnings, middles, and ends. Because of the complexity of these phenomena, one can become stuck at many different points along the experience continuum. Therefore, the value of a diagnostic tool is to help the clinician discover the point of difficulty for the patient and intervene at the correct place to maximize awareness, understanding, and change.

Gestalt therapists, because of their process perspective, risk overlooking the possibility that their in-the-moment assessments are in fact diagnoses. To avoid this oversight, what is needed is a recognition of the nature of diagnosis within the Gestalt framework and a healthy inclusion of aspects of more traditional diagnostic approaches. This latter recommendation addresses the pitfall mentioned earlier of the therapy being too fixed in the here and now without an acknowledgment of the patient's habitual behavior patterns. Therefore, it is useful to broaden the Gestalt diagnostic perspective by borrowing from other therapeutic disciplines (see Delisle, 1991; Yontef, 1988). Ultimately, however, regardless of how one defines diagnosis, it is crucial to remember that is merely a tool for change. Its purpose is not to burden the patient or therapist with constricting and irremediable labels but to facilitate the patient's awareness, growth, and health.

## HOW DO GESTALT THERAPISTS DIAGNOSE?

Traditionally, Gestalt therapists have diagnosed by paying attention to the phenomenon in the moment. At some point an aspect of behavior becomes interesting, something stands out, and a pattern emerges. This pattern might lead to a diagnostic statement such as, "The patient appears to be retroflecting" (constricting his or her emotions). The remaining therapeutic work in the session might be focused on that retroflection. This form of diagnosis is valuable for a number of reasons: first, the behavior is readily observable; second, the techniques outlining how to work with retroflections are clearly articulated and straightforward; and, third, the diagnosis defines a piece of therapeutic work that can often be satisfactorily completed in one therapy session. It should be pointed out that Gestalt therapists do not have a single way to deal with the phenomenon of someone who characteristically—that is, more often than is usual—retroflects energy when faced with stressful situations. Furthermore, we do not have a theory for predicting if the constant work on retroflections will result in some enduring change by affecting the ground of the individual.[1] The ground consists of the traces of experience, history, and physiology contained in larger, deeper grooves out of which lively figures spring forth. This ground must ultimately be affected if a person is to experience a more permanent change.

## THE EXPERIENCE CYCLE AND CHARACTER

Healthy, organized functioning can be defined by breaking down figure formation and destruction into an "experience cycle" (Zinker, 1977), which is illustrated in Figure 19.1. The crosshatched portion represents emotional

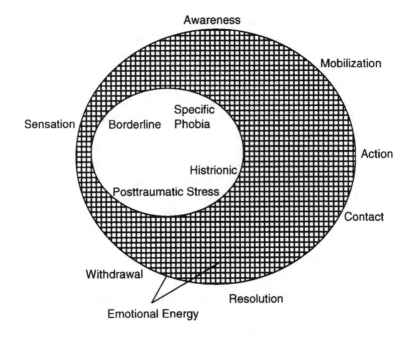

**FIGURE 19.1.** Experience cycle.

energy, which is a physiological response to stimulation. Emotional energy builds in intensity from sensation to contact and then recedes through the withdrawal stage. Individual phases are placed around the outside of the outer circle, and various disorders are placed along the inside of the inner circle. Their placement corresponds to the hypothesized original areas of blockage and distortion. It should be noted that this schema is a beginning attempt at integrating the cycle and DSM-IV diagnostic categories and rests on the following assumptions:

1. The stages of the experience cycle are in fact artificial demarcations of a continuous, flowing unit of experience; thus, the phases are overlapping.

2. Competence is directly related to the skills and abilities needed to articulate and complete each stage satisfactorily (Zinker & Nevis, 1981). Ultimately, being able to complete a cycle, to create and destroy a figure with clarity, defines healthy functioning (Wallen, 1957).

3. Although the cycle was originally intended to describe momentary experience, it can be extended to encompass larger periods of time.

4. The stages of the cycle reflect a developmental progression. The earlier in the cycle the disturbance occurs, the more the experience tends to (a) consist of very old ingrained patterns, (b) be primarily physiologically as opposed to behaviorally influenced, and (c) be less observable to others and thus less amenable to therapeutic change.

5. A disturbance at one stage of the cycle will affect all remaining stages.

6. Although one might intervene at later stages of the cycle with some success, chronic, habitual behavior can be changed ultimately only by intervening at the phase where the disturbance originally occurred.

7. The intervention(s) must occur many times before any long-lasting changes can occur.

8. When working as therapists, we are able to utilize direct observation to "see" the patient move through the middle stages of the cycle where emotion is highest, that is, mobilization, action, and contact. Therefore, our understanding of the patient's experience during the other stages is usually inferred from self-reports. Thus, most patient difficulties are originally noticed as an inability to mobilize emotion, move toward action, or make contact. Much of therapeutic work involves pinpointing other phases that present difficulty and helping the patient develop skills and resources to move through and successfully complete these phases.

9. Although we recognize the difference between personality and neurotic disturbances, for purposes of illustration we are not distinguishing between them. This is in keeping with the DSM-IV: "The coding of Personality Disorders should not be taken to imply that their pathogenesis or range of appropriate treatment is fundamentally different from that for the disorders coded on Axis 1" (American Psychiatric Association, 1994, p. 26).

10. For the purpose of this chapter, we are ignoring relationship patterns as a primary vehicle for assessing blockage and distortion (see Evans, 1994). In fact, Gestalt therapy places much emphasis on here-and-now dialogue as well as the developing relationship between therapist and patient (see Melnick, 1997).

## INDIVIDUAL PHASES OF THE CYCLE

*Sensation/Awareness.* The first phase of the cycle, sensation/awareness, involves all experiences taken in by the senses. The individual must be able to sort out an awareness from the vast array of internal and external stimuli impinging on the senses. Sensations consist of everything one sees, touches, hears, smells, and tastes and include all of the physiological, proprioceptive, and kinesthetic sensations. Completion of this phase results in the ability to articulate a clean awareness, that is, one upon which to accurately build as well as one that reflects with accuracy the sensory experience of the individual.

*Mobilization.* The second phase is mobilization. As an awareness is defined, an individual's interest and emotional energy begin to grow, ultimately organizing a want, a desire. Thus, competing figures recede into the background as emotional energy is invested in a dominant content (Zinker & Nevis, 1981; Zinker, 1994). The task of this phase is to form a sharply delineated figure out of a rich and varied ground.

*Movement or Action.* The third phase, the movement or action stage, is built on sensation/awareness and mobilization. Since this is the first stage that is clearly obvious to others, blockage in the previous two stages will most likely be evident here. This stage involves the ability to move toward an attractive object or away from an unattractive one.

*Contact.* The fourth phase of the cycle is contact. According to Zinker and Nevis (1981), contact "is the fruit of the movement/ action phase. Wants or concerns have been melded into a newly created whole—a whole which is different from its parts" (p. 10). Strong contact is based on a clear awareness supported by ample emotional energy. Contact also produces and enhances emotional arousal. This stage continues the sharpening of a compelling figure. The contact phase, too, is largely observable to others.

*Resolution/Closure.* The fifth phase, resolution/closure, involves review, that is, a summarizing, reflecting, and savoring of one's experience and meaning making. It involves both an appreciation of what has been and a regretting of what could not be. This is a slow stage because most of the emotional energy has been drained from the figure and the person is psychologically positioning him-/herself to let go, to withdraw, and ultimately to turn to a new sensation.

*Withdrawal.* The final stage, marking the end of the cycle before a new one begins, is withdrawal. It is a period during which one's boundaries are drawn closer and emotional energy used in contacting the environment is minimal. Many in our action-oriented society might perceive this phase as boring and thus miss the significance of this integrating stage. Both resolution/closure and withdrawal are primarily internal in nature and not easily observed by others.

The experience cycle is more than an abstract theoretical framework—it has practical utility. It is able to describe behavioral phenomena discussed by other theories in a way that not only makes sense but also leads to effective intervention. In the following four subsections we hope to demonstrate this. First, four popular diagnostic categories from DSM-IV (American Psychiatric Association, 1994) will be outlined. After each description, they will be discussed using the framework of the experience cycle. Last, interventions that arise naturally from the theoretical description will be articulated.

## The Sensation/Awareness Stage: Borderline Personality Disorder

Borderline personality disorder, as described in DSM-IV, is an example of blockage at the sensation/awareness level. Diagnostic criteria are outlined in Table 19.1.

**TABLE 19.1. DSM-IV Diagnostic Criteria for Borderline Personality Disorder**

A pervasive pattern of instability of interpersonal relationships, self-image, and affects, and marked impulsivity beginning in early childhood and present in a variety of contexts, as indicated by five (or more) of the following:

(1) Frantic efforts to avoid real or imagined abandonment. **Note:** Do not include suicidal or self-mutilating behavior covered in Criterion 5).

(2) A pattern of unstable and intense interpersonal relationships characterized by alternating between extremes of idealization and devaluation.

(3) Identity disturbance: markedly and persistently unstable self-image or sense of self.

(4) Impulsivity in at least two areas that are potentially self-damaging (e.g., spending, sex, substance abuse, reckless driving, binge eating). **Note:** Do not include suicidal or self-mutilating behavior covered in Criterion 5).

(5) Recurrent suicidal behavior, gestures, threats, or self-mutilating behavior.

(6) Affective instability due to a marked reactivity of mood (e.g., intense episodic dysphoria, irritability, or anxiety usually lasting a few hours and only rarely more than a few days).

(7) Chronic feelings of emptiness.

(8) Inappropriate, intense anger or difficulty controlling anger (e.g., frequent displays of temper, constant anger, recurrent physical fights).

(9) Transient, stress-related paranoid ideation or severe dissociative symptoms.

*Note.* From American Psychiatric Association (1994, p. 654). Copyright 1994 by the American Psychiatric Association. Reprinted by permission.

As one can surmise from these diagnostic criteria, the borderline patient cannot maintain a stable emotional response to input, whether internal or external. Whether this is caused by the distorted intake of sensations, the inability of an individual to code sensory stimuli into a manageable form, or the overloading of stimuli that interferes with figure formation is of much theoretical debate. What is certain is that some individuals cannot easily tolerate, manage, or translate these sensory stimuli into acceptable and manageable forms and figures.

One result is high emotional lability and acontextual responses to stimulation. To use Gestalt terminology, the ground available to the borderline patient is nonsupportive, resulting in an inability to tolerate more than minimal stimulation.

It should be pointed out that sensations are difficult for all of us. Most of our sensory appetites are too large for what is organismically acceptable, and thus we have to learn management techniques. However, most people do not have to deal with the variability, range, and enormous distortion of sensation with which people who are characteristically bound in this phase must contend.

The therapeutic work with a borderline patient is to help with the management of sensations by lowering and limiting them at both an internal and external level. Once sensation is manageable, awareness can emerge and movement through the cycle can continue.

In psychotherapy, the task is to teach these patients to manage sensations by lowering input—or, when this is impossible and stimulus overload occurs, by draining the mobilized energy through supportive and nondestructive forms of expression. The first task involves learning to slow down the input in order for the individual to run less of a risk of being flooded. Sensations need to be made smaller in order to form a figure that can be satisfactorily completed. This is accomplished by helping patients focus on their experience and label it accurately.

Techniques that increase sensations, such as the use of the empty chair, are potentially dangerous (From, 1984), as are confrontational, behavioral, and paradoxical interventions that tend to produce added or ambiguous sensory input. Another major therapeutic mistake would be to teach borderline patients management or repertoire expansion techniques that assume that their sensory mechanisms are working properly. The basic problem is not one of inadequate behavioral repertoires.

When flooding occurs, the therapeutic work involves teaching the patient to drain energy in a nondestructive way. Stimulus overload can be minimized in this instance by a therapeutic stance of "soft, clean contact." It is here that the concept of soothing is important. If the therapist becomes upset—for example, becomes mobilized or increases his/her sensations—it will add to the patient's already excessive stimulation. The therapist must learn to keep internal stimulation low by self-soothing and ultimately by teaching the patient soothing techniques. (It is interesting that this approach to the treatment of borderline patients is consistent with that articulated by the self-theorists and outlined by Tobin, 1982, and Yontef, 1983.) However, unlike self-theorists, and as stated earlier, Gestalt theorists do not believe it is necessary to hypothesize a specific cause, for example, a form of inadequate mothering, in order to prescribe an intervention.)

## Mobilization-Specific Phobia

The second phase of the experience cycle occurs with the generation of emotional energy around sensation. If the energy gets trapped in the body and there is no muscle release, anxiety occurs. The way that the individual deals with this trapped emotional energy has historically been labeled psychoneurosis and, more recently, anxiety disorder. DSM-IV lists within this category such disorders as obsessive–compulsive disorder, panic disorder, and various phobias such as agoraphobia and specific phobia. One can also add to these a vast array of psychosomatic problems that result from this chronic blocking of emotional energy.

To illustrate mobilization dysfunction, specific phobia has been chosen. The characteristics are outlined in Table 19.2.

**TABLE 19.2. DSM-IV Diagnostic Criteria for Specific Phobia**

A. Marked and persistent fear that is excessive or unreasonable, cued by the presence or anticipation of a specific object or situation (e.g., flying, heights, animals, receiving an injection, seeing blood).

B. Exposure to the phobic stimulus almost invariably provokes an immediate anxiety response, which may take the form of a situationally bound or situationally predisposed Panic Attack. **Note:** In children, the anxiety may be expressed by crying, tantrums, freezing, or clinging.

C. The person recognizes that the fear is excessive or unreasonable. **Note:** In children, this feature may be absent.

D. The phobic situation(s) is avoided or else is endured with intense anxiety or distress.

E. The avoidance, anxious anticipation, or distress in the feared situation(s) interferes significantly with the person's normal routine, occupational (or academic) functioning, or social activities or relationships, or there is marked distress about having the phobia.

F. In individuals under age 18 years, the duration is at least 6 months.

G. The anxiety, Panic Attacks, or phobic avoidance associated with the specific object or situation is not better accounted for by another mental disorder, such as Obsessive–Compulsive Disorder (e.g., fear of dirt in someone with an obsession about contamination), Posttraumatic Stress Disorder (e.g., avoidance of stimuli associated with a severe stressor), Separation Anxiety Disorder (e.g., avoidance of school), Social Phobia (e.g., avoidance of social situations because of fear of embarrassment), Panic Disorder with Agoraphobia, or Agoraphobia without History of Panic Disorder.

*Note.* From American Psychiatric Association (1994, pp. 410–411). Copyright 1994 by the American Psychiatric Association. Reprinted by permission.

Phobias involve either the investment of too much emotion around an apparently appropriate figure (a person will not visit the South because of a fear of poisonous snakes) or the mobilization of emotion around an apparently inappropriate object (a person avoids all heights but has no experience with trauma connected with them). In the second case, the sensation is given the incorrect meaning because the individual cannot tolerate the correct labeling of earlier sensations. (For example, sensation and affect generated by heights might be similar to those the individual first experienced as a young child when her/his parents would fight.) The labeling of a sensation is one way in which meaning is given to experience. Phobia involves the avoidance of the accurate meaning that could lead to a completion of the cycle that is appropriate to the sensation. Instead, a distorted (symbolic) or incorrect meaning is given to the sensation.

Phobias are maladaptive because they do not lead to satisfactory completion. They do, however, often serve to discharge or deflect emotion, thus temporarily controlling it so that the individual can tolerate it. For example, as stated above, one may label certain sensations associated with intimacy (increased heartbeat, tightness in the chest, sweaty palms, etc.) as "fear of heights." This incorrect attribution of meaning allows the individual to function in a relatively anxiety-free manner as long as heights are avoided. However, if therapy produces the understanding that these sensations are attached to an avoidance of intimacy, then the patient is faced with a conflicting duality. Now it is possible to move toward emotional closeness with another, but only with an awareness of the heightened tension that such intimacy may create.

The two major manifestations of phobias are a distorted or exaggerated response to an appropriate object to be feared (e.g., a poisonous snake) that is generalized well beyond the object and a distorted or exaggerated response to a metaphorical, symbolic, or psychologically linked object that has little or no correlation with the appropriate sensation. Treatment involves the symbolic or in vivo matching of the correct events or patterns with the stimulus so that completion can occur. Since much of what we call psychotherapy deals with the above, it might be best to categorize the approaches briefly.

Certain techniques lead to diminution of anxiety so that the person can reexperience the situation and attach the correct meaning to the sensation. These include many desensitization and cognitive approaches. Others, such as meditative and breathing techniques, help the individual to tolerate the sensations so that a less distorted meaning can emerge. Still other approaches provide support so that people do not have to bear their pain and anxiety alone, thus helping them complete the cycle. In the United States, the financial, psychological, and ideological support that our society is beginning to provide for Vietnam veterans and victims of sexual and psychological abuse are examples of this support. It should be noted that if a specific meaning emerges but the behavior does not change and the anxiety does not diminish, then the patient may be diagnosed as suffering from posttraumatic stress disorder, which is described in a later subsection.

In summary, to move through the mobilization stage of the cycle means to express the blocked emotional energy so that a contactful figure that may lead to completion can be created. As with other stages, the work must be done over and over again in order for the emotional energy to be available for the generation of appropriate and adequate contact. The Gestalt approach allows the therapist to draw from a wide range of techniques to craft a procedure that fits both the patient and the symptomatology (Melnick, 1980).

## Contact Phase: Histrionic Personality Disorder

The fourth stage of the experience cycle occurs when awareness, supported by appropriate emotional energy, results in a flexible and meaningful meeting of the self and the environment, usually in the form of an other. To meet phenomenologically implies that not only do I see but also I am seen; that not only do I speak in order to reach you but also I am heard. In the moment, each notices that the two individuals together are qualitatively different, a "we" that is different from either alone.

Disturbance of contact results in experiences that do not fit within the range of "good enough," but rather are too little or too much for a specific environmental context. An example is a hug that either has too little energy or is not warm enough or is inappropriately passionate given the environmental situation. Either extreme is jarring and incompatible and does not result in a joining experience. Both extremes are contextual disturbances in that the evaluation of too little or too much is made in relation to the other, to the self, to the situation, to the total phenomenological field. The expression "too little energy," which typically involves the pulling back from another, has been historically labeled as retroflection, whereas "too much energy" has been traditionally called hysterical or histrionic.

It should be noted that disturbances of contact, rather than reflecting characterological issues, might instead be a function of inadequate behavioral repertoires. (Repertoire evaluation can also occur at the third phase, movement or action, which was discussed earlier.) Traditionally, inadequate repertoires have been analyzed and increased by education, including behavior modification. Furthermore, the increasing and refinement of repertoires had, until recently, generally not been considered as falling within the domain of psychotherapy. However, if the therapeutic dilemma is not one of inadequate repertoires but, instead, one of fixed repertoires that limit and narrow a person's ability to make contact with the environment, then the behaviors do fall within the diagnostic guidelines of disorders.

Histrionic personality disorder is an example of disturbance of the contact boundary, as described by DSM-IV. Diagnostic criteria are outlined in Table 19.3.

**TABLE 19.3. DSM-IV Diagnostic Criteria for Histrionic Personality Disorder**

A pervasive pattern of excessive emotionality and attention seeking, beginning in early adulthood and present in a variety of contexts, as indicated by five (or more) of the following:

(1) Is uncomfortable in situations in which he or she is not the center of attention
(2) Interaction with others is often characterized by inappropriate sexually seductive or provocative behavior
(3) Displays rapidly shifting and shallow expression of emotions
(4) Consistently uses physical appearance to draw attention to self
(5) Has a style of speech that is excessively impressionistic and lacking in detail
(6) Shows self-dramatization, theatricality, and exaggerated expression of emotion
(7) Is suggestible, i.e., easily influenced by others or circumstances
(8) Considers relationships to be more intimate than they actually are

*Note.* From American Psychiatric Association (1994, pp. 657–658). Copyright 1994 by the American Psychiatric Association. Reprinted by permission.

The stereotypical model of histrionic functioning is that of the flamboyant actor. This stereotype is often true for the histrionic character, wishes to be seen, heard, appreciated, and applauded but is not very interested in others in more deep, complex ways. Thus, if a therapist attempts to prematurely create for the patient a more contactful experience, the therapist may encounter indifference at best and difficulty at worst.

The emotional energy in histrionic patients is inner determined, undisciplined, and exaggerated, and does not keep in tune with the environmental field. They are perpetually in action without benefit of an accurate awareness. Thus, the existential work with histrionic people is to help them bear the truth of their overly large existence. They are fated to take up a lot of room, to say a lot, and to do a lot. Even though they may suffer from an energy disturbance, it would be a mistake to attempt directly to teach them to be aware of or change their energy. Histrionic people are only minimally interested in awareness, for it complicates life and makes it less exciting.

Thus the dilemma for the therapist is how to help these patients slow down as well as become interested in the environmental field. Experiments that deal directly with slowing down the action, such as reading a menu completely before ordering food or counting to 10 before acting, may be utilized. Further, having the patient learn to go inward before acting heightens the probability that the forthcoming action may be truly contactful. Thus, directing the patient to notice tension, breathing, and so on might ultimately lead to a slowing down of movement.

To help these patients trade in their wish for simplicity for a more complex orientation to the world is difficult at best. However, experiments that teach them to notice environmental contexts, including other people, are beneficial. Examples include having the patient ask the therapist questions as well as notice and articulate physical and psychological boundaries.

## Demobilization Phase: Posttraumatic Stress Disorder

The last stage will be labeled demobilization, as it incorporates both the resolution/closure and withdrawal stages of the experience cycle previously discussed. The purpose of demobilization is to allow for the absorption of an experience into the ground of the individual, principally by making meaning of it, so that it will not be elicited inappropriately.

As with other stages of the cycle, when there is a synergy between the experience of the individual and the individual's capacity to deal with it, demobilization proceeds in a smooth and graceful manner. The person is able to disengage from the experience, to chew it over, and absorb and digest it. Ultimately, the individual becomes somehow different and wiser in a subtle way. If the experience is too charged to be easily absorbed into the ground, then a form for expelling or using up the excess emotional energy must be initiated. If this is not done, then the old figure will not be properly integrated and will have a perpetually distorting and disproportionate effect on the current and future experience of the individual.

This need to demobilize is a complex process that has been largely ignored by Western society as well as by Gestalt therapists. Society supports a cultural bias against demobilization by underestimating the amount of time needed to understand and integrate experiences. Among Gestalt therapists there is often a bias against "talking about" experiences. Furthermore, as a culture we do not value aloneness and movement inward. When one mobilizes, it is movement outside the skin toward contact. However, demobilization involves a movement inward to a nonpublic place where one may be alone.

Gestalt therapists, too, have ignored and had difficulty in articulating the demobilization process. In the past, it has been taught as a less significant part of the experience cycle than in fact it is. The difficulty in understanding this process is connected with its largely intrapsychic nature. As indicated previously, it is harder for others to see. Thus, like the sensation stage of the experience cycle, the process of the individual must often be inferred rather than actually observed.

Furthermore, demobilization is often unpleasant. When the event is large and negative, the experience is a grief reaction. Thus, demobilization is associated with death, illness, divorce, and defeat. However, demobilization is also a positive process, such as falling off to sleep, dreaming, fantasizing, and celebrating.

Hypothetically, demobilization can be broken down into four substages: *turning away, assimilation, encountering the void*, and *acknowledgment*. By describing the experience cycle as reflecting larger experiences in the life of the individual, one expands beyond the original definition of the cycle as a description of present experiences. Describing demobilization in terms of substages should, we hope, be useful despite the distorting and stretching of the cycle experience.

The first substage involves either a turning away or a being turned away from a figure in which energy is still invested (e.g., respectively, stopping drinking; death of a spouse). The need of parents in our society to diminish their interest in their children as the children grow older is a common experience of turning away. The relationship begins in confluence and progresses into the stage where the child introjects the parents' ideas and values. In some cultures, children may continue to introject for much of their lives, but in Western society, which values autonomy and independence, an increasing psychological separation between parent and child is preferred. For children to develop integrity—that is, to experience boundaries cleanly and clearly—they must detach from parents and create other interests. As a child leaves, so must the parents distance themselves, or they will be faced with one of two equally sad alternatives: either a hard rupturing of the child–adult boundary resulting in mutual trauma, or a type of deadly confluence that restricts developmental maturation. One aspect of maturity is the capacity to move away from a boundary gently.

To turn away when one still has energy invested requires much support. It can come in many ways, in the form of either self-generated or external support. To be self-supportive, to rely only on one's own resources, is difficult and runs contrary to the natural inclination to move toward energized objects in the environment. Not only does self-support incorporate an intellectual and emotional introjection of values, it also includes an invoking of an internalized rhythm sadly absent for many in our society. For to have faith, to hold one's hand, to gently rock and talk softly to oneself, to soothe oneself—this ultimately involves the introjection of good nourishing parenting.

The generation of external support often involves placing oneself within a structure that provides highly detailed procedures for leading one's life while in the process of turning away. Therefore choice, as well as temptation, is minimized. Examples of this type of structure are Alcoholics Anonymous and similar organizations that deal with addictive behaviors. These organizations articulate both the techniques for and the potential pitfalls in the turning-away process.

Another external option utilized in turning away involves the creation of a large and compelling figure to which to transfer unspent emotional energy. Love on the rebound and some born-again religious conversions are examples of this type of figure substitution. The problem with moving quickly toward something large and captivating is that it does not allow for the next substage of the demobilization process, assimilation, to occur. Consequently, little is ultimately learned, and the person may be doomed to skip from one love or religious experience to another.

Assimilation involves a chewing over of the experience in order to drain emotional energy. The process is difficult for many therapists in that the work may appear redundant and boring. Furthermore, because our society underestimates the amount of time necessary to chew over experience, patients may be faced not only with doing the hard work but also with having to deal with the embarrassment engendered by the intensity of feelings and the surprisingly long time that their interest remains. It is the therapist's task to normalize the experience and support the process. However, if a patient's restlessness with the duration and intensity of feelings is joined by the therapist's boredom, blockage may ensue.

The third substage, encountering the void, can be terrifying. Our society does not value or provide much training for the experience of feeling emptied of interest, of caring, of figures. The void consists of a segment in time when nothing matters. Often we avoid it by creating artificial engagements such as self-talk and noncontactful activities. Ultimately, it is the fear of the unknown that keeps many locked into either painful or nonnourishing figures. And it is this inability to turn from the old, the painful, and the nonnourishing to the unknown that is a precondition for many of the "addictions" so prevalent in our society today such as workaholism, love addiction, and codependency.

The fourth substage, acknowledgment, involves a soft, low emotional energy and an owning of how the experience has changed the individual. It is during this time that individuals are able to articulate the learnings, both good and bad, from the experience as well as to express and live out the changes in their lives. Thus the patients have gained a piece of wisdom and are able to interact with the environment in a fresh and more profound manner.

An example of an instability to demobilize can be found in posttraumatic stress disorder (PTSD). Criteria are outlined in Table 19.4. The first therapeutic task in the demobilization of PTSD involves helping patients accept that a turning away must occur. Once this acknowledgment takes place, then the work of draining the interest can begin. However, since trauma can be mesmerizing, we must help patients acknowledge both sides: that they both wish to lose interest and wish to stay interested in the traumatic event.

A second therapeutic task involves helping patients find forms through which they can express their feelings in a small way. These forms usually involve repetitive actions that cause no harm. Talking is the primary method utilized as a form of "doing" without a large mobilization. The patient must feel supported in the expression of a feeling without an external outcome or without an aim to change anything.

When demobilization from powerful events associated with PTSD is dealt with, sadness is often elicited naturally as the seasons of the year and anniversaries trigger affect-laden memories and sensations. When the sadness is evoked, the task is then to softly talk through the events. However, the therapist may get stuck and experience difficulty in helping patients move beyond the traumatizing event. There are several possible reasons for this. The first is pacing. Demobilization is a slow process that must be supported. The therapist must struggle to not become impatient or judgmental regarding the redundancy and amount of time involved. Second, patients will sometimes become frightened by emotions that are engendered. It is the therapist's job to provide adequate support for the patient to tolerate the emotional arousal as well as to help keep the emotions at a level that can be absorbed into the individual's ground. Third, patients may have an inadequate repertoire with which to drain the energy. To "sing the blues," protest, light a candle, or plant a flower are rituals that are socially sanctioned for dealing with trauma and can be used to expand patients' repertoire.

Lastly, the therapist must carefully monitor his/her own interest. One must learn to be interested just enough. Too little interest will not provide enough support, and too much interest on the part of the therapist will generate energy that fuels the patient's attachment and prevents demobilization. When demobilization is being worked on, a real danger is created if the therapist is more interested than the patient.

**TABLE 19.4. DSM-IV Diagnostic Criteria for Posttraumatic Stress Disorder**

A. The person has been exposed to a traumatic event in which both of the following were present:
   (1) The person experienced, witnessed, or was confronted with an event or events that involved actual or threatened death or serious injury, or a threat to the physical integrity of self or others.
   (2) The person's response involved intense fear, helplessness, or horror. **Note:** In children, this may be expressed instead by disorganized or agitated behavior.

B. The traumatic event is persistently reexperienced in one (or more) of the following ways:
   (1) Recurrent and intrusive distressing recollections of the event, including images, thoughts, or perceptions. **Note:** In young children, repetitive play may occur in which themes or aspects of the trauma are expressed.
   (2) Recurrent distressing dreams of the event, including images, thoughts, or perceptions. **Note:** In children, there may be frightening dreams without recognizable content.
   (3) Acting or feeling as if the traumatic event were recurring (includes a sense of reliving the experience, illusions, hallucinations, and dissociative flashback episodes, including those that occur on awakening or when intoxicated). **Note:** In young children, trauma-specific reenactment may occur.
   (4) Intense psychological distress at exposure to internal or external cues that symbolize or resemble an aspect of the traumatic event.
   (5) Physiological reactivity on exposure to internal or external cues that symbolize or resemble an aspect of the traumatic event.

C. Persistent avoidance of stimuli associated with the trauma and numbing of general responsiveness (not present before the trauma), as indicated by three (or more) of the following:
   (1) Efforts to avoid thoughts, feelings, or conversations associated with the trauma.
   (2) Efforts to avoid activities, places, or people that arouse recollection of the trauma.
   (3) Inability to recall an important aspect of the trauma.
   (4) Markedly diminished interest or participation in significant activities.
   (5) Feeling of detachment or estrangement from others.
   (6) Restricted range of affect (e.g., unable to have loving feelings).
   (7) Sense of a foreshortened future (e.g., does not expect to have career, marriage, children, or a normal life span).

D. Persistent symptoms of increased arousal (not present before a trauma), as indicated by two (or more) of the following:
   (1) Difficulty falling or staying asleep.
   (2) Irritability or outbursts of anger.
   (3) Difficulty concentrating.
   (4) Hypervigilance.
   (5) Exaggerated startle response.

E. Duration of the disturbance (symptoms in Criteria B, C, and D) is more than one month.

F. The disturbance causes clinically significant distress or impairment in social, occupational, or other important areas of functioning.

*Note.* From American Psychiatric Association (1994, pp. 428–429). Copyright 1994 by the American Psychiatric Association. Reprinted by permission.

It should be pointed out that we are describing an ideal, for one can never demobilize fully. If one is lucky, most figures will naturally be assimilated into background and the remaining energy will be used in a productive way.

The last substage of demobilization is an acknowledgment of the process. If patients have learned well, they will know something that they never knew before. If demobilization has proceeded correctly, patients will be able to answer the question: "How am I different?"

In sum, the work in dealing with problems in demobilization is to help the individual create small experiences to reduce the level of emotional arousal. The danger is in creating a remobilization experience. It should be pointed out that, as with other stages of the cycle of experience, an inability to demobilize might be a function of the person's inability to experience or integrate sensations, to mobilize, or to make contact. If this is the case, then the work must include dealing with these other aspects of the cycle.

## SUMMARY

In this chapter a basic human dilemma is posed: How is one to know and describe another? To answer that query, the issues faced by Gestalt therapists in attempting to meaningfully diagnose and assess patients and the Gestalt experience cycle and its utilization for describing character have been discussed. Finally, an effort has been made to fit a few common DSM-IV diagnoses into the paradigm of the experience cycle as well as to prescribe appropriate methods of intervention.

Diagnosis is an art as well as a science, for its purpose, after all, is to provide a useful model of experience. As Gleick (1987) so aptly writes:

> The choice is always the same. You can make your model more complex and more faithful to reality, or you can make it simpler and easier to handle. Only the most naive scientist believes that the perfect model is the one that perfectly represents reality. Such a model would have the same drawbacks as a map as large and detailed as the city it represents, a map depicting every park, every street, every building, every tree, every pothole, every inhabitant, and every map. Were such a map possible, its specificity would defeat its purpose: to generalize and abstract. Mapmakers highlight such features as their clients choose. Whatever their purpose, maps and models must simplify as much as they mimic the world. (p. 279)

In retrospect, this attempt at mapmaking is but a rough beginning filled with contradictions and exceptions. But this is how it should be, for Gestalt therapy is phenomenologically based theory grounded in the celebration of the uniqueness of the individual.

## ACKNOWLEDGMENTS

Portions of this chapter were originally published in Melnick and Nevis (1992). Copyright 1992 by Gardner Press. Reprinted by permission.

## NOTE

1. Historically, Gestalt therapy held an implicit assumption that increasing awareness and changing behavior in the present would lead to permanent change. How this was to be accomplished has remained somewhat vague. This belief has been challenged by a number of contemporary Gestalt therapists (e.g., see Melnick, 1997; Wheeler, 1991).

## REFERENCES

American Psychiatric Association. (1994). *Diagnostic and statistical manual of mental disorders* (4th ed.). Washington, DC: Author.

Delisle, G. (1991). A Gestalt perspective of personality disorders. *British Gestalt Journal, 1*, 42–50.

Evans, K. (1994). A review of "Diagnosis: The struggle for a meaningful paradigm," by J. Melnick and S. M. Nevis. *British Gestalt Journal, 3*, 40–41.

From, I. (1984). Reflections on Gestalt therapy after thirty-two years of practice: A requiem for Gestalt. *Gestalt Journal, 7*, 4–12.

Gleick, J. (1987). *Chaos.* New York: Viking.

Huckabay, M. (1992). An overview of the theory and practice of Gestalt group process. In E. Nevis (Ed.), *Gestalt therapy: Perspectives and applications* (pp. 303–330). New York: Gardner Press.

Kraus, M. (1989). Beyond homeostasis: Toward understanding human systems. *Gestalt Institute of Cleveland Review, 3*(2), 1–7.

Melnick, J. (1980). The use of therapist imposed structure in Gestalt therapy. *Gestalt Journal, 3*, 4–20.

Melnick, J. (1997). Welcome to *Gestalt Review. Gestalt Review, 1*, 1–8.

Melnick, J., & Nevis, S. M. (1992). Diagnosis: The struggle for a meaningful paradigm. In E. Nevis (Ed.), *Gestalt therapy: Perspectives and applications* (pp. 57–77). New York: Gardner Press.

Parlett, M. (1991). Reflections on field theory. *British Gestalt Journal, 1*, 69–81.

Parlett, M. (1993). Towards a more Lewinian Gestalt theory. *British Gestalt Journal, 2*, 115–120.

Polster, E., & Polster, M. (1973). *Gestalt therapy integrated.* New York: Brunner/Mazel.

Tobin, S. (1982). Self-disorder, Gestalt therapy and self psychology. *Gestalt Journal, 5*, 3–44.

Tobin, S. (1985). Lacks and shortcomings in Gestalt therapy. *Gestalt Journal, 8*, 65–71.

Wallen, R. (1957). *Gestalt therapy and Gestalt psychology.* Paper presented at the Ohio Psychological Association annual meeting, Cleveland.

Wheeler, G. (1991). *Gestalt reconsidered.* New York: Gardner Press.

Yontef, G. (1983). The self in Gestalt therapy: Reply to Tobin. *Gestalt Journal, 6*, 55–70.

Yontef, G. (1988). Assimilating diagnostic and psychoanalytic perspectives into Gestalt therapy. *Gestalt Journal, 11*, 5–32.

Zinker, J. (1977). *Creative process in Gestalt therapy.* New York: Brunner/Mazel.

Zinker, J. (1994). *In search of good form.* San Francisco: Jossey-Bass.

Zinker, J., & Nevis, S. M. (1981). *The Gestalt theory of couple and family interactions.* Working paper, Center for the Study of Intimate Systems, Gestalt Institute of Cleveland.

# IV

\*\*\*\*\*

# CONCLUSION

# 20

\*\*\*\*\*

# Experiential Therapy
## *IDENTITY AND CHALLENGES*

Leslie S. Greenberg
Germain Lietaer
Jeanne C. Watson

## IDENTITY

### Key Elements

Experiential therapy consists of those approaches that, within the context of a facilitative human relationship, focus on awareness and the evocation and symbolization of experience in awareness. Experiential therapy thus recognizes both the power of the understanding relationship and the importance of differential forms of experience promoting interventions in facilitating therapeutic change. The quality of the bond between participants as well as collaboration on the tasks and goals of therapy are thus seen as essential in creating a therapeutic alliance. The alliance in experiential therapy is constituted by a warm empathic bond, collaboration on the goal of increasing awareness, and deepening of experience and agreement to engage in tasks that promote the resolution of specific in-session emotional problems (Watson & Greenberg, 1988).

The relational bond is seen as involving three main healing ingredients; first, a more transcendent aspect, the human presence of the therapist, witnessing and validating the other's humanness; second, a set of more explicit facilitative attitudes that create a safe working environment; and, third, a set of specific interpersonal processes that are facilitative of growth and promote psychological healing. The "I–thou" relationship involving such elements as presence, commitment to dialogue, and nonexploitiveness, as well as the Rogerian triad of empathy, positive regard, and congruence, best describes the general nature of the relationship. A relational bond of this type is seen as both confirming the client as an authentic source of experience and as providing the optimal context for helping the client to attend to and become aware of preverbal experience and to communicate and explore it without fear of evaluation. The facilitative relationship, in addition to being curative in and of itself, thus provides a safe environment for working on particular problems. Finally, not only does the relationship serve as a confirming environment and as a context for specific forms of intrapsychic work, but it is itself also a medium for specific corrective interpersonal processes. Thus certain forms of work on the relationship between client and therapist are also seen as mutative.

In addition to the above ingredients of a "healing" relationship, facilitating work on particular therapeutic tasks is seen as a core ingredient of experiential therapy. The most global task of experiential therapy is that of deepening clients' experiencing. This involves helping clients attend to feelings in order to make sense of experience in a manner that helps them solve emotional problems. More specific tasks are also engaged in. These tasks, such as resolving puzzling problematic reactions or splits between parts of the self, also involve deepening experiencing in particular ways. Resolving problematic reactions, for example, involves deepening experiencing by facilitating specific processes such as identifying elements of the stimulus situation that trigger problematic reactions and realizing the subjectivity of one's own construals, while resolving splits involves deepening experiencing through such processes as identifying internal criticisms and accessing primary needs. The specific tasks thus all involve deepening experiencing, but each one involves a variety of processes for achieving this in different problem contexts.

## Image of Human Nature and Functioning

An existential view of human nature, one that sees existence as preceding essence, provides the unifying common ground for experiential approaches. People are seen as active agents in the construction of their own realities, and choice is seen as the final arbiter in human functioning. Individuals are seen as being born morally neutral, with a penchant for both health and sickness and both good and bad. What is essential, however, is that people are seen as having innate worth, the ability to know the difference between good and evil, and the capacity to choose between them. Free will thus is the foundational principle, and therapy involves facilitation of the actualization of the potential for good. Health is seen as arising from the integration of polarities, and the attainment thereby of internal harmony, equilibrium, and the creation of coherent meaning.

Experiential theory of personality in addition proposes a process model of the self. The self is seen as a dynamic experiential system in a continual process of self-organization. This replaces a more static, structural view—of a self-concept determining behavior. Experiential theory is dialectically constructivist in nature, emphasizing that change is an inherent aspect of all systems, that meaning is created by human activity, is created in dialogue, is constrained by a bodily felt emotional experience, and ultimately is created by synthesis of experience and symbol (Greenberg, Rice, & Elliott, 1993; Greenberg & Pascual-Leone, 1995). Emotional experience thus is seen as both creating and being created by its conscious symbolization and expression. This view thus casts us as creators of the self we find ourselves to be. In addition, experiential therapy, by adopting a relational view of functioning, sees the self as coming into existence on the border between inside and outside, between organism and environment, by a synthesis of bodily experience, symbol, and the confirmation of another.

Flowing from this foundation, emotional experience, although seen as a basically healthy resource, is viewed as capable either of providing healthy adaptive information based on the biologically adaptive emotion system or, in certain instances, of becoming maladaptive through learning and experience. The most basic process for the individual in therapy is thus one of reflecting on and evaluating for him-/herself what is healthy and what is maladaptive. Therapy then involves facilitating awareness of the adaptive and the healthy for use as a guide, and understanding and transformation of that which is unhealthy and maladaptive. Awareness involves symbolization of bodily felt meaning. Transformation is achieved by exposing symbolized maladaptive experience to newly accessed and symbolized adaptive, internal experience (other parts of the self) and to new corrective interpersonal experience. Transformation thus comes by (1) integrating maladaptive experience (such as worthlessness or shame) with adaptive internal resources (such as anger at violation and pride in self) to form a new more balanced whole (such as self-worth and assertiveness) and (2) having corrective emotional experiences with the therapist that will act to disconfirm pathogenic beliefs about others (such as "If I am weak, others will be scornful") and about self ("If I am weak I will disintegrate"). In addition to these two specific sources of change, the therapist's ongoing attunement to affect, confirmation of that which is healthy and more adaptive, and focus on internal resources and new possibilities is seen as leading to a strengthening of the client's self.

## Goals

The general goals of treatment are to promote more fluidic and integrative self-organizations. The therapy focuses on the whole person; that is, it is person-centered rather than problem or symptom focused. But within this holistic focus, determinants of different types of self dysfunction are focused on. Thus a change in the manner of functioning of the whole self as well as changes in particular problems in self-organization, and the attendant cognitive–affective processing problems, are recognized as important. For example, a client may be seen as changing her/his manner of functioning by becoming more empathic to the self and being able to symbolize bodily felt experience, as well as changing in a specific domain by resolving unfinished business with a significant other. The identification of particular types of self or interpersonal problems promotes the development in therapy of a treatment focus on these problems within a holistic approach. This focus emerges in a co-constructive process over the course of treatment. Thus treatment, in addition to promoting self acceptance and a strengthening of the self, aims at solving particular problems of self-organization that emerge in treatment.

## BASIC PRINCIPLES OF PRACTICE

The basic principles of practice discussed in Part II of this volume suggest that empathy, awareness of relational experience that emerges in treatment with the therapist, dialogue, experiential focusing, meaning creation, promoting agency, and translating in-session change to extra-sessional behavior are all defining principles of an experiential approach. In experiential therapy empathy is seen as a complex cognitive–affective process of entering into another's worldview, understanding as well as being with the other, in order to help the person regulate affect and co-construct new meaning. In addition to being empathic, when the therapist's experience of the client in the session or the client's experience of the therapist becomes problematic, this is used as a marker for communicating about what is occurring interpersonally between the client and therapist. Congruence and immediacy have always been a part of an experiential approach, but with a shift to a more interpersonal view these are now used explicitly to deal with different types of relational issues. Thus the use of relational skills that focus on metacommunicating about the relationship are becoming more important in the practice of experiential therapy, especially in longer-term treatments.

However, focusing on clients' internal experience—helping them to symbolize it and create new meaning—continues to be the central task in a task-oriented therapy in which different processes are promoted at different times to aid experiential processing. The experiential processes that are facilitated range from symbolizing a bodily felt sense, to evoking memories, to letting an intense feeling form, to expressing feelings, to reflecting on experience to create meaning. The client in addition is seen as an active agent engaging in these processes, and in-session therapy tasks are *done by* clients rather than *done to* them. In experiential therapy the dichotomy between the attitudes of the therapist and the use of techniques finally is transcended. Both tasks and bonds are seen as aspects of relating. Without appropriate attitudes, techniques are empty forms, and without method, one is not able to offer optimal facilitation. Finally, while it is the process in the session that remains the central focus of an experiential form of treatment, some emphasis is placed on translating in-session change into extra-session change. Homework and practice, especially of the type that helps increase awareness and consolidate change, thus are used, and therapists also pay attention to how to promote therapeutic experience *between* sessions.

## Assessment and Case Formulation

The experiential therapies have always favored responding to the whole person over assessing dysfunction and diagnosing disorder. This has been done out of a belief that a diagnostic stance serves to destroy a person's humanity and interferes with the therapist's ability to relate to the other as a person. Just as, for example, one would not label one's spouse as having an avoidant personality disorder without severely damaging the nature of the relationship and effecting one's stance toward one's spouse, so one would not wish to objectify one's client in this manner. Believing as we do that clients are experts on their own experience, our concerns with the disempowering effects of therapists taking a more knowing stance have led us to try not to define the content of their experience, nor to direct them to deal with particular material on which we have predetermined they need to focus. We thus have eschewed case formulation and content directiveness.

This eschewing of formulation and diagnosis, however, has led the experiential tradition into a type of unintended uniformity assumption—that all people are alike and all shall be treated in the same way. This has led critics to view the experiential approaches as lacking in differential diagnosis and differential intervention. In addition, it has led to the view that experiential approaches are not relevant for people with major disorders and only relevant for people with general problems in living, self-esteem difficulties, and milder forms of psychological distress.

Part of the problem is that the basic process orientation in this approach, the orientation that has led to its opposition to diagnosis, has never been fully articulated, nor has it been fully appreciated or understood by critics more familiar with medical or psychological assessment-oriented perspectives. In the latter more structural view diagnosis is seen as a necessary precursor of correct choice of treatment. A process perspective (Whitehead, 1929), however, starts from a radically different premise, one that sees flux and change as the basic nature of reality. From a process perspective a structural form is simply a momentary state. Rather than seeing a person's problems as based on a preexisting enduring structure that one needs to diagnose before treating, a different procedure is followed. The problem is seen instead as being constituted by current forms of self-organization that block the healthy process of being in flux. In this view the best way to promote change is to access maladaptive forms that block healthy functioning and influence the processes that produce and maintain them in order to facilitate natural movement and new directions.

In addition, a process perspective that involves responding to the current state rather than to a prediagnosed, presumed stable state, does not promote uniform responding. Far from it. Rather, it involves great sensitivity to momentary differences and great variation in response to perceived differences. It is this focus on moment-by-moment variation, rather than on stability and enduring patterns, that leads a process-experiential approach to not adopting traditional assessment, which is viewed as too static and not sufficiently transactional. The process view thus promotes differential moment-by-moment intervention to different moments in the client's experiential flux. Process and flux in experience is thus figural over stability and enduring form in the personality. This view has promoted sensitivity to the person's unique moments of concrete experience rather than to identifying dysfunctional patterns across situations. In addition, experience is seen as too context dependent to warrant expenditure of much effort on highlighting stable characteristics over time. Thus people are not viewed as being any particular way independent of context, but rather are seen as being in a constant process of self-organizing in relation to their interpersonal contexts.

What has been lacking in this process view, however, is the articulation of a comprehensive process diagnostic system that specifies important momentary states and processes that are recognized and responded to differentially in successful treatment. The exclusive focus on fluidic process, with little attention to problematic states, was important historically as an antidote to overly rigid diagnostic and prescriptive views. However, as empathy, awareness, and recognition of the value of facilitative in-session processes have become more universally recognized and integrated into general approaches to therapy, the intensity of this opposition has become less necessary. Experiential therapy now needs to find ways to integrate more structural points of view that recognize stability and patterns of human experience into its process theory and practice. One of the clearest research findings is that the client variable is the one most predictive of outcome (Lambert & Hill, 1994), suggesting that regardless of the context there is something about clients themselves that is very important in treatment.

Consistent with a phenomenological process-oriented view, experiential therapists have recently begun to capture differences between people by describing the differences in their in-session experiential states. They have begun to specify different ways in which to intervene with these different states (Greenberg et al., 1993; Gendlin, 1996; Toukmanian, 1992; see also chapters in Part III of this volume) and have proposed a process form of case formulation (Goldman & Greenberg, 1995, 1997). This type of process-sensitive approach provides a process-diagnostic and process-directive form of treatment that will become the hallmark of a modern experiential psychotherapeutic methodology. In this approach the therapist uses process diagnosis as a key tool and is seen as an expert not on *what* a client experiences but on *how* to differentially facilitate optimal client processes at particular times. Therapists thus offer expertise on what methods will help exploration of particular states. Therefore they are at times process directive, facilitating different kinds of exploratory processes, whereas at other times they are purely responsive, being empathically attuned and checking their understanding.

In this process-diagnostic, process-directive approach, in addition to identifying markers of specific intrapersonal processing difficulties, such as problematic reactions, splits, unfinished business, and an unclear felt sense (Greenberg et al., 1993), markers of relational difficulties that it is important to address have begun to be identified. These markers may be based on the therapist's internal experience of the client and on an identification of transactional patterns. For example, a marker of a relational problem based on the therapist's internal experience arises when he/she notices that his/her own unconditionality, or ability to listen and accept, is breaking down. This marks an opportunity for greater facilitative transparency designed to deal with the breakdown in acceptance. Other important relational markers, based on identifiable client in-session performances that have already begun to be investigated, are ruptures in alliances, moments of misunderstanding, and moments of shame from lack of therapist attunement (Safran & Muran, 1996; Rhodes, Geller, Elliott, & Greenberg, 1995; Wheeler, 1996, 1997).

Rennie (1998) also has recently provided indicators as to when therapists might consider a process identification—identifying the current processing activity the client is engaged in—in order to help the client increase awareness of her/his processing. Process identification involves facilitating clients in becoming aware of "how" they are processing in favor of an empathic response to "what" they feel and mean. If, for example, we find ourselves losing interest or feeling we have heard all this before, "in much the same old way," we might want to ask what activity our client is currently engaged in, or comment in a validating way that we "have the feeling you may be going around and around and feeling like you are not really getting any further ahead." Comments such as these are designed to stimulate clients' awareness of and reflection on their current style of processing. A process identification of this kind, like a Gestalt awareness experiment, may have the effect of shaking up the process a little.

## Differential Treatment of Different Disorders

The chapters in Part III of this volume on the experiential treatment of different disorders, on depression, posttraumatic stress disorder, anxiety disorders, psychosomatic disorders, sexual abuse, borderline personality disorder, and dissociative and psychotic processes all offer examples of well-articulated experiential treatments of specific disorders.

What characterizes all the chapters in this volume on differential treatment is that they are based on the experience-near study of the processes in which these clients engage in therapy and the specification of therapist interventions that seem most helpful for these states. This sets the criterion for what makes a differential approach to disorder *experiential*. An experiential approach to differential treatment will first and foremost be based on a study of the actual *in-therapy current processes* of people with that type of problem rather than on the nature of the problem as a structural entity. An experiential approach thus involves a study of the in-session nature of the disturbing experiential states and processes in that disorder, the in-therapy processes of change in these states, and the type of therapist interventions that facilitate these changes. The chapters on differential treatment in this volume will be reviewed below to highlight this approach to differential treatment.

In Chapter 10 Greenberg, Watson, and Goldman argue, from a process-experiential perspective, that certain commonalities do appear to exist in depressive experience and that certain types of problematic in-session states characteristically emerge in clients in treatment for depression. Therapists are encouraged to be alert to these states. Rather than imposing preconceptions on what is causing depression, therapists are encouraged to assess current determinants of depression—that is, states—and to be differentially responsive to different types of markers of these states as they occur. The therapist does not decide a priori what the client needs to explore in order to be helped, nor is the therapist simply a companion to the client's exploratory processes. Rather, the therapist is an active collaborator in determining the therapeutic focus, helping to recognize certain problematic states and offering his/her expertise in the type of exploratory processes that might be helpful. In addition to providing a marker-guided, process-directive form of intervention, Greenberg et al. provide a theoretical model of the depressogenic process that emphasizes the importance of emotional memories in depression and suggest that these need to be evoked and then reorganized. This is done by accessing the individual's growth capacities and adaptive feelings and needs to challenge the maladaptive depression-producing emotion schemes.

In Chapter 11 Elliott, Davis, and Slatik, in presenting their process-experiential approach to posttraumatic stress disorder (PTSD), start from the basis of a phenomenological description of people's experience of trauma. Their identification of the experience of three "world-moments," the pre-, during, and postvictimization moments, informs their treatment. They show us how understanding the characteristic experience in this disorder can be used to help the therapist understand more deeply and respond differentially to the client's unique experience. Rather than using descriptions and theories of the disorder, as preconceptions into which to fit clients, the descriptions and theories are used as ways of better understanding clients' experience when and if that pattern arises. Having different views on the disorders thus is not necessarily prescriptive constricting and dehumanizing, nor does it have to lead a therapist to imposing these views on the client. It is the way differential diagnoses are used that will make these understandings compatible with an experiential approach that is seeking to access the persons vast pool of internal resources for growth and change. When assessment and differential understanding promotes deeper, quicker understanding and differential ways of facilitating the type of exploration most helpful for the current experiential state, it does not have to place theoretical blinders on therapists views nor distortions on the clients experience.

Note that in their treatment of PTSD, Elliott et al. find some types of experiential states and tasks that are different from those that arise in depression, as well as some of the same types. This indicates that a differential approach to these two disorders is helpful and that therapists will benefit by being alerted to the potential relevance of different types of tasks to different types of disorders. Thus, for example, in dealing with flashbacks in PTSD, renarrating traumatic episodes is most helpful in order to symbolize traumatic affective experience in words. This form of intervention would not be relevant or helpful in depression unless trauma were involved. In depression, focusing on self-criticism and dependence and loss may be most helpful. In addition, the type of work with emotion may differ with clients with the two types of problems: trauma clients may need to symbolize underregulated preverbal emotional experience, whereas depressed clients may need to access unacknowledged or overregulated feelings. Thus we see that different emotional resolution process and different therapeutic tasks may be more relevant to people in particular states and that similar states are likely to be more prevalent in particular populations.

Turning to Wolfe and Sigl's treatment of general anxiety disorders in Chapter 12, we see that these authors look at the specific emotional processing difficulties that characterize anxiety disorders to inform treatment. Based on a view that the dynamics of self-experience involves two major processes, the interruption of experience and the relentless reflexivity of attention, the authors identify specific forms of self-dysfunction in anxiety. These range from the dysfunctional content of specific self-beliefs, through the existence of discrepancies between self-beliefs and either self-standards or immediate self-experience, to attempts to escape a dreaded or hated self. Wolfe and Sigl then suggest the use of different experiential techniques to address each specific form of self-pathology. Thus, similar to the process experiential view above, this approach favors the use of differential intervention for different current processing difficulties and defines specific processing difficulties that are most relevant and prevalent for a specific type of disorder—in this case, anxiety.

Sachse (Chapter 13), in his specific form of client-centered therapy for clients with psychosomatic disorders, finds that a tendency to avoid facing and coping with negative aspects of self is characteristic of this population's process in therapy. This approach again is based on the study of the treatment of this type of population and the development from this of a particular theoretical view of the particular disturbance and a set of interventions most appropriate for these disturbances. Treatment with this population, Sachse suggests, needs to be more confrontive. Therapists need to identify the types of avoidant processing the client is engaging in and offer them alternative forms of processing. Only after helping these clients to become aware of their processing is there a shift to focusing back on deepening their experiencing and clarifying their contents. Again we see a treatment based on the facilitation of differential processing as important in this disorder. Currently this treatment is conceptualized as occurring in different phases in which each phase is marked by a particular style of processing. In addition, markers of particular processing states and appropriate interventions are identified.

Using a psychodramatic approach to treat sexual abuse, in Chapter 14 Hudgins presents a model of reexperiencing trauma. In order to prevent retraumatization, she emphasizes the need for safety in doing such reexperiencing work. We see a hoped-for similarity in her approach to that of Elliott et al. (Chapter 11) in dealing with trauma. In both chapters the authors promote reexperiencing and the bringing of the traumatic memories under greater conscious control. We see too how much this differs from say, Sachse's more confrontive approach of bringing psychosomatic clients' manner of avoidant processing to awareness. The different populations clearly require different processes. Thus each treatment of the above disorders differentially applies the basic principles of an experiential approach such as relational empathy and congruence, as well as promotion of client awareness and experiencing, but does the latter in different ways within different populations.

In working with personality disorders the relational process comes more into focus. In Chapter 15 Eckert and Biermann-Ratjen offer a client-centered treatment of people with borderline personality disorders in which they see a particular relational stance, unconditional positive regard or validation, as crucial for this population. In terms of etiology they see threat to the self as resulting quite naturally in the rage that so characterizes this population and suggest that it is the lack of unconditional positive regard that produces the threat to self and that its presence is the central curative agent in therapy. In addition to emphasizing the role of unconditional regard in their treatment, they give us certain markers and optimal responses for particular processes of special concern, such as splitting into good and bad, integrating love and hate, and of seeing the clients' parents in a more balanced way. Again the general approach is applied to specific population by identifying the specific type of processes associated with this population's in-therapy performance and experience.

Warner shows us in Chapter 16 how empathic attunement and confirmation of experience is crucial in helping people with dissociative experiences and recommends that we welcome and be empathic to the different parts of the personality as they emerge. In Chapter 17 Prouty presents an approach to working with psychotic and retarded patients' experience that focuses on restoring psychological contact necessary for psychotherapy with these contact-impaired people. He postulates that contact is the first and necessary precondition of psychotherapy and defines work on establishing contact as a stage of pre-therapy. He offers specific kinds of responses, such as contact reflections, and specific types of contact functions and behaviors that need to be established, thereby providing us with a uniquely novel way of viewing and being with people who are having hallucinations.

All the above experiential approaches to different disorders are characterized by sharing the common principles of experiential therapy. They focus on present experiencing in the context of a facilitative relationship and focus more specifically on the nature of the disordered experience characteristic of the specific class of disturbance with which they are working. No longer is experiential therapy to be seen as a uniform therapy without differential interventions for different disorders. Rather, it should be seen as having a variety of methods, ranging from empathic responding to feeling, through talking about the relationship, to the use of enactments, and a specific set of relational stances ranging from supportive, through disclosing, to confrontational that are differentially applied to different experiential states on the basis of what is most likely to promote particular kinds of processes most helpful at that time. These processes range from awareness of current processing activities, through symbolizing affect, to making sensor contact with reality and doing homework.

## CHALLENGES

### Psychopathology

A major challenge in the next century will be the development of a more complex theory of psychopathology. Major current views of psychopathology are based on singular views such as incongruence (Rogers, 1951), interruptive processes (Perls, Hefferline, & Goodman, 1951), or blocks to process (Gendlin, 1962). These will be replaced by a more multifaceted view of dysfunction that will incorporate but go beyond them. The process of developing a theory of psychopathology is represented in this volume by Chapter 18 of Speierer and Chapter 19 of Nevis and Melnick.

Speierer, using the idea of congruence as a central organizing principle, suggests that disorder can be broken into three large categories on the basis of the kind of incongruence operating. The three groupings are organic dispositional incongruence, psychosocial incongruence, and life-event-based incongruence. According to this view it is psychosocial forms of incongruence that are most suited to a person-centered, process-oriented, experiential therapy. This is an initial differential scheme that tackles the issue of diagnosis by first breaking down the whole domain of the treatment-seeking population into those most suitable for referral to psychotherapy and those most suitable for medical or other psychosocial interventions. It is most useful for screening out people who might be treated in a large medical facility and/or who have organic and social circumstances that do not make experiential therapy the treatment of choice. Speierer further attempts to show how traditional diagnostic categories fit into this framework, placing (for example) autism into the organic/dispositional category, most depression and anxiety into the psychosocial category, and loss of a limb into the life-events category. This is a useful molar discrimination to make. In addition he suggests that the actualizing tendency at times can become dysfunctional, introducing the important idea that experiential therapy will have to develop a more differentiated view of the growth tendency and will need to devise ways of discriminating when to facilitate people's ability to rely on it and when and how to facilitate transforming loss or absence of actualizing capacities.

In Chapter 19 on diagnosis, Melnick and Nevis approach the issue essentially by offering a process-diagnostic view of assessment. They suggest the Gestalt experience cycle as a means of identifying problems in current functioning. Describing various types of blocks and distortions in this cycle, they make an initial attempt at associating different disorders with these at different points in the cycle. This type of thinking presents an initial attempt at linking Gestalt views to DSM categories. In our view the identification of certain processes with certain contact disturbances is promising as an idea. However, rather than identifying nosological groups with disturbances at one point in the cycle as Melnick and Nevis have done, we suggest that it would be better to see each type of disorder as involving a variety of specific types of disturbance at different points in the cycle. Thus rather than identifying PTSD with demobilization alone, as they have done, this disorder might be seen as involving distortion at the sensation/awareness level and possibly problems at other points, as well as in the demobilization phase. This would allow therapists to focus on multiple processes as they arise in the moment in any individual but still to be able to uniquely characterize different disorders according to the pattern and predominance of certain types of processes. This approach would keep a process perspective in the foreground but still link it to traditional diagnosis.

The challenge of the coming century will be to more fully develop a dialectical stance that helps us transcend the dichotomy between structure and process and between following and leading. We will need to synthesize more static, traditional diagnoses, as well as content-based case formulation with radical moment-by-moment process views to achieve more fluid process-diagnostic assessments, more marker-guided process-directive forms of responding, and more collaborative methods of attaining a focus of treatment. An additional need and benefit of recognizing enduring dysfunctional forms in people's functioning and the willingness to articulate our views with DSM diagnosis will be a greater possibility of dialoguing with colleagues of different orientations about psychopathology and an increased ability of meshing with traditional treatment systems that use standardized diagnostic category systems.

The dilemma of an experiential approach to pathology lies in how to respect the individual and respond to the whole person, and how to attend to common or universal aspects of certain kinds of emotional difficulties and states. General states such as depression, anxiety, and trauma, or types of patterns of processes such as avoidant functioning, inability to maintain stable relationships, and obsessive or compulsive functioning, do appear to exist. As we have said, the solution originally adopted—of taking a purely process view of functioning and emphasizing therapists' attitudes as the major component of treatment—led to a type of uniformity myth that all practice is the same. Experiential therapy was seen as suggesting that all people deal with highly similar problem determinants. The phenomenological emphasis on the uniqueness of each person's experience paradoxically resulted in a type of view that the same therapeutic process applied to all. We need to transcend the dichotomy between labeling people, and in so doing losing sight of them, and simply focusing on momentary experience, thereby losing sight of the reoccurring processes that differentiate different types of disorder.

It appears to us that the process-oriented way of categorizing and codifying differences that we have termed process diagnosis moves the emphasis from what a person is like to what a person is doing in the session. Focusing on the state or processes a person is currently engaged in with the therapist in the session allows one to identify blocks to healthy functioning without categorizing the person as a whole as dysfunctional. Thus we need to talk about depressive, anxious, and borderline processes, not people. This would acknowledge that all people engage in processes such as self-criticism, catastrophic expectation, and splitting the good and the bad, and that all have to find ways of dealing with these. People can become more or less repetitive and rigid in the processes they engage in both internally and interactionally. To the degree that people lose flexibility their behavior and experience is restricted into a narrow range of options. Thus they become predictable. New episodes produce repetitive experience and behavior that can become maladaptive patterns. Treatment ought to help melt rigidity and restore people's ability to make more flexible contact with the world.

## Research

A further challenge for the new millennium will be to rejuvenate the empirical investigation of experiential therapy. A renewal of joint academic effort, focused particularly on empirical research, is needed to help put this approach back on a firm footing. For example, Wolfus and Bierman (1996) have recently demonstrated the effectiveness of experiential therapy for violent men. They have run 22 successful groups in a program called "Relating without Violence" and have demonstrated the effectiveness of these groups. Teusch, Böhme, and Gastpar (1997) recently reported a comparison of a client-centered group treatment of panic and agoraphobia with the same treatment plus behavioral exposure. Both treatments were effective in reducing symptoms. Although the combined treatment was superior on a few indices for a short period there was no difference between groups at 1-year followup. More research of this nature on different experiential therapy programs is needed. Not only more research but also increased scholarly communication by means of journals and national and international meetings will be important in reviving this approach.

Research should involve discovery oriented, qualitative, and descriptive research, as well as more traditional clinical trials and verification-oriented research. A pluralistic approach to research of this type, including both more hermeneutic, human science methods and more positivist, physical science methods, is necessary to create different strands of investigation (Toukmanian & Rennie, 1992). It will be the tying together of these different strands that will create the strongest bond of human knowledge. Pluralistic methods that combine study of subjective experience and observable behavior, thereby integrating both meaning and reliable measurement, will help create a shared view of what leads to change in psychotherapy. This will help us both to understand how change occurs and to demonstrate the effectiveness of experiential therapy. This will result in our ultimately being able to relate process to outcome to establish what processes promote change.

Additional research is needed on the general nature of facilitative relating and about when specific forms of relating are most helpful. Further research is needed to clarify the nature of empathy, therapist presence, and psychological contact. More specific markers of relationally based opportunities for specific forms of relating also need to be specified and optimal ways of responding to them investigated. Markers such as client hostility toward or challenging of the therapist, or client moments of fragile dependence or insecurity that lead to deep anxiety at separation from the therapist, all need to be clearly specified. Features of optimal forms of responding to these relational markers also need to be rigorously delineated. We need to know when it is best to be empathic and when we need to go beyond empathy to meta-communicate or confront.

## Training

Training will also need to be based more on research findings, thereby facilitating the integration of research and practice. One of the strongest research findings to date is that the relationship with the therapist is the best predictor of outcome. In training we thus need to find a balance between facilitating development of basic relational attitudes and the personal awareness and growth that promotes them, on the one hand, and more technical training in differential intervention, on the other. In addition, therapists need to be trained in working with different populations and in how to respond to different in-session client states in these populations. Thus therapists will be taught, for example, that in response to an attack, especially by people with borderline rage, recognizing what they themselves did and understanding what was experienced as hurtful by their clients, and not defending themselves or escalating the situation, will lead to healing of alliance ruptures. Similarly they will be taught how to best respond to moments of fragile dependence and insecurity when dependent clients feel that they cannot leave the session or maintain themselves without the therapist. They will learn how empathy with the client's fear of disintegration and isolation leads to a firming up of the client's self and how providing structure, coping skills, and transitional experiences (and objects) helps people deal with the separation difficulty. They will learn too that being congruent is crucial when their empathy fails.

Training in the identification of already investigated states, such as unresolved bad feeling toward a significant other and problematic reactions, and in the appropriate interventions need to be provided. This should be supplemented with training in the clear definition and investigation of other states, such as those that indicate a readiness for allowing of painful emotion, promoting of self-soothing, awareness of avoidance, and opportunities for integrating good and bad feelings. Means of training students to seemlessly integrate these specific forms of responding with an overall ability to be present will be developed, such that, like fine concert pianists, their final performance will be a holistic integration of explicit skill and tacit knowledge into an artistic rather than a technical accomplishment.

## Integration

Finally, integration of various approaches under an umbrella identity of experiential therapy will be necessary to create a new third force. This will include the major approaches identified here, client-centered, existential, and Gestalt, and other experiential approaches such as focusing-oriented therapy, the body therapies, bioenergetics, feeling–expressive therapy, feminist therapy, logotherapy, psychodrama, and reevaluation therapy. This integrated force will then be strong enough to stand alongside cognitive and dynamic approaches as a recognized alternative. Once an experiential therapy identity has been established by an integration of diverse subgroups under a common framework, the task of exploring commonalities and differences with cognitive and dynamic therapies can begin. Then, from a strong base and with a secure identity, experiential therapy will be able to enter a dialogue with other orientations. Experiential therapy will be able to make a stronger contribution to these other approaches and will be more able to learn from them, aiding in the quest for an ultimately unified, non-school-based approach to treatment. Until the time of an integrated approach to the treatment of psychological problems has been developed, experiential therapists need a strong identity based on the study of good practice. We have attempted, in this book, to lay the groundwork for this.

## REFERENCES

Gendlin, E. T. (1962). *Experiencing and the creation of meaning: A philosophical and psychological approach to the subjective.* New York: Free Press of Glencoe.

Gendlin, E. T. (1996). *Focusing-oriented psychotherapy: A manual of the experiential approach.* New York: Guilford Press.

Goldman, R., & Greenberg, L. S. (1995). A process-experiential approach to case formulation. *In Session, 1*(2), 35–51.

Goldman, R., & Greenberg, L. S. (1997). Case formulation in process-experiential therapy. In T. D. Eells (Ed.), *Handbook of psychotherapy case formulation.* New York: Guilford Press.

Greenberg, L. S., & Pasqual-Leone, J. (1995). A dialectical constructivist approach to experiential change. In R. Neimeyer & M. Mahoney (Eds.), *Constructivism in psychotherapy.* Washington, DC: American Psychological Association Press.

Greenberg, L. S., Rice, L. N., & Elliott, R. (1993). *Facilitating emotional change: The moment-by-moment process.* New York: Guilford Press.

Lambert, M., & Hill, C. (1994). Assessing psychotherapy outcomes and processes. In A. Bergin & S. Garfield (Eds.), *Handbook of psychotherapy and behavior change.* New York: Wiley.

Perls, F. S., Hefferline, A., & Goodman, P. (1951). *Gestalt therapy.* New York: Dell.

Rennie, D. (1998). *Person-centred counseling: An experiential approach.* New York: Sage.

Rhodes, R., Geller, J., Elliott, R., & Greenberg, L. S. (1995, June). *Misunderstanding events.* Panel presentation at a meeting of the Society for Psychotherapy Research, Berkeley, CA.

Rogers, C. R. (1951). *Client-centered therapy.* Boston: Houghton Mifflin.

Safran, J., & Muran, J. (1996). The resolution of ruptures in the therapeutic alliance. *Journal of Consulting and Clinical Psychology, 64,* 447–458.

Teusch, L., Böhme, H., & Gastpar, M. (1997). The benefits of an insight-oriented and experiential approach on panic and agoraphobic symptoms. *Psychotherapy and Psychosomatics, 66,* 293–301.

Toukmanian, S. (1992). Studying the clients' perceptual process and their outcomes in psychotherapy. In S. Toukmanian & D. Rennie (Eds.), *Psychotherapy process research: Paradigmatic and narrative approaches.* Newbury Park, CA: Sage.

Toukmanian, S., & Rennie, D. (1992). *Psychotherapy process research: Paradigmatic and narrative approaches.* Newbury Park, CA: Sage.

Watson, J., & Greenberg, L. (1988). The therapuetic alliance in short-term humanistic and experiential therapies. In J. Safran & J. C. Muran (Eds.), *The therapeutic alliance in brief psychotherapy.* Washington, DC: American Psychological Association Press.

Wheeler, G. (1996). Shame in two paradigms of psychotherapy. *British Gestalt Journal, 4*(2), 76–85.

Wheeler, G. (1997). Self and shame: A Gestalt approach. *Gestalt Review, 3,* 221–224.

Whitehead, A. (1929). *Process and reality.* Cambridge, UK: Cambridge University Press.

Wolfus, B., & Bierman, R. (1996). An evaluation of a group treatment program for incarcerated male batterers. *International Journal of Offender Therapy and Comparative Criminology, 40*(4), 318–333.

# Index